D1228893

SAVING WOMEN'S LIVES

Strategies for Improving Breast Cancer Detection and Diagnosis

Committee on New Approaches to Early Detection
and Diagnosis of Breast Cancer

National Cancer Policy Board

Board on Science, Technology, and Economic Policy
Policy and Global Affairs Division

Janet E. Joy, Edward E. Penhoet, and Diana B. Petitti, *Editors*

INSTITUTE OF MEDICINE *AND*
NATIONAL RESEARCH COUNCIL
OF THE NATIONAL ACADEMIES

THE NATIONAL ACADEMIES PRESS
Washington, D.C.
www.nap.edu

THE NATIONAL ACADEMIES PRESS 500 Fifth Street, N.W. Washington, DC 20001

NOTICE: The project that is the subject of this report was approved by the Governing Board of the National Research Council, whose members are drawn from the councils of the National Academy of Sciences, the National Academy of Engineering, and the Institute of Medicine. The members of the committee responsible for the report were chosen for their special competences and with regard for appropriate balance.

Support for this project was provided by the Apex Foundation, the Breast Cancer Research Foundation, the Carl J. Herzog Foundation, Mr. Corbin Gwaltney, Mr. John Castle, the Josiah Macy Jr. Foundation, the Kansas Health Foundation, and the National Cancer Institute. This study was supported, in part, by Contract No. N01-OD-4-2139, TO #110 between the National Academy of Sciences and the National Cancer Institute. Any opinions, findings, conclusions, or recommendations expressed in this publication are those of the author(s) and do not necessarily reflect the view of the organizations or agencies that provided support for this project.

Library of Congress Cataloging-in-Publication Data

Saving women's lives : strategies for improving breast cancer detection and diagnosis / Committee on New Approaches to Early Detection and Diagnosis of Breast Cancer, National Cancer Policy Board, Board on Science, Technology, and Economic Policy, Policy and Global Affairs Division ; Janet E. Joy, Edward E. Penhoet, and Diana B. Petitti, editors.
p. ; cm.
Includes bibliographical references and index.
ISBN 0-309-09213-2 (hardcover)
1. Breast—Cancer—Diagnosis. 2. Breast—Cancer—Government policy—United States. 3. Breast—Cancer—Prevention. 4. Medical screening.
[DNLM: 1. Breast Neoplasms—diagnosis. 2. Mammography. 3. Mass Screening. 4. Research. WP 870 S267 2004] I. Joy, Janet E. (Janet Elizabeth), 1953- II. Penhoet, Edward E. III. Petitti, Diana B. IV. National Cancer Policy Board (U.S.). Committee on New Approaches to Early Detection and Diagnosis of Breast Cancer. V. National Research Council (U.S.). Policy and Global Affairs. VI. National Research Council (U.S.). Board on Science, Technology, and Economic Policy.
RC280.B8S28 2004
616.99′449075—dc22

2004022343

Additional copies of this report are available from the National Academies Press, 500 Fifth Street, N.W., Lockbox 285, Washington, DC 20055; (800) 624-6242 or (202) 334-3313 (in the Washington metropolitan area); Internet, http://www.nap.edu.

For more information about the Institute of Medicine, visit the IOM home page at: **www.iom.edu.**

Copyright 2005 by the National Academy of Sciences. All rights reserved.

Printed in the United States of America.

Cover designed by Beth Schlenoff.

THE NATIONAL ACADEMIES
Advisers to the Nation on Science, Engineering, and Medicine

The **National Academy of Sciences** is a private, nonprofit, self-perpetuating society of distinguished scholars engaged in scientific and engineering research, dedicated to the furtherance of science and technology and to their use for the general welfare. Upon the authority of the charter granted to it by the Congress in 1863, the Academy has a mandate that requires it to advise the federal government on scientific and technical matters. Dr. Bruce M. Alberts is president of the National Academy of Sciences.

The **National Academy of Engineering** was established in 1964, under the charter of the National Academy of Sciences, as a parallel organization of outstanding engineers. It is autonomous in its administration and in the selection of its members, sharing with the National Academy of Sciences the responsibility for advising the federal government. The National Academy of Engineering also sponsors engineering programs aimed at meeting national needs, encourages education and research, and recognizes the superior achievements of engineers. Dr. Wm. A. Wulf is president of the National Academy of Engineering.

The **Institute of Medicine** was established in 1970 by the National Academy of Sciences to secure the services of eminent members of appropriate professions in the examination of policy matters pertaining to the health of the public. The Institute acts under the responsibility given to the National Academy of Sciences by its congressional charter to be an adviser to the federal government and, upon its own initiative, to identify issues of medical care, research, and education. Dr. Harvey V. Fineberg is president of the Institute of Medicine.

The **National Research Council** was organized by the National Academy of Sciences in 1916 to associate the broad community of science and technology with the Academy's purposes of furthering knowledge and advising the federal government. Functioning in accordance with general policies determined by the Academy, the Council has become the principal operating agency of both the National Academy of Sciences and the National Academy of Engineering in providing services to the government, the public, and the scientific and engineering communities. The Council is administered jointly by both Academies and the Institute of Medicine. Dr. Bruce M. Alberts and Dr. Wm. A. Wulf are chair and vice chair, respectively, of the National Research Council.

www.national-academies.org

COMMITTEE ON NEW APPROACHES TO EARLY DETECTION AND DIAGNOSIS OF BREAST CANCER

EDWARD E. PENHOET (*Chair*), Director, Science and Higher Education Programs, Gordon and Betty Moore Foundation, San Francisco, CA

DIANA B. PETITTI (*Vice Chair*), Senior Scientific Advisor, Health Policy and Medicine, Kaiser Permanente Southern California, Pasadena, CA

MARTIN D. ABELOFF, Director, Sidney Kimmel Comprehensive Cancer Center at Johns Hopkins, Baltimore, MD

COLIN B. BEGG, Chairman, Department of Epidemiology and Biostatistics, Memorial Sloan-Kettering Cancer Center

M. KATHLEEN BEHRENS, General Partner, RS & Co. Venture Partners IV, L.P. RS Investments, San Francisco, CA

RICHARD BOHMER, Assistant Professor, Harvard Business School

CHRISTINE BRUNSWICK, Vice President, National Breast Cancer Coalition, Washington, DC

SANJIV S. GAMBHIR, Director, Molecular Imaging Program at Stanford, Stanford University, Stanford, CA

ROBERT A. GREENES, Professor, Radiology and Health Sciences & Technology, Harvard Medical School, Brigham and Women's Hospital, Boston, MA

JEFFREY R. MARKS, Associate Professor, Department of Surgery, Duke University Medical Center, Durham, NC

BARBARA J. McNEIL, Ridley Watts Professor and Head, Department of Health Care Policy, Harvard Medical School; Professor of Radiology, Brigham and Women's Hospital, Boston, MA; Head of Department of Health Care Policy, Harvard Medical School, Boston, MA

DAVID C. MOWERY, Professor, Walter A. Haas School of Business, University of California, Berkeley, CA

ETTA D. PISANO, Chief of Breast Imaging, Department of Radiology, University of North Carolina Hospitals, Chapel Hill, NC

GLENN D. STEELE, President and CEO, Geisinger Health System, Danville, PA

KIRBY G. VOSBURGH, Associate Director, Center for Integration of Medicine and Innovative Technologies (CIMIT), Cambridge, MA

WILLIAM C. WOOD, Chief of Surgery, Emory University Hospital, Atlanta, GA

Consultants

LAURA J. ESSERMAN, Director, Carol Franc Buck Breast Care Center, University of California, San Francisco, CA

LANCE A. LIOTTA, Chief, Laboratory of Pathology, National Cancer Institute, Bethesda, MD

LARRY NORTON, Deputy Physician-in-Chief and Director of Breast Cancer Programs, Memorial Sloan-Kettering Cancer Center, New York, NY

Study Staff

JANET E. JOY, Study Director

ROGER C. HERDMAN, Director, National Cancer Policy Board

JAMES J. DANIERO, Research Associate

ELIZABETH J. BROWN, Research Assistant

MARY ANN F. PRYOR, Project Assistant

ANIKE L. JOHNSON, Administrative Assistant

Reviewers

This report has been reviewed in draft form by individuals chosen for their diverse perspectives and technical expertise, in accordance with procedures approved by the National Research Council's (NRC's) Report Review Committee. The purpose of this independent review is to provide candid and critical comments that will assist the institution in making its published report as sound as possible and to ensure that the report meets institutional standards for objectivity, evidence, and responsiveness to the study charge. The review comments and draft manuscript remain confidential to protect the integrity of the deliberative process. We wish to thank the following individuals for their review of this report:

Mina J. Bissell, Life Science Division, Lawrence Berkeley National Laboratory, Berkeley, CA

Steven R. Cummings, Research Institute at the California Pacific Medical Center, University of California, San Francisco, CA

Alan M. Garber, Center for Health Policy and Center for Primary Care and Outcomes Research, Stanford University, Stanford, CA

Lawrence H. Miike, Former Commissioner of Hawaii Department of Health, Honolulu, HI

Barbara S. Monsees, Mallinckrodt Institute of Radiology, St. Louis, MO

Charles B. Wilson, Health Technology Center, San Francisco, CA

Although the reviewers listed above have provided many constructive comments and suggestions, they were not asked to endorse the conclusions or recommendations nor did they see the final draft of the report before its release. The review of this report was overseen by **Paul D. Cleary, Ph.D., Professor of Health Care Policy, Harvard Medical School and Maureen Henderson, O.B.E., M.D., Emeritus Professor of Epidemiology and Medicine, University of Washington.** Appointed by the NRC and Institute of Medicine, they were responsible for making certain that an independent examination of this report was carried out in accordance with institutional procedures and that all review comments were carefully considered. Responsibility for the final content of this report rests entirely with the authoring committee and the institution.

Acknowledgments

Progress in the fight against breast cancer has benefited enormously from the efforts of thousands of volunteers who have worked to raise awareness, money, and provide support to women with breast cancer. This report has likewise benefited enormously from the generous efforts of volunteers. In addition to committee members who volunteered their time and tremendous efforts, dozens of other experts volunteered their time either through formal presentations or through informal contacts with the study staff. Those who made formal presentations to the committee are listed in the workshop agendas in Appendix B. The following people provided technical comment on draft sections of the report: Nananda Col, David Feigal, Charles Finder, Joseph Hackett, Barbara Monsees, David Pwinica-Worms, Barbara Rimer, Mary Ropka, Alan Rosenberg, Mitchell Schnall, Karen Sepucha, Robert A. Smith, and Sean Tunis. Their expert counsel was much appreciated and invaluable. Kim Adcock, Leonard Berlin, and David Page, Laszlo Tabar, and Earl Steinberg provided critical reference material or shared their unpublished work. Pam Butler and Priscilla Butler were a treasure trove of information and shared many analyses related to workforce issues done by the American College of Radiology.

In addition to outside experts, Sharyl Nass, Maria Hewitt, and Jill Eden, study directors at the National Cancer Policy Board, were always generous and insightful in their advice about the many different issues related to the study. Elizabeth McCarthy and Jennifer VanRoeyen, both interns at the Institute of Medicine (IOM) for several months during the early stages of the study, did wonderful jobs of researching and developing background material for the study. Elizabeth Brown had been on the IOM staff for only a few months and proved outstanding in her ability at filling in the many information holes that remained in the late stages of the report. James Daniero, the research associate throughout the study, was entrusted with an extraordinary amount of responsibility for the research, development, and production of this report. He has been dedicated and resourceful in solving countless challenges that arose during the course of the study—from coping with record-setting blizzards in the midst of committee meetings to preparing essential background materials while supervising the multitude of production and administrative tasks associated with the study. As much as he has provided exemplary staff support, he has been a pleasure and privilege for all to work with.

Roger Herdman, director of the National Cancer Policy Board, was always available for consultation and always provided wise and thoughtful perspectives on all matters of health policy and technology. His support at every stage of this project is enormously appreciated.

Alison Mack and Margie Patlak, consulting writers for various sections of the report, were wonderful colleagues who provided input to the study above and beyond their writing contributions. Jennifer Otten, Janice Mehler, and Bill McLeod of the IOM each provided wonderful assistance at different stages of the study, and all consistently went above and beyond the call of duty to help shepherd the study through the Academy process. Special thanks to Janet Joy for her tireless efforts in preparing this report on behalf of the committee and for her many contributions to obtaining and synthesizing the evidence that is the basis for the recommendations.

The committee also gratefully acknowledges Margaret E. Mahoney and Carol Richards who were instrumental in enlisting support for this report and whose vision led to its genesis.

Acronyms

AAMC	Association of American Medical Colleges
ACE	Angiotensin-Converting Enzyme
ACR	American College of Radiology
ACRIN	American College of Radiology Imaging Network
ACS	American Cancer Society
AHRQ	Agency for Healthcare Research and Quality
AIDS	Acquired Immunodeficiency Syndrome
ALLHAT	Antihypertensive and Lipid Lowering Treatment to Prevent Heart Attack Trial
AMA	American Medical Association
ASRT	American Society of Radiologic Technicians
BCCPTA	Breast and Cervical Cancer Prevention and Treatment Act
BCS	Breast-conserving surgery
BI-RADS®	Breast Imaging Reporting and Data Systems
CABG	Coronary Artery Bypass Surgery
CAD	Computer-Assisted Detection
CDC	Centers for Disease Control and Prevention
CLIA	Clinical Laboratory Improvement Amendment
CMS	Centers for Medicare and Medicaid Services
CPT	Current Procedural Terminology
CT	Computed Tomography

DCIS	Ductal carcinoma in situ
DICOM	Digital Imaging and Communications in Medicine
DMIST	Digital Mammography Imaging Screening Trial
DoD	Department of Defense
EDRN	Early Detection Research Network
EIS	Electrical Impedance Scanning
FDA	Food and Drug Administration
GAO	Government Accounting Office
HDC/BMT	High-dose chemotherapy/Bone marrow transplant
HHS	Health and Human Services
HIPAA	Health Insurance Portability and Accountability Act
ICBIO	Interagency Council on Biomedical Imaging in Oncology
IDE	Investigational Device Exemption
IOM	Institute of Medicine
IRB	Institutional Review Board
LOH	Loss of Heterozygosity
MQSA	Mammography Quality Standards Act
MRI	Magnetic Resonance Imaging
NCI	National Cancer Institute
NCICB	National Cancer Institute Center for Bioinformatics
NDMA	National Digital Mammography Archives
NHSBSP	National Health Service Breast Screening Programme
NIBIB	National Institute of Biomedical Imaging and Bioengineering
NIH	National Institutes of Health
NINR	National Institute of Nursing Research
NSABP	National Surgical Adjuvant Breast and Bowel Project
PCR	Polymerase Chain Reaction
PDQ	Physician Data Query
PET	Positron Emission Tomography
PHI	Protected Health Information
PMA	Premarket Approval
PPV	Positive Predictive Value
PSA	Prostate Serum Antigen

QUADAS   Quality Assessment of Diagnostic Accuracy

RDOG   Radiology Diagnostic Oncology Group
ROC   Receiver Operating Characteristic
RT   Radiologic Technician

SEER   Surveillance, Epidemiology, and End Results
SPECT   Single-emission Photon Emission Computed Tomography
STAR   Study of Tamoxifen and Raloxifene
STARD   Standards for Reporting of Diagnostic Accuracy

USPSTF   U.S. Preventive Services Task Force

VNPI   Van Nuys Prognostic Index

WHO   World Health Organization

The National Academies is pleased to acknowledge that a gift in support of this project was made in honor of Sallie Nicholls, Beth Weibling, Jane Carlson Williams, Bonnie Main, and Amy McGraw, and in memory of Joan Morgan and Mabel Frost McCaw.

Contents

List of Boxes, Figures, and Tables

BOXES

FIGURES

TABLES

Executive Summary

The outlook for women with breast cancer has improved significantly since 1989 as the mortality rate has declined steadily, a decline attributed both to earlier detection through wider use of mammography screening and to improved treatments. Yet breast cancer remains a major problem, second only to lung cancer as a leading cause of death from cancer for women. This year over 200,000 new cases will be diagnosed and about 40,000 women—most diagnosed in earlier years—will die from the disease.

As their basic understanding has improved, researchers have discovered that breast cancer is far from simple. The disease has many forms that follow many pathways. Some are swift and lethal while others may never progress. Unfortunately, the tools available today cannot distinguish between the small pre-invasive lesions that will become lethal and those that will not. Consequently, most breast cancers are treated as if they were destined to be lethal and many women undergo difficult treatments, such as mastectomy, radiation, and chemotherapy, that might never have been needed.

Current treatments for breast cancer range from the relatively simple, but daunting, procedure known as lumpectomy, which removes cancerous and surrounding breast tissues, to the modified radical mastectomy in which an entire breast and the adjacent lymph nodes are excised. Both may be accompanied by chemotherapy and/or radiation therapy. None of these treatments, however, is guaranteed to save a woman's life, and, because so little is understood about the cellular mechanisms and processes that govern cancer progression, no one can predict with certainty which patients will be "cancer survivors" after treatment.

To date, no way to prevent breast cancer has been discovered and experience has shown that treatments are most effective when a cancer is detected early, while still small and contained and before it has spread to other tissues. Those two facts suggest that, at the present time, improving early detection and diagnosis is the most effective way to continue reducing the toll from breast cancer.

Several years ago an Institute of Medicine (IOM) and National Research Council (NRC) committee examined the array of promising detection and diagnostic technologies then in various stages of development, and concluded that mammography, while far from perfect, was still the best choice for screening the general population to detect breast cancer at early and treatable stages. Their findings and recommendations were published in 2001 in *Mammography and Beyond: Developing Technologies for Early Detection of Breast Cancer*.

For a variety of reasons, many women do not undergo regular screening. These reasons include limited availability of screening in some areas, inadequate insurance coverage, and misunderstanding of the value of screening. Also, some women are so afraid of breast cancer they choose not to be screened. Others find the procedure painful. The fact that mammography does not work equally well for all women, especially those with dense breast tissue, is a further complication.

In addition, the potential for false-positive and false-negative results remains high. Studies suggest that, due to a lack of sensitivity leading to false-negative findings, mammography screening may miss as many as 1 in 6 tumors. At the other extreme, the risk of a false-positive result is about 1 in 10, meaning that about 1 in 10 suspicious findings on a screening mammogram are false alarms. About three-quarters of suspicious areas biopsied as a result of a mammogram turn out to be benign—though only after a woman has endured the fear that she has breast cancer and borne the costs and discomfort of additional medical procedures.

In 2002, the IOM and NRC named a second committee to examine which of the approaches identified in *Mammography and Beyond* held the greatest promise for improving early detection and diagnosis. In addition, this group was asked to both identify and recommend ways to overcome and/or circumvent barriers to the development, evaluation, and, finally, incorporation into clinical practice of those strategies with the greatest potential.

Charged with developing a rational and workable framework for the early detection and diagnosis of breast cancer, the committee was also given the broader, and in some ways more formidable, challenge of improving the understanding of both the media and the general public of the public health issues that both underlie and impede the development of new approaches, including the role of regulatory policies and insurance coverage.

With *Mammography and Beyond* as a starting point, the committee identified several potential approaches: broader access to and use of mammography, better quality mammography, or the development of new technologies. They concluded that for the immediate future, broader and better use of mammography holds the greatest potential to save lives.

Even the most promising of the new technologies, committee members determined, will probably lead only to incremental improvements in existing technologies, and will not replace them. Indeed, finding ways to ensure those incremental advances are integrated into existing systems holds more immediate promise for improving outcomes for breast cancer patients than attempts to isolate a single new technology that might replace mammography. Important avenues of research and development for exciting technologies, such as biological markers of cancer and molecular profiling, although still in their infancy, are especially promising as diagnostic tools.

Simply identifying promising technologies, even those proven through extensive clinical trials, would have no value unless those technologies are suitable for and adopted in clinical practice so they become available to the women who might benefit. Because most clinical trials for cancer detection are designed to evaluate a single technology and do not provide information that might help physicians choose which competing approaches would most benefit patients, the questions asked of new technologies should be which should be used and when, not which is best. As the committee reminded, breast cancer is a complex disease that passes through numerous critical stages, each requiring different tools for detection and diagnosis, and demanding different sets of decisions.

The first decision, of course, is whether a woman decides to be screened for breast cancer, a decision that depends, in part, on a woman's perception of her own breast cancer risk, which is often distorted. For many women, the very topic of breast cancer provokes confusion and dread. Many women overestimate their risk of getting and dying of breast cancer before the age of 50, a finding mirrored in the many magazine articles that suggest a significant risk of breast cancer in younger women. Much of their information comes from news reports and advertisements in the mass media, and more recently the Internet, which tend to emphasize dramatic, unusual, and extreme examples rather than balanced and factual presentations.

Extensive, and sometimes inaccurate, media coverage of recent controversies about the effectiveness of screening mammography has contributed to public confusion about the value of mammography, its role in breast cancer detection, and the ages at which it is most likely to be beneficial.

Also, glowing reports of "medical breakthroughs" and "promising" technologies that have not been submitted for approval or even tested in patients add another layer of confusion and uncertainty.

Physicians face different kinds of decisions. When confronted with an abnormal mammogram, they must decide which technology will provide the most expedient and reliable result and, then, how much faith to put in that result. At present, they receive little research-based guidance about emerging technologies, which combinations of technologies, and which approaches would be most effective for certain groups of patients.

The committee included clinicians involved in breast cancer screening, detection, and treatment; experts in cancer and molecular biology; those with expertise in clinical studies, as well as those involved with the development, evaluation, and adoption of medical technology and with experience in health care administration.

To supplement their own considerable expertise, members held a number of background workshops and heard from a range of technology developers, researchers, and leaders of clinical studies designed to improve systems for early detection and diagnosis. They also discussed the many issues involved in assessing new medical technologies with senior staff at the federal agencies and with representatives of private insurance groups, all the groups that act as gatekeepers for medical technology.

Based on this information and their lengthy deliberations, the committee identified four major categories for recommendations aimed at improving early detection and diagnosis of breast cancer: improve current application of screening mammography; integrate biology, technology, and risk models to develop new screening strategies; improve the environment for research and development; and improve the implementation and use of new technologies. The detailed rationale and supporting data for each category are in the body of the report. A brief summary of pertinent findings, together with the recommendations, follows (recommendations are also listed separately in the box at the end of this summary).

IMPROVE CURRENT APPLICATION OF SCREENING MAMMOGRAPHY

A growing shortage of radiologists who specialize in reading mammograms, coupled with an imbalance between the closures and openings of screening facilities, has created unacceptable delays in some parts of the country. At the same time the number of false-positive readings appears to be increasing, possibly due to increasing defensive medicine in reaction to the frequency of malpractice litigation.

Improving screening practices to reduce the number of false positives could reduce the costs of additional testing by an estimated $100 million per year, in addition to eliminating the mental anguish and the possible need for a biopsy for thousands of women and also cutting unnecessary waiting time. Though no one knows the actual costs of settling malpractice suits, since so many are settled out of court, these settlements are thought to contribute to the ever-escalating costs of malpractice insurance for radiologists who read mammograms, a trend that discourages physicians from entering the profession.

Given these, and other, factors, the committee sought ways to optimize the productivity of radiologists who interpret mammograms and, at the same time, improve their accuracy. They looked toward the experience of other countries, notably the United Kingdom, and their organization of screening services. Although differences in the number of "excess" biopsies due to false-positive readings were difficult to assess, for even within the United States significant regional variations exist, committee members did identify elements in the programs of some European countries, as well as Canada and Australia, that could be useful in the United States, which has limited national or regional standards or programs for breast cancer screening. For instance, in the United Kingdom radiologic technologists, who are not physicians, are trained to meet national certification standards, and have proven comparable in accuracy and speed to radiologists.

Also, the British National Breast Cancer Screening Program invites every woman for a screening mammogram, which is paid for through the National Health Service—but only at three-year intervals. In the United States, the recommended screening interval is one year, which is likely to detect more cancers, but women do not get screened unless they are referred by health care providers or refer themselves. Many women are never screened because they lack adequate, if any, insurance coverage. That group tends to include underserved women in lower socioeconomic groups in whom breast cancer may not be detected at an early stage when still treatable.

A program that might be adapted by health care providers in the United States is the European Code Against Cancer which stresses that screening should be done within integrated breast care centers that have quality assurance programs. Another model is Britain's National Health Service Breast Screening Program, which has developed national quality assurance standards and a quality assurance network though which programs are regularly monitored, with results measured against established targets. In the United States no organization collects or monitors data to promote high performance levels and guidelines are only voluntary. (The Mammography Quality Standards Act [MQSA] requires facilities in the United States to collect quality data for internal use, but does not require the facilities to use the data in any specific or documented approach for quality improvement.)

In Sweden and the Netherlands, which both report low rates of false positives, screening takes place in outlying centers and diagnosis and workup takes place in centralized facilities. Great Britain has developed a quality assurance self-assessment program, the only one of its kind in the world, which, while voluntary, is used by 90 percent of that nation's radiologists to identify weaknesses and improve interpretive skills.

By contrast, in the United States screening services are rarely integrated within a comprehensive breast cancer center, and typically separated from treatment, counseling, and support services. The MQSA addressed the technical quality of mammograms, but does not require standards to improve delivery of services and quality of interpretation, or quality assurance and a continuing education program intended to enhance the accuracy of interpretation.

To improve services in the United States, the committee recommended:

Health care providers and payers should consider adopting elements of successful breast cancer screening programs from other countries. Such programs involve centralized expert interpretation in regionalized programs, outcome analysis, and benchmarking. (Recommendation A1)

At this time, one of the few regulations directly relating to the quality of interpretation in the United States requires physicians who interpret mammograms to read a minimum of 960 exams in a 24-month period, which averages out to 480 per year. By comparison, breast imaging specialists in the United Kingdom are required to read at least 5,000 each year.

A number of technologies under development have potential to improve the quality and accuracy of mammography interpretation. These include such technologies as computer-aided detection (CAD), which does not replace interpretation by a radiologist but can highlight areas of concern for further review by the radiologist. The greatest value of CAD may prove to be its potential to increase the performance level of general radiologists to that of those who specialize in breast imaging.

Too, the shortage of mammography personnel may actually impede the kinds of innovation that would improve their efficiency for experts are needed to both assess and properly use these new technologies.

To address these issues the committee recommended:

Breast imagers and technology developers should work in collaboration with health care providers and payers to improve the overall quality of mammographic interpretation by: (Recommendation A2)

- **adopting and further developing practices that promote self-improvement of breast imagers, but that do not jeopardize the workforce; and**
- **developing technologies, such as CAD, that have the potential to improve quality, and expanding their use once they have been validated.**

In addition to the inconsistent quality of mammographic interpretation, some experts believe the growing shortage of breast imagers might soon create a crisis in access to high-quality mammography services. This shortage, coupled with an imbalance between the closures and openings of screening facilities, has created delays of several months in some parts of the country. One approach to address this shortage would be to train physician assistants, or physician extenders, a practice that has helped to alleviate shortages and reduce the workload for physicians in other medical specialties. The judicious use of physician extenders could raise the productivity of the limited number of radiologists who interpret screening mammograms. The committee does not suggest that physician extenders should interpret diagnostic mammograms or that screening mammograms should be interpreted solely by a physician extender, rather they would work to expand the capacity of radiologists.

The MQSA stipulates that mammograms are to be interpreted only by a physician specifically certified in mammography. The Act does not, however, preclude other personnel from examining the mammograms that are *also* interpreted by certified physicians. Although not widely appreciated and rarely practiced, it would in fact be permissible within the provisions of the MQSA to have nonphysician personnel examine mammograms—as long as a certified physician signed the mammogram report indicating that he or she had interpreted it. This suggestion that physician extenders could be enlisted to help read mammograms could thus offer women a more thorough examination than is currently typical of most mammography facilities where mammograms are viewed only by a single breast imager.

The potential for alleviating the shortage prompted the committee to recommend:

> To expand the capacity of breast screening programs, mammography facilities should enlist specially trained nonphysician personnel to prescreen mammograms for abnormalities or double-read mammograms to expand the capacity of breast imaging specialists. (Recommendation A3)

INTEGRATE BIOLOGY, TECHNOLOGY, AND RISK MODELS TO DEVELOP NEW SCREENING STRATEGIES

The wide-ranging levels of risk for breast cancer have important implications for screening and detection. Most guidelines in the United States now recommend annual mammograms for every woman over the age of 40, but the ability to better classify women according to their risk levels—whether high, normal, or low—could allow a more individualized approach to screening. For example, most women would gain no medical benefit from screening before the age of 40 or from twice-yearly screening, though a small minority of women might benefit.

Finding techniques that permit such classification will demand a better and more precise understanding of risk factors. To date, the most significant risk factors are age and gender. The widely used "Gail model" identified five risk factors: age, age at menarche, age at first live birth, number of prior breast biopsies, and the number of first degree relatives with breast cancer. Based on data from the Breast Cancer Detection Demonstration Project conducted in the 1970s and involving 200,000 women, the model has proven highly accurate at predicting the numbers of women within various age and risk groups who will develop cancer within the next five years, but it is only moderately accurate at predicting which individual women will develop the disease.

Another limitation of the Gail model is that it does not include genetic risk factors. Risk assessments for women with BRCA genetic mutations have been developed from retrospective analyses of risks in the relatives of carriers from high-risk families. The accuracy of these analyses has been questioned as population-based studies indicate the risk may be substantially lower. Also risk assessments for carriers have not taken into account the other risk factors used in the Gail model.

The committee believes that individual screening strategies are crucial to improving the early detection of breast cancer and that accurate risk assessment is an essential step toward the eventual development of individualized screening strategies.

Therefore:

Researchers and technology developers should focus their efforts on developing tools to identify those women who would benefit most from breast cancer screening. Such tools should be based on individually tailored risk prediction techniques that integrate biologic and other risk factors. (Recommendation B1)

The combination of established risk factors with more comprehensive genetic risk profiles will require the development of mathematical models to relate genetic predictors, biological expression, natural course of disease, and responses to treatment in order to:

- Elucidate the natural course of disease progression and identify disease subgroups with distinctive risk profiles and treatment susceptibilities;
- Identify aspects of the models where further research and data collection are needed;

- Provide guidance to technology developers as to the types of technologies that will be most useful, including the required performance characteristics.

The current biological revolution has introduced a new era in cancer detection. Considerable progress has been made in identifying biomarkers for cancer and developing aggregate profiles of breast cancer in specific genes and proteins. Already the theoretical promise of this progress is being realized in animal models.

Yet the novel diagnostic tests of genomics and proteomics, despite their tantalizing potential, must be developed with a goal of clinical usefulness and, ultimately, value to the patient. These tests may prove much too complex for routine screening if they provide too much information, not too little. It is difficult, for instance, to validate tests that provide hundreds of thousands of results for each specimen, as opposed to single-result tests, but without such validation the tests will be of limited value.

Another possible drawback to these tests may be their lack of specificity; they may be able to detect cancer, but not be able to identify the type of cancer or location. Because of this, their first useful clinical applications may be to monitor therapeutic response and recurrence, and not as screening tools. Even as individual biomarkers for cancer are identified, blood tests to screen women who are symptom free and at normal risk may be meaningless based on a one-time measurement.

Further in the future, there exists the potential for individualized management of each case based on specific molecular characteristics. The development of a profile of deranged cellular circuitry in each cancer patient may allow the tailoring of therapy to meet the individual molecular profile, the microenvironment of the specific tumor and the cancer. Instead of single targets and single therapeutic agents, multiple targets may be used. Instead of waiting for a therapeutic response or signs of recurrence, those targets can be monitored, through the use of molecular imaging or serum proteomics.

Fulfilling the promise of molecular imaging and the potential of biological markers for breast cancers and other cancers will require substantial funding as well as collaborations between molecular biologists and scientists from many disciplines. Their joint goal must be to achieve the rational design of new diagnostic tools, establish their importance and utility, and adopt them for clinical use. These tools must meet safety and effectiveness criteria as well as evidence-based standards. Assistance from all parts of the system, from payers, providers, and patients, will be needed to ensure that innovative technology becomes integrated as part of the existing system.

To achieve maximum potential from innovative technologies, the committee further recommended:

> **Technology innovators, including basic scientists, should work with clinicians, health systems experts, and epidemiologists from the earliest stages of development in order to increase the likelihood of creating clinically useful tools for the early detection of breast cancer.** (Recommendation B2)

Because understanding the implications of risk plays an important role in breast cancer, the committee gave considerable attention to the problems involved with risk communication. Their concerns included finding better ways to communicate the notions of absolute and relative risk—no easy task, at best—both to individual women and to members of the public, including the news media.

Better tools are needed for communicating risk to help health care providers—the physicians, nurses, and counselors who work directly with patients—communicate more effectively with patients. Conversely, better tools are needed for patients and the public, specifically including the media, so they will have greater understanding of the material.

Many physicians do not communicate risk effectively and far too often patients either fail to recognize or are reluctant to admit their confusion. As more accurate predictive tools are identified and as individual risk profiles are developed, the need for such tools will become even more pressing.

To address this, the committee recommends:

> **Research funders, including the National Cancer Institute (NCI) and private foundations, should develop tools that facilitate communication regarding breast cancer risk to the public and to health care providers.** (Recommendation B3)

IMPROVE THE ENVIRONMENT FOR RESEARCH AND DEVELOPMENT

A number of groups, including the IOM and NRC's *Mammography and Beyond* committee and the NCI's Breast Cancer Research Progress Group have established priorities for breast cancer research. These include the identification of biomarkers, molecular analysis of the transition from pre-invasive to invasive disease, and the need for extensive databases so data can be assimilated and exploited for maximum benefit. These priorities, which the committee believes are appropriate, are reflected in the research portfolios of NCI, Department of Defense (DOD), and private funders. In addition, the committee members concluded that the "discovery research" that lays the foundation for innovative technologies is proceeding well, with promising developments that reflect these priorities on the horizon.

But a frustrating and considerable time lag occurs between the identification and development of a promising technology and the testing and experience that shows whether the promise will be achieved and the technology will prove useful. The fact that no system exists for the assessment of new technologies—aside from post-marketing surveillance which only detects product failures and does not assess performance once in use—means that there is no way to compare or evaluate the clinical effectiveness of technologies once they are on the market, a process that would require either long-term clinical studies or the collection, evaluation, and comparison of data.

Because so many more new technologies make it to the market than prove clinically useful, the committee sought ways to identify technologies that are not only feasible but will actually improve health or the delivery of health care services. These efforts ought to involve collaborative efforts among technology developers, not-for-profit organizations (including professional societies), advocacy groups, private health care payers, and provider organizations working together toward such joint goals as adopting and setting standards for assessment and adoption of new technology.

To achieve this goal, the committee recommended:

The National Institutes of Health, Agency for Healthcare Research and Quality (AHRQ), and Centers for Medicaid and Medicare Services (CMS) should collaborate to establish programs and centers (which may be virtual) that bring together expertise and funding to enable a more comprehensive approach to technology assessment and adoption. (Recommendation C1)

- **These efforts should involve collaboration with technology developers, not-for-profit organizations (including professional societies), advocacy groups, private health care payers, and provider organizations.**
- **Experimentation with innovative organizational structures for the centers should be encouraged.**
- **Adoption of standards for collecting and sharing data should be a priority.**

Clinical studies are expensive, typically costing millions of dollars in addition to the time and effort of participating patients, physicians, and nurses, but such studies are essential to the successful evaluation and adoption of new treatments and technologies. Too many clinical studies fail to provide useful data or to answer the basic question of whether a new technology improves health outcomes. That reflects an underlying problem with study design. Because of the costs involved, considerable attention should be given to avoiding poor study design, eliminating unintentional bias, and standardizing data collection.

These studies depend on the willing participation of the public and many researchers have noted a growing reluctance to participate, especially in studies that involve genetic testing and the collection of biological materials. Some of this reluctance has been attributed to fears that results of these tests could be misused by employers and by health and life insurance companies to discriminate against those with existing or potential problems.

With implementation of regulations under the Health Insurance Portability and Accountability Act of 1996 (HIPAA), other problems have emerged. The act was created for many reasons, among them to ensure the privacy and confidentiality of health information and make the transfer of health data more efficient. While the law was not intended to hinder research, it has changed the way health plans, clearinghouses, and providers handle personal health information and the way researchers share information.

The potential impact on research may prove far-reaching, especially on population-based research that requires broad and unbiased access to the medical records of health providers. The law also threatens the establishment of large databanks and makes it difficult to link data gathered in different institutions or to do studies that require long-term follow-up, which will be virtually impossible if all data have to be deidentified. While the Association of American Medical Colleges has established a network and database to monitor and document the impact of the law on research, uncertainty about the impact and interpretation of this very complex and lengthy law has already led to delays in research and has complicated the grant and contract process.

The concerns of committee members about the impact of this law, with its potential to impede efforts to improve the detection and diagnosis of breast cancer, led them to recommend that:

> **Professional societies should work together with women's health organizations to identify barriers to participation in studies (especially those that require provision of biologic specimens) and ways in which those barriers might be overcome. (Recommendation C2)**

> - **A public education campaign should be undertaken to inform the public, particularly under-represented groups, of the merit of participation in research studies that require the involvement of healthy volunteers and the donation of biologic specimens for genetic analysis.**
> - **Advocacy groups and women's health organizations should participate in design and execution of public education about clinical trials.**

This could be a collaborative effort, and might include the NCI and the American Cancer Society (ACS).

- The Department of Health and Human Services (CHHS) should join with private entities in monitoring the effect of the HIPAA Privacy Rule on the pace of research progress.

Breast cancer advocacy groups and women's health organizations have played very important roles in raising public awareness and generating support for efforts to reduce the toll from breast cancer. They could work with other groups such as NCI and ACS on a campaign to educate the public about the merit of participating in research studies that depend on healthy volunteers and the donation of biological materials for genetic analysis. They should also particularly target under-represented groups whose participation in such research is essential to reducing health care disparities based on race and ethnicity.

Further addressing concerns about the unintended consequences of the HIPAA privacy rule, the committee called upon the Department of Health and Human Services to work with the private sector in efforts to monitor its impact on the pace of research progress.

IMPROVE THE IMPLEMENTATION AND USE
OF NEW TECHNOLOGIES

Several disquieting facts suggest the urgent need to improve both the implementation and use of new technologies: many cancer detection technologies that have been proposed and developed have proved to be of no value to patients; approval by the Food and Drug Administration (FDA), which evaluates a technology for safety and effectiveness, is no guarantee the technology will be used.

Perhaps most important, though, is the pivotal role of insurance coverage, which poses a classic "Catch 22" dilemma for most new technologies. Federal and private insurers do not pay for new procedures and technologies until their role in improving outcomes for patients has been documented, but until these same procedures and technologies have been widely used outside of a research setting—which generally means someone must pay for their use—it is almost impossible to demonstrate how well a technology does, or does not, perform in actual use.

Contrary to public perceptions, only about 10 percent of new technologies that do make it to the market have undergone the kinds of clinical testing that demonstrate safety and effectiveness. Others have been approved because they have been judged to be similar to technologies already on the market and certain kinds of genetic and diagnostic tests, especially those performed in laboratories and not intended for direct sale, are not reviewed by FDA.

The rising costs of product development and the expense of clinical trials, coupled with uncertainty about the outcome of FDA review, have become significant roadblocks to the development of innovative technologies, particularly by small and start-up companies with limited financial resources. Recently FDA has worked to help reduce costs and expedite the review process, trying to work more closely with those groups who have little experience with FDA. How effective this approach will prove is still uncertain.

Based on their review, committee members concluded additional steps were needed, not only to expedite the assessment and to document the effectiveness of new procedures but also, once proven, to promote wider use in clinical practice. For instance, conditional coverage could help document which new technologies do improve the outlook for patients if data collection and evaluation are required. Then, if a technology failed to meet expectations, coverage could be withdrawn, but there is a caveat—experience has shown the near impossibility of eliminating coverage once it has been provided. Therefore, the committee does not recommend conditional coverage without careful analysis of feasible mechanisms for implementation.

Promoting wide use of new technologies that do prove beneficial poses other challenges, as well. Private practitioners need to learn how to use these procedures and incorporate them into their practices effectively. Studies have shown that strategies such as lectures and distribution of reading materials do little to change the way physicians practice medicine.

Current NIH efforts that include workforce training and efforts to translate research into practical applications and develop clinical research networks beyond academic settings address this problem.

The committee's strong conviction that basic research needs to be integrated with technology development and assessment prompted the following recommendation:

> **Breast cancer research funders, such as the NIH, DOD, and private foundations, should support research on screening and detection technologies that encompasses each aspect of technology adoption from deployment to application, and should include monitoring of use in practice.** (Recommendation D1)

- This will involve identification of optimal combinations and sequencing of breast cancer detection technologies.
- Research funders and private foundations should model and assess changes in practice and organization change that would optimize the benefit of new technology (including risk assessment).

This recommendation includes the identification of optimal combinations and sequencing of breast cancer detection technologies as well as developing models for, and then assessing, changes in practice and organization that would optimize benefits from new technologies, including risk assessment.

The committee further recommended:

The NIH, the AHRQ, and other public and private research sponsors should collaborate with health systems, providers, and payers to support research that would monitor clinical use of technologies to identify potential failures, as well as opportunities for improvement, with particular attention to: (Recommendation D2)

- how appropriately the technologies are being utilized,
- their impact on clinical decision making, and
- their impact on health outcomes.

Summary of Recommendations

A. Improve Current Application of Screening Mammography

A1. Health care providers and payers should consider adopting elements of successful breast cancer screening programs from other countries. Such programs involve centralized expert interpretation in regionalized programs, outcome analysis, and benchmarking.

A2. Breast imagers and technology developers should work in collaboration with health care providers and payers to improve the overall quality of mammographic interpretation by:

• Adopting and further developing practices that promote self-improvement of breast imagers, but that do not jeopardize the workforce.

• Developing technologies, such as computer aided detection, that have the potential to improve quality, and expanding their use once they have been validated.

A3. To expand the capacity of breast screening programs, mammography facilities should enlist specially trained nonphysician personnel to prescreen mammograms for abnormalities or double-read mammograms to expand the capacity of breast imaging specialists.

B. Integrate Biology, Technology, and Risk Models to Develop New Screening Strategies for Breast Cancer

B1. Researchers and technology developers should focus their efforts on developing tools to identify those women who would benefit most from breast cancer screening. Such tools should be based on individually tailored risk prediction techniques that integrate biologic and other risk factors.

B2. Technology innovators, including basic scientists, should work with clinicians, health systems experts, and epidemiologists from the earliest stages of development in order to increase the likelihood of creating clinically useful tools for the early detection of breast cancer.

B3. Research funders, including the NCI and private foundations, should develop tools that facilitate communication regarding breast cancer risk to the public and to health care providers.

C. Improve the Environment for Research and Development of New Technologies for Breast Cancer Detection

C1. The NIH, AHRQ, and CMS should collaborate to establish programs and centers (which may be virtual) that bring together expertise and funding to enable a more comprehensive approach to technology assessment and adoption.

- These efforts should involve collaboration with technology developers, not-for-profit organizations (including professional societies), advocacy groups, private health care payers, and provider organizations.

- Experimentation with innovative organizational structures for the centers should be encouraged.

- Adoption of standards for collecting and sharing data should be a priority.

C2. Professional societies should work together with women's health organizations to identify barriers to participation in studies (especially those that require provision of biologic specimens) and ways in which those barriers might be overcome.

- A public education campaign should be undertaken taken to inform the public, particularly under-represented groups, of the merit of participation in research studies that require the involvement of healthy volunteers and the donation of biologic specimens for genetic analysis.

- Advocacy groups and women's health organizations should participate in design and execution of public education about clinical trials. This could be a collaborative effort, and might include the NCI and the ACS.

- The DHHS should join with private entities in monitoring the effect of the HIPAA Privacy Rule on the pace of research progress.

D. Improve the Implementation and Use of New Technologies

D1. Breast cancer research funders, such as the NIH, DoD, and private foundations, should support research on screening and detection technologies that encompasses each aspect of technology adoption from deployment to application, and should include monitoring of use in practice.

- This will involve identification of optimal combinations and sequencing of breast cancer detection technologies.

- Research funders and private foundations should model and assess changes in practice and organization change that would optimize the benefit of new technology (including risk assessment).

D2. The NIH, AHRQ, and other public and private research sponsors should collaborate with health systems, providers, and payers to support research that would monitor clinical use of technologies to identify potential failures, as well as opportunities for improvement, with particular attention to:

- how appropriately the technologies are being utilized,

- their impact on clinical decision making, and

- their impact on health outcomes.

1

Introduction

The outlook for women with breast cancer has improved in recent years. Because of the combination of improved treatments and the benefits of mammography screening, breast cancer mortality has decreased steadily since 1989.[2] And yet, closer scrutiny reveals a complicated picture. Some breast cancers are lethal, and each year about 40,000 women and 400 men die from breast cancer in the United States. Others are not fatal, and some women diagnosed with breast cancer will needlessly undergo mastectomies, chemotherapy, and radiation. But no one knows which breast cancers are destined to be lethal and which are not, because too little is known about the cellular processes that determine cancer progression, and the diagnostic tools used today cannot distinguish small pre-invasive lesions that will progress from those that will not. For now, all breast cancers must be viewed as if they may be fatal. This means treatments for invasive breast cancer that range from uncomfortable (lumpectomy) to grueling (chemotherapy, radiation, and mastectomy), none of which guarantees a cure.

Although therapy for breast cancer has improved over the years, it is clear that there are no reliable ways of preventing this cancer. It is also clear that treatments are generally more effective when breast tumors are small and localized than when they are large and have already invaded other tissues. Even the drastic measure of undergoing a double mastectomy will substantially reduce the risk but will not completely eliminate the possibility of developing breast cancer. The limited methods for preventing and treating breast cancers leave early detection as the most promising approach for reducing morbidity and mortality from breast cancer.

A SAFETY NET

Mammography is a safety net that saves thousands of lives each year, yet thousands more slip through that net (see Box 1-1). Many women who would benefit from mammography do not undergo regular screening. Others who do undergo regular screening develop breast cancers that were not detected by their mammography exam. Additionally, then there are others whom screening mammography is unlikely to benefit, such as those who have no access to treatment or whose breast cancer is unresponsive to treatment even when detected early.

The goal of screening for breast cancer is not to detect all breast abnormalities; the goal is to prevent deaths from breast cancer. Thus the benefits of mammography depend on the availability of effective treatment. Despite the common misconception, screening mammography does not benefit women by reducing their risk of breast cancer, but rather by reducing mortality through detecting breast cancer at earlier and more treatable stages.

BOX 1-1
Millions of Women Do Not Receive Annual Mammograms

In 2002, approximately 60.5 percent of women aged 40 to 64 received mammograms in the United States. Based on U.S. Census Bureau data for 2002, this means that:

- 27.7 million women aged 40 to 64 received mammograms that year, and
- 18.1 million women aged 40 to 64 did *not* receive mammograms.

An estimated 15,300 women aged 40 to 64 died of breast cancer in 2003.

The risk of breast cancer rises steeply with age, but the use of mammography screening increases much less with age. Approximately 63.8 percent of women 65 and over received mammograms in the United States in 2002. Based on Census Bureau data for 2002, this means that:

- 13.3 million women 65 and over received mammograms that year, and
- 7.5 million women 65 and over did *not* receive mammograms.

An estimated 23,000 women over 65 died of breast cancer in 2003.

It is generally several years from the time a lethal breast cancer is first detected and the time of death. In most cases, women who die of breast cancer in a particular year are not the same women who receive a screening mammogram or even are first diagnosed that year.

SOURCE: U.S. Census Data for July 2003; Cancer Prevention and Early Detection Facts and Figures, ACS 2004.

Although mammography saves lives, it is not perfect. Depending on the study, the sensitivity of screening mammography ranges from 83 to 95 percent, which means that as many as 17 percent of cancer cases may go undetected by mammography. As many as three-quarters of the breast lesions that are biopsied in the United States as a result of a suspicious mammogram are benign.[9,11] More effective approaches to the early detection and diagnosis of breast cancer would go a long way toward improving the care of women concerned about their risk of breast cancer—both by reducing the number of false alarms and unnecessary biopsies and by decreasing the number of cases that go undetected.

BEYOND MAMMOGRAPHY

There are several potential ways to improve detection of breast cancer: more widespread use of mammography, better quality mammography, or development of new technologies. Of these three, greater use of mammography, as it now exists, even though it remains an imperfect screening technology, would likely save the most lives in the short run.

Although a number of new technologies are poised to expand the suite of current options, most advances are likely to be incremental improvements in existing technologies. The most significant technology changes to be adopted in clinical practice since 2001, when the Institute of Medicine and the National Research Council's *Mammography and Beyond* report was published, have been improvements in existing technology. Four new digital mammography systems[a] and three new systems for computer-aided detection[b] were approved by the Food and Drug Administration and are all on the market now. Thus far, the accuracy of digital mammography has been shown to be equivalent to, but not superior to, traditional film-screen mammography, although clinical studies are still under way.[14]

There have also been changes relevant to breast cancer detection that are only indirectly related to technology developments. First, the sense of crisis concerning the shortage of breast imagers has deepened, and mammography facilities continue to close. Second, the Health Insurance Portability and Accountability Act Privacy Rule took effect in April 2003 and is a source of great concern to those conducting certain types of clinical studies. Third, the extent to which ductal carcinoma in situ (DCIS) cases are overtreated remains unclear, but the most recent data suggest that until it is

---

[a]Senographe 2000D (GE Medical Systems), MAMMOMAT (Siemens Medical Systems), SenoScan (Fisher Imaging), and Selenia (LORAD).

[b]MammoReader (Intelligent Systems Software), Second Look (iCAD), and ImageChecker (R2 Technology).

possible to predict the outcome of individual cases of DCIS, the wisest course for mammographically detected DCIS is full diagnostic workup and treatment. Another change since the publication of *Mammography and Beyond* is that the storm over Goetzsche and Olsen's criticism of the value of screening mammography has largely subsided. Every expert organization that has reviewed their critique together with other published data has concluded that the evidence indicates that screening mammography saves lives.

Other promising new technologies might improve the early detection and diagnosis of breast cancer, but none are ready for widespread clinical use. Some are based on advances in imaging technology, others on advances in molecular biology, and still others on a combination of both. Certain innovations might someday allow the stages in the traditional care pathway to be telescoped. For example, a blood test that identified cancer risk might also detect active cancer, if present, thereby creating a direct link between prescreening and diagnosis. Another blood test might determine that a woman's risk of breast cancer is so low that yearly mammograms might not be necessary.

INVESTING IN RESEARCH

Fostering the invention and early stage development of medical technology is essential and depends on the nurturing of basic medical research. With the possible exception of AIDS, breast cancer research receives more funding than any other disease—due, in no small part, to the long-standing and tireless efforts of breast cancer activists. The National Cancer Institute (NCI) currently supports more research projects and clinical studies for breast cancer than for any other type of cancer.[c] In addition to the National Institutes of Health (NIH), breast cancer research is supported by private health charities and the Department of Defense (DoD), which together provide more than $300 million per year, for a total of roughly $800 million per year. By comparison, NCI spent $311 million on prostate cancer and the DoD's Medical Research Program spent $85 million for a total of just under $400 million.

The committee believes that current priorities for basic research are appropriate. The investment in basic research over the past few decades has yielded a wealth of knowledge that supports the invention of a rich array of powerful new technologies—from imaging devices that can display the activity of individual cell types to assays that can simultaneously measure

---

[c]According to the NCI website, 2,932 breast cancer projects and 112 clinical trials are supported. In comparison, the average for all 56 types of cancer (or aspects of cancer) listed by NCI is only 8 clinical trials and 276 projects.[17]

the activity of thousands of genes or proteins, among others. But considerable time elapses between the development of a promising technology and determining whether its promise can be realized.

Inevitably, more exciting new technologies are announced than are proven useful in clinical practice. Although basic research enables the development of early stage technologies, different strategies are needed to identify which technologies are truly feasible and add clinical value by improving people's health or the delivery of health care services. This involves large-scale, well-designed multicenter clinical trials. However, clinical trials have historically received substantially less support from NIH than basic research.

Even when technologies have been shown to offer clinical benefit, they add no value until they are adopted in clinical practice and used effectively. It is often many years from the time when early adopters, or leading-edge clinicians, adopt new technologies and when those technologies become widely and effectively used in the larger health care community. The likelihood that an innovation will be adopted into clinical practice depends not only on its performance characteristics, but also on the capacity of health care organizations to integrate it effectively into their practices. Indeed, effective application of new advances in medicine is a serious bottleneck in improving patient care and a source of concern to the medical community.[12,24] Balas and Boren estimated that the interval between discovery and application for innovations has been an average of 17 years.[3] The committee believes it is also important to analyze which new technologies are adoptable in clinical practice. This would entail a more comprehensive approach to technology assessment than is commonly practiced.

An immediate challenge lies in ensuring that incremental advances deliver the greatest possible value to patients. This will require the development of systems to permit evidence-based choices among suites of evolving options. The key to improving the detection and diagnosis of breast cancer is, therefore, not necessarily to focus on the single emerging technology that is the most deserving of support, but rather on the systems that provide the best possible health outcomes for breast cancer patients.

In many cases, some approaches or technologies are better than others under certain circumstances, but they are rarely better in all circumstances. The challenge lies in knowing what to use when. Most clinical studies for cancer detection are designed to evaluate a single new technology and do not provide the data that permit evidence-based choices among different options or how to sequence those options to maximize overall efficiency and effectiveness.[d] Rather than evaluating each technology only on its own,

---

[d]There are some notable exceptions such as the research being done by Mitch Schnall, Keith Paulsen, and their colleagues.

it must be considered in the overall context of clinical practice. There is a critical need for evidence that will support rational integration of different approaches to breast cancer detection and that will consider the organizational issues.

SCOPE OF THIS STUDY

This study is a sequel to *Mammography and Beyond,* released by the Institute of Medicine (IOM) and the National Research Council (NRC) in 2001. The committee that produced that study was asked to (1) review existing technologies and (2) identify promising new technologies for breast cancer detection technologies. They were also asked to analyze the steps in medical technology development relevant to breast cancer detection technologies, including the policies that influence technology adoption.

The previous committee thus provided an overview of current and near-term technologies for breast cancer detection and outlined the long and arduous path from invention to adoption of new technologies (Table 1-1). The present committee reviewed the conclusions and recommendations in *Mammography and Beyond,* endorses them, and agrees that they should be supported. Indeed, several of them already have been implemented. Because the present committee decided not to repeat the previous committee's excellent work, this report does not attempt a comprehensive review of current and emerging breast cancer detection technologies, nor does it provide an in-depth analysis of medical technology development.

TABLE 1-1 Imaging Technologies for Breast Cancer Reviewed in *Mammography and Beyond*

Technology	Description	FDA approved*
Film-screen mammography	The standard x-ray technique	Yes
Full-field digital mammography	Digital version of x-ray technique	Yes
Ultrasound	Forms images by reflection of megahertz frequency	Yes
Magnetic resonance imaging (MRI)	Forms images using radio emissions from nuclear spins	Yes

Both were covered in the previous report. However, an overview of current technologies that are under development for breast cancer detection is important background for this report and is provided in Appendix A. This report also builds on the work of the previous committee by analyzing what improvements or innovations in breast cancer detection and diagnosis will have the greatest impact on reducing the toll of breast cancer, and what can be done to foster those improvements (see the statement of task in Box 1-2). Where there is overlap between the two reports, this committee relied most heavily on information published after the *Mammography and Beyond* report was written. Roughly 80 percent of all references were published in 2000 or later. (Although *Mammography and Beyond* was published in 2001, the final draft was submitted in 2000.)

Attention is focused on near-term improvements that could be accomplished within 5 to 15 years. A single breakthrough technology that will revolutionize the early detection of breast cancer is not likely in the next few years, and in any case, like other technologies that might change the landscape further in the future, it is unpredictable. The committee did not identify specific devices, protocols, or procedures that should be most encouraged, because that should be determined by evidence based on carefully designed studies. In the meantime, it is important to apply current knowledge more effectively to develop systems that will ensure access to new technologies as soon as they are ready—that is, when they have been demonstrated to be safe, effective, and to add value to the tools already available to improve breast cancer outcomes.

Routine use	Infrequent use	Clinical data suggests a role for . . .	Clinical data not yet available
Screening and Diagnosis			
Screening and Diagnosis			
Diagnosis		Screening	
	Diagnosis	Screening	

continued

TABLE 1-1 Continued

Technology	Description	FDA approved*
Scintimammography	Sense tumors from gamma-ray emission of radioactive pharmaceutical	Yes
Thermography	Seeks tumors by infrared signature	Yes
Electrical impedance imaging	Maps the breast's impedance with low-voltage signal	Yes
Optical imaging	Localizes tumors by measuring scattered near-infrared light	
Electrical potential measurement	Identifies tumors by measuring potentials at array of detectors on skin	
Positron emission tomography	Forms images using emission from annihilation of positrons from radioactive pharmaceuticals	Yes
Novel ultrasound techniques	Includes compound imaging, which improves resolution; 3D and Doppler imaging	
Elastography	Uses ultrasound or MRI to infer the mechanical properties of tissue	
Magnetic resonance spectroscopy	Analyzes tissue's chemical makeup using radio emissions	
Thermoacoustic computed tomography	Generates short sound pulses within breast using RF energy and constructs a 3D image from them	
Microwave imaging	Views breast using scattered microwaves	
Hall-effect imaging	Picks up sonic vibrations of charged particles exposed to a magnetic field	
Magnetomammography	Senses magnetic contrast agents collected in tumors	

*Most of these technologies are approved for uses other than screening. Also, strictly speaking some devices are "approved" and others are "cleared" (see Chapter 6 for discussion of FDA device approval).

Routine use	Infrequent use	Clinical data suggests a role for . . .	Clinical data not yet available
		Diagnosis	
		Diagnosis	
		Diagnosis	
		Diagnosis	
		Diagnosis	
			Screening and diagnosis
			Screening and diagnosis
			Screening and diagnosis
			Screening and diagnosis
			Screening and diagnosis
			Screening and diagnosis
			Screening and diagnosis
			Screening and diagnosis

Adapted from table in IEEE Spectrum. http://www.spectrum.ieee.org/pubs/spectrum/0501/cancert1.html [Accessed August 28, 2003].

BOX 1-2
Statement of Task

The committee will (a) consider which of the existing and evolving approaches hold the greatest promise for improving the early detection and diagnosis of breast cancer and (b) analyze the degree to which different stages in the development of innovative medical technologies might act as bottlenecks, particularly for those technologies that promise to improve the early detection of breast cancer. Strategies to improve the efficiency of those steps will be identified and evaluated, with the goal of accelerating the flow of the most promising new approaches from the conceptual stage to clinical practice.

In addition to recommending strategies to enhance the discovery, development, and dissemination of approaches to the early detection and diagnosis of breast cancer, a fundamental and overarching goal of this study will be to improve the understanding of the media and the general public about the public health issues underlying the development of new approaches.

Specific tasks include:

1. Develop a framework for examining new technologies for the early detection and diagnosis of breast cancer. This includes:

    • Identifying the defining principles of effective new detection and diagnostic approaches.
    • Identifying technological, financial, and regulatory obstacles to the development and use of these detection and diagnosis options in clinical practice.

2. Consider the role of regulatory and coverage policies in the development of medical innovations, particularly those relevant to early detection and diagnosis of breast cancer. Related tasks include:

    • Consider modifications to the FDA review processes that might facilitate new technology development.
    • Consider coverage approval mechanisms that could accommodate the various developmental stages of new technologies. Possibilities include modular, interim, or conditional approval strategies.
    • Examine the impact of current health care payment systems on the development and clinical application of new and innovation medical technology.
    • Consider what role, if any, cost-effectiveness considerations should play in the development and regulation of new medical technologies.

The committee believes the lives of many women could be saved by adopting several key strategies, including:

1. improving the organization of breast cancer screening and the interpretation of mammograms,

2. developing more individually tailored approaches to the early detection of breast cancer, and

3. focusing on how different technologies can be optimally integrated into clinical practices, instead of evaluating only the performance characteristics of individual technologies.

All of these steps should be supported by evidence, which unfortunately is not always the case in the adoption of new technologies into clinical practice.

The challenge of developing and integrating the "right" medical technologies so that patients receive the best possible treatment applies to all fields of medicine—especially where early detection is as important to health and survival as it is in breast cancer. Thus this report should be of interest to all those who are concerned with the development and application of medical technologies. Its primary audiences, however, are those working to reduce the toll of breast cancer through early detection, including breast cancer activists and women's health organizations; breast cancer researchers; technology developers; clinicians such as breast imagers, primary care physicians, and oncologists; federal, state, and private research sponsors; and those who regulate medical technologies through the FDA, Centers for Medicare and Medicaid Services (CMS), private payers, and Congress. (CMS manages the Medicare program, which is historically the largest health care payer in the United States.)

This study also seeks to improve the understanding of the media and the public about the public health issues underlying the development of new approaches. The committee tackled this goal in two ways: first, by explaining commonly misunderstood concepts in cancer screening—particularly the standards of evidence for screening technologies and the analysis of risk—and second, by reviewing some of the problems and consequences of media coverage of medical advances, especially those related to breast cancer.

PUBLIC EXPECTATIONS ARE HIGH

Public expectations for reducing the toll of breast cancer are high, and the public has a seemingly insatiable appetite for news about breast cancer, as indicated by the frequency of that topic in magazines with large female readerships.[7,25] Undoubtedly this need for news is partially because breast cancer is the disease that women fear most.[16]

The mass media, both news and advertising, are the main sources of health information for many Americans.[18] Unfortunately, there is considerable evidence that the media portray breast cancer unrealistically, and that women's perceptions of their risk of having breast cancer and dying from it—and, not coincidentally, of the benefits of various tests and treatments for breast cancer, including mammography—are similarly skewed.[5,7,22]

New treatments or technologies are often presented in the media as "breakthroughs" that promise unqualified advances.[5] Even though breakthrough technologies are rare and unpredictable, media reports encourage the hope that such a technology for breast cancer detection is lurking in the shadows. In fact, virtually all medical technology development has its roots in basic research, and the world of research is so well-lit by the pressure to publish that there are few, if any, dark corners in which important technology advances lie hidden. Moreover, the technical backgrounds of members of the committee responsible for this report including surgery, radiology, molecular biology, imaging, physics, information technology, and epidemiology should ensure sufficient access to events in the research and development community to assure readers that the committee is not overlooking truly promising new developments.

Risk in the Media

Research indicates that women tend to overestimate their lifetime risk of developing and dying from breast cancer, and particularly the likelihood of that happening before age 50 (reviewed by Burke and colleagues).[1,4,6,7,13,15,19] Many women mistakenly believe that their short-term risk of breast cancer diminishes with age.[8,10,20] Investigating the media as a possible source of such misperceptions, Burke and his colleagues examined 172 vignettes illustrating women's experiences with breast cancer that appeared in a broad sample of popular U.S. magazines over a four-year period.[7] The age distribution of women in the vignettes was almost the reverse of the actual age distribution of breast cancer (Figure 1-1). Nearly half of the vignettes featured women diagnosed with breast cancer before age 40; such women account for only about 5 percent of breast cancer cases. Yet, the vignettes rarely referred to women age 60 or above with breast cancer, which is when the majority of cases occur.[4,10]

Gripping stories that generate fear of breast cancer in young women may also increase demand for tests and treatments perceived to improve the chances of surviving this disease. Hundreds of articles and television stories in the early 1990s portrayed high-dose chemotherapy (which included bone marrow transplantation) as the only hope for patients with advanced breast cancer, despite a lack of evidence that this risky and expensive procedure actually extended survival.[5] In the mid-1980s, about 100 women per year received high-dose chemotherapy; in 1994, more than 4,000 of these procedures were performed. Similarly, deceptive marketing of MRI for breast cancer screening played on women's desire for an "accurate" test (Box 1-3).

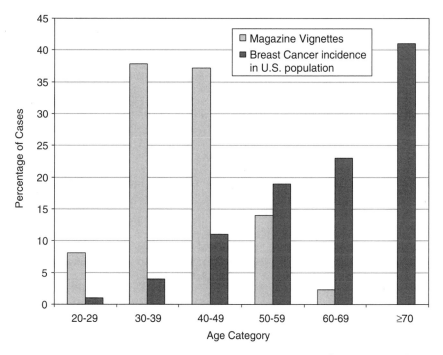

FIGURE 1-1 Personal stories in women's magazines overrepresent the incidence of breast cancer in younger women and underrepresent it among older women.[7]

Reports of "Breakthroughs" Are More Prevalent Than Actual Breakthroughs

The sense of exaggerated risk surrounding breast cancer provides fertile ground for the marketing of tests and treatments promising to reduce that risk, such as MRI screening.[21] Blood tests, imaging technology, even cancer care and surgical products are increasingly marketed directly to consumers. Many of these direct-to-consumer advertisements encourage readers' fear so as to promote the advertised product or service.

Another problematic form of marketing occurs indirectly through media reports of medical developments while they are still "works in progress,"[5] such as press releases discussing the content of articles at the time of their publication in medical journals[26] and research abstracts from scientific meetings. A scientific meeting is a forum for scientists to present works in progress, and nearly half of that work remains unpublished[23]— typically, because the results could not be replicated, or they were too inconclusive to pass peer review. Lisa Schwartz and her colleagues tracked

---

BOX 1-3
Misleading Marketing of MRI for Breast Cancer Screening

Aggressive marketing of MRI for breast cancer screening by AmeriScan™ incensed breast imagers for years because the manufacturer exaggerated the accuracy of the technology in a widely distributed series of Internet, television, radio, and newspaper ads. The original ad claimed 100 percent accuracy, although—with pressure from the FDA—that was revised to "almost 100 percent." Even that is an overstatement because most people presume that accuracy includes both specificity and sensitivity. Although the sensitivity of MRI is very high, specificity is relatively low and MRI does not reliably detect microcalcifications.

Although some breast MRI applications are supported by the literature, screening is not one of them. MRI has been proven effective for uses such as evaluating women with breast implants that may have ruptured. It is also used for women known to have breast cancer to evaluate the extent of tumors prior to surgery, or after surgery to monitor response to treatment.

After several years of outcry among breast imagers, the Medical Board of California and the San Francisco District Attorney's Office jointly filed a lawsuit in San Francisco Superior Court on October 23, 2003, against the founder and medical director of AmeriScan.™ Less than two weeks later, AmeriScan™ announced its closure.

---

the outcome of presentations at high-profile scientific meetings that received mass media coverage and found that in as many as one in four of these presentations the findings were never published—which means that they were never subjected to peer review, or they were and failed. Even press releases of published material can be unreliable. A study of press releases issued by leading medical journals found that the releases routinely failed to mention study limitations or industry funding, and often presented data in formats that exaggerated findings.[26]

STUDY PROCESS

This study was carried out by a committee on which all major areas of breast cancer detection were represented, including breast cancer screening, diagnosis, and treatment; clinical trials expertise; cancer and molecular biology; medical technology development and evaluation; health care administration; and technology innovation and adoption. The committee supplemented its expertise through several workshops, which were organized as information-gathering, brainstorming sessions (see Appendix B for

Workshop Agendas). Committee members heard from technology developers representing small and large companies and from researchers developing some of the most innovative systems for early detection of breast cancer, including a variety of imaging, biological, and computer technologies. The committee also heard from the leaders of several of the most important clinical studies aimed at improving systems for the early detection of breast cancer. Finally, the committee heard from senior staff at the federal agencies that regulate the availability of new medical technologies, as well as representatives of private insurance, who also serve as gatekeepers. The committee has made extensive use of relevant published review papers, and referred back to the original papers only if the review failed to include all of the pertinent data.

A series of reports on breast cancer have been produced by, or under the aegis of, the IOM and NRC's National Cancer Policy Board. These reports include *Mammography and Beyond: Developing Technologies for the Early Detection of Breast Cancer* (2001), *Meeting Psychosocial Needs of Women with Breast Cancer* (2004), and *Improving Mammography Quality Standards* (in progress, 2004). As part of that series, this report explores ways of improving early detection and diagnosis of breast cancer in women through developing better technologies and advancing their introduction and application, and educating women and other interested stakeholders about mammography and other detection modalities. The ultimate objective of this and all the other studies is better care and better outcomes for women with breast cancer and their families.

ORGANIZATION OF THIS REPORT

Chapter 2 covers the basic principles of effective screening. These principles are well established, but they are confused so often in the media and even in some of the scientific literature that it is important to review them here. Many controversies over mammography have been entwined with debates over the appropriate interpretation of data from screening studies. Often what the public remembers most is only that "mammography is debatable," even after the overwhelming majority of experts have concluded that the preponderance of data clearly supports the value of mammography. In addition, because there has been so much discussion about the importance of weighing the benefits and harms of screening mammography, and yet so little discussion about the actual harms, this chapter reviews the reported harms of mammography. Finally, because the increased frequency of DCIS diagnoses and treatment are cited so often as a negative consequence of widespread mammography screening, the DCIS dilemma is reviewed.

Chapter 3 explores strategies for improving mammography screening. Many of these strategies involve new approaches to organizing mammography services, with an emphasis on improving the quality of mammographic interpretation and the critical need for breast imaging specialists. Existing technologies that can compensate for the technical limitations of mammography are also discussed.

Chapter 4 discusses what is known about breast cancer risk factors, how risk perception is often confused, and how improved knowledge about breast cancer risk factors could be used to develop individualized strategies for breast cancer detection. The committee believes that better tools for understanding breast cancer risk will be invaluable for reducing breast cancer mortality.

Chapter 5 reviews the status and challenges of biologically based technologies for the detection and diagnosis of breast cancer. Undoubtedly such technologies hold the key to improving our understanding of breast cancer biology and should be pursued, but for the most part, these technologies have not yet been validated for the early detection of breast cancer and are still in their infancy.

Chapter 6 tackles the challenges inherent in translating research results and early stage inventions into clinically useful applications. For much of technology development, this is the weak link where so many technologies fail to realize their initial promise. This process is not merely bureaucratic although it may seem so to the public. Rather, it is a dynamic, research-driven transition between the "possibly useful" and the "truly useful." Methodological issues and federal agencies and programs that support this process are also described. Countless technologies that were believed initially to be major advances turn out to offer no benefit and may even harm patients. This stage represents the difference between belief-based medicine and evidence-based medicine.

Chapter 7 deals with the final, and possibly most neglected, phase in the development and application of new technologies—namely, that of ensuring that the technologies improve patients' health. Without consideration of this phase, which includes how technologies are best used to complement each other, new technologies will fall short in saving women's lives.

Finally, Chapter 8 summarizes the committee's main findings and recommendations for developing new strategies for breast cancer detection and diagnosis.

REFERENCES

1.   Alexander NE, Ross J, Sumner W, Nease RF Jr, Littenberg B. 1996. The effect of an educational intervention on the perceived risk of breast cancer. *J Gen Intern Med* 11(2):92-97.

2.   American Cancer Society. 2001. *Breast Cancer Facts and Figures 2001-2002*. Atlanta, GA: American Cancer Society.

3.   Balas E, Boren SA. 2000. Managing Clinical Knowledge for Health Care Improvement. Bemmel J, McCray AT, Editors. *Yearbook of Medical Informatics: Patient-Centered Systems*. Stuttgart, Germany: Schattauer Verlagsgesellschaft mbH. Pp. 65-70.

4.   Black WC, Nease RF Jr, Tosteson AN. 1995. Perceptions of breast cancer risk and screening effectiveness in women younger than 50 years of age. *J Natl Cancer Inst* 87(10):720-731.

5.   Brownlee S. 2003, August 3. Health, Hope and Hype: why the media oversells medical "breakthroughs." *The Washington Post*.

6.   Bunker JP, Houghton J, Baum M. 1998. Putting the risk of breast cancer in perspective. *BMJ* 317(7168):1307-1309.

7.   Burke W, Olsen AH, Pinsky LE, Reynolds SE, Press NA. 2001. Misleading presentation of breast cancer in popular magazines. *Eff Clin Pract* 4(2):58-64.

8.   Dolan NC, Lee AM, McDermott MM. 1997. Age-related differences in breast carcinoma knowledge, beliefs, and perceived risk among women visiting an academic general medicine practice. *Cancer* 80(3):413-420.

9.   Elmore JG, Nakano CY, Koepsell TD, Desnick LM, D'Orsi CJ, Ransohoff DF. 2003. International variation in screening mammography interpretations in community-based programs. *J Natl Cancer Inst* 95(18):1384-1393.

10.   Fulton JP, Rakowski W, Jones AC. 1995. Determinants of breast cancer screening among inner-city Hispanic women in comparison with other inner-city women. *Public Health Rep* 110(4):476-482.

11.   Institute of Medicine and National Research Council. 2001. *Mammography and Beyond: Developing Technologies for the Early Detection of Breast Cancer*. Washington, DC: National Academy Press.

12.   Institute of Medicine. 2003. *Exploring Challenges, Progress, and New Models for Engaging the Public in the Clinical Research Enterprise: Clinical Research Roundtable Workshop Summary*. Washington, DC: The National Academies Press.

13.   Lavelle K, Charlton A. 1998. Women's perception of risk of cancer. *BMJ* 317(7157):542.

14.   Lewin JM, Hendrick RE, D'Orsi CJ, Isaacs PK, Moss LJ, Karellas A, Sisney GA, Kuni CC, Cutter GR. 2001. Comparison of full-field digital mammography with screen-film mammography for cancer detection: results of 4,945 paired examinations. *Radiology* 218(3):873-880.

15.   McCaul KD, Branstetter AD, O'Donnell SM, Jacobson K, Quinlan KB. 1998. A descriptive study of breast cancer worry. *J Behav Med* 21(6):565-579.

16.   MORI Medicine & Science Research. 2002, October 17. Women See Family History Not Old Age as Greatest Breast Cancer Risk [MORI is an approved survey firm for the British National Health Service]. Accessed May 13, 2003. Web Page. Available at: http://www.mori.com/polls/2002/breakthrough.shtml.

17.   National Cancer Institute. Cancer Research Portfolio. 2003. Accessed June 1, 2004. Web Page. Available at: http://researchportfolio.cancer.gov/.

18.   Phillips KP, Kanter EJ, Bednarczyk B, Tastad PL. 1991. Importance of the lay press in the transmission of medical knowledge to the scientific community. *N Engl J Med* (325):1180-1183.

19.   Pilote L, Hlatky MA. 1995. Attitudes of women toward hormone therapy and prevention of heart disease. *Am Heart J* 129(6):1237-1238.

20.   Press N. 1995. *Survey, Orange County Region 10 California State Breast Cancer Early Detection Partnership Program (BCEDP)*. Sacramento, CA: California Department of Health.

21. Schwartz LM, Woloshin S. 2002. Marketing medicine to the public: a reader's guide. *JAMA* 287(6):774-775.

22. Schwartz LM, Woloshin S. 2002. News media coverage of screening mammography for women in their 40s and tamoxifen for primary prevention of breast cancer. *JAMA* 287(23):3136-3142.

23. Schwartz LM, Woloshin S, Baczek L. 2002. Media coverage of scientific meetings: too much, too soon? *JAMA* 287(21):2859-2863.

24. Sung NS, Crowley WF Jr, Genel M, Salber P, Sandy L, Sherwood LM, Johnson SB, Catanese V, Tilson H, Getz K, Larson EL, Scheinberg D, Reece EA, Slavkin H, Dobs A, Grebb J, Martinez RA, Korn A, Rimoin D. 2003. Central challenges facing the national clinical research enterprise. *JAMA* 289(10):1278-1287.

25. Wells J, Marshall P, Crawley B, Dickersin K. 2001. Newspaper reporting of screening mammography. *Ann Intern Med* 135(12):1029-1037.

26. Woloshin S, Schwartz LM. 2002. Press releases: translating research into news. *JAMA* 287(21):2856-1858.

2

Benefits and Limitations of Mammography

Mammography is possibly the most intensely scrutinized and debated medical procedure of our time, but there is virtually no disagreement on two points. First, there is no other breast cancer screening tool that has a better combination of sensitivity and specificity. Second, as practiced today, mammography could be better. This chapter reviews the basic features of, and factors involved in, effective mammography screening and its benefits and limitations.

SCREENING VERSUS DIAGNOSIS

Mammography has two main uses, screening and diagnosis, and there are important medical and economic differences between the two. *Screening mammography* is an x-ray-based procedure applied to a woman who has no signs or symptoms of breast disease and is used for the early detection of breast cancer. The ultimate purpose of screening is not to detect breast cancer at an early stage, but to save lives. An added benefit of screening is that small, screen-detected tumors might be effectively treated with less aggressive and harsh regimens than larger tumors. *Diagnostic mammography* (also called problem-solving mammography) uses the same x-ray-based procedure but is tailored by the radiologist for specific patients' signs or symptoms. This procedure is designed to diagnose previously observed signs or symptoms of breast disease in a man or woman, or to determine the presence or absence of breast cancer in someone with a personal history of breast cancer or biopsy-proven breast disease.

The fundamental tenet of screening for any disease is that finding the disease before symptoms develop enables detection at a less advanced stage, and that initiating treatment at that time will reduce the adverse effects of the disease.[43]

The World Health Organization (WHO) outlined the principles of effective screening in 1968 and they are as true today as they were then. In their simplest form, the WHO screening guidelines encompass five key points, each of which applies to breast cancer and mammography:

- The disease being screened is serious and prevalent,
- The test is sensitive and specific,
- The test is well tolerated,
- The test is inexpensive, and
- The test changes therapy or outcome.

The implications of these principles are that the disease must be prevalent enough *within* the population or subpopulation being screened to warrant testing individuals who show no signs or symptoms of the diseases. The value of different screening schedules and/or different technologies are likely to be different for different subpopulations, and the determination of optimal strategies requires careful study. Methodological challenges and studies currently under way are discussed in Chapter 6.

STANDARDS OF EVIDENCE

The value of a screening tool is determined by the relationship between the nature of the disease being screened and the performance characteristics of the screening tool. Sensitivity and specificity are the two most commonly cited measures of a screening or diagnostic test, but the more informative measure is the positive predictive value, which incorporates both sensitivity and specificity (see Box 2-1a and 2-1b).

Sensitivity refers to the proportion of true-positive results; this is calculated by dividing the number of breast cancer cases that were detected by the total number of breast cancer cases in the population tested, which equals the sum of those that were detected plus those that were missed. Estimates of the sensitivity of screening mammography from different studies range from 83 to 95 percent.[72]

Specificity refers to the proportion of true-negative results, or tests that correctly indicate that a woman does not have breast cancer among screened women without breast cancer. Mammography specificities generally fall in the range of 90 to 98 percent.[72] In other words, the risk of a false-positive mammogram is about 1 in 10. Two studies suggest that among women who receive annual mammograms for 10 years, half will have at least one suspi-

---

BOX 2-1a
Screening Terminology

Mammographic Result	Condition	
	Breast Cancer Present	Breast Cancer *Not* Present
Negative findings (No Abnormalities Detected)	False Negative	True Negative
Positive findings (Abnormality Detected)	True Positive	False Positive

Sensitivity (Se) refers to the proportion of true-positive results, or tests that correctly indicate a woman has breast cancer.

> Se = TP / (TP + FN)
> *where TP = True Positives and FN = False Negatives*
> *(TP + FN) = Total number of cancer cases*

Specificity (Sp) refers to the proportion of true-negative results, or tests that correctly indicate that a woman does not have breast cancer.

> *Sp = TN / (TN + FP)*
> *where TN = True Negatives and FP = False Positives*
> *(TN+FP) = Total number of cancer-free cases*

Positive Predictive Value (PPV) refers to the probability that a patient with a positive test actually has the disease.

> PPV = TP / (TP + FP)
> *where TP = True Positives and FP = False Positive*
> *(TP+FP) = Total number of abnormal, or positive, mammograms*

---

cious finding leading to additional tests, such as diagnostic mammography, ultrasound, or biopsy, but that are later shown to be false alarms.[12,21]

Positive predictive value measures the probability that a patient with a positive (abnormal) test result actually has the disease. The higher the positive predictive value, the lower the number of false-positive results. Predictive value is determined by the sensitivity and specificity of the test, and the prevalence of disease in the population being tested. (Prevalence is defined as the proportion of persons in a defined population at a given point in time with the condition in question.) The more sensitive a test, the less likely it is that an individual with a negative test will have the disease and thus the greater the negative predictive value. The more specific the

BOX 2-1b
Hypothetical Screening Results

	Condition	
Mammographic Result	Breast Cancer Present	Breast Cancer *Not* Present
Negative findings (No Abnormality Detected)	4 False Negatives	9,600 True Negatives
Positive findings (Abnormality Detected)	36 True Positives	400 False Positives

In this example, the prevalence of breast cancer is 4%. Sensitivity is 90% and specificity is 96%.

Overall, this results in a positive predictive value of 8%.
This example assumes that out of 10,000 women who were screened, 436 had abnormal findings, 36 cancers were confirmed by biopsy, and the mammograms of 4 women appeared normal despite the presence of cancer.

test, the less likely an individual with a positive test will be free from disease and the greater the positive predictive value.

When the prevalence of disease in those without signs or symptoms is low, the positive predictive value will also be low, even using a test with high sensitivity and specificity. For such rare diseases where there will be few true positives, a large proportion of those with positive screening tests inevitably will be found not to have the disease upon further diagnostic testing (Box 2-1b). One way to increase the positive predictive value of a screening test is to target the screening test to those at high risk of developing the disease, based on considerations such as demographic factors, medical history, or occupation. For example, mammograms are recommended for women over age 40, because that population has a higher prevalence of breast cancer.

Because the ultimate purpose of screening is to save lives by detecting cancer sufficiently early for effective curative treatment to be administered, screening effectiveness must be measured in terms of reduction in cancer mortality. However, because the death rate from breast cancer in "healthy" women who qualify as participants in a screening trial is relatively low (around 1/10 of 1 percent per year) it requires many thousands of women to be followed for many years before there are sufficient numbers of deaths from breast cancer to evaluate the impact of screening with adequate statistical power. Indeed, the mammography trials that have been conducted have involved a total of more than half a million participants. Methodological issues in cancer screening trials are reviewed in Chapter 6.

MAMMOGRAPHY UNDER FIRE

In what has been described as "the journalistic equivalent of shouting fire in a crowded theater," *The New York Times* published a review in 2001 of a scientific article disputing the value of mammography, thereby igniting a year-long controversy whose ramifications continue. The basis of the controversy was a review conducted by Peter Gotzsche and Ole Olsen of the Nordic Cochrane Center in Copenhagen.[39,74] Although both Gotzsche and Olsen are listed as authors on the primary papers and worked at the Nordic Cochrane Center, Olsen left in 2001 and Gotzsche is the lead proponent of the claims. They argued that several of the key mammography screening trials were scientifically flawed and concluded that there was no evidence of benefit from mammography. The first screening trial of mammography was initiated in 1963. Since then, seven have been carried out in four countries.[a] Most reported reductions in breast cancer mortality and more than a dozen countries have established breast cancer screening programs.

Gotzsche and Olsen's analysis has been reviewed since then by a series of expert groups, including the Global Mammography Summit and the International Agency for Research on Cancer of the WHO, who met specifically to review these criticisms (Box 2-2). These and numerous other reviews concluded that many of Gotzsche and Olsen's criticisms were unsubstantiated, and the remaining deficiencies in the screening trials were judged not to invalidate the trials' findings that screening mammography reduces breast cancer mortality.[73] Gotzsche and Olsen's critique was based on judgments of the quality of the screening studies, but those judgments were based on misreading of the data and the literature.[36,37] As is often the case, the eruption of a medical controversy receives more media attention than its resolution, and these expert reviews received relatively little media attention. It is thus not surprising that some members of the public continue to believe, incorrectly, that there is debate among the experts about whether screening mammography saves lives.

---

[a]In one trial, conducted in Canada, the data were separated for women in their 40s and 50s, so this is sometimes considered two trials, for a total of eight screening mammography trials.

BOX 2-2
After the Storm: Expert Reviews of
Mammography Screening Trials

Physicians Data Query (PDQ) *January 2002*

The PDQ is an independent panel of cancer experts that regularly reviews evidence on cancer and prepares information for the National Cancer Institute (NCI). The PDQ posts its reports on the NCI website, but is independent of the NCI and does not issue guidelines or make official recommendations. It supported Gotzsche and Olsen's criticism of mammography and concluded that "screening for breast cancer does not affect overall mortality, and that the absolute benefit for breast cancer mortality appears to be small."

International Agency for Research on Cancer of the WHO *March 2002*

The group, consisting of 24 experts from 11 countries, concluded that trials have provided sufficient evidence for the efficacy of mammography screening of women between 50 and 69 years. The reduction in mortality from breast cancer among women who chose to participate in screening programs was estimated to be about 35 percent. For women aged 40-49 years, there is only limited evidence for a reduction. The quality of the trials that were used to make these evaluations was carefully assessed. The working group found that the effectiveness of national screening programs varies due to differences in coverage of the female population, quality of mammography, treatment, and other factors. Organized screening programs are more effective in reducing the rate of death from breast cancer than sporadic screening of selected groups of women.

Global Summit on Mammographic Screening *June 2002*

In response to the uncertainty over the efficacy of breast screening, a Global Summit on Mammographic Screening was organized at the European Institute of Oncology in Milan. The Summit was planned in association with the WHO, European Commission, American Cancer Society, U.S. Centers for Disease Control and Prevention, American Italian Cancer Foundation, European Society for Medical Oncology, American Society of Clinical Oncology, and International Union Against Cancer.

The design and recent results from the seven randomized trials were presented and discussed in detail. Some of the criticisms put forward by Gotzsche and Olsen were discarded as being wrong; others had been addressed by new analyses and

Although the debate on the benefits of mammography focused on the validity of the first seven clinical screening trials, these are only part of the evidence. A series of studies conducted in community settings that are more comparable to actual clinical practice have supported the conclusions of those earlier clinical screening trials.[27] Overall, the evidence indicates that shown to be of minor significance. The remaining minor considerations did not detract from the conclusion that screening mammography reduced the mortality from breast cancer in women receiving an invitation to be screened in well-organized clinical trials: The reduction in breast cancer mortality appeared to be between 21 and 23 percent, according to recent estimates. Those participating fully could expect greater benefit.

There was unanimity that with the current evidence from randomized trials, taking full account of any limitations to their methodology, there were no grounds for stopping on-going screening programs or planned programs.

The group also stated that mammographic screening is only one step in the total management of the woman with breast cancer. This goal can only be attained through rigorous, high-quality screening, diagnosis, and treatment.

United States Preventive Services Task Force (USPSTF) *September 2002*

The USPSTF is an independent panel of experts in primary care and prevention that systematically reviews the evidence of effectiveness of clinical preventive services and develops recommendations for their use.

The USPSTF concluded that the criticisms made against the Swedish trials by Gotzsche and Olsen are misleading and scientifically unfounded. "We found the same flaws [as Gotzsche and Olsen]," says Janet D. Allan, vice-chair of the task force and dean of the School of Nursing at the University of Texas Health Science Center in San Antonio. "They interpreted the flaws as being fatal flaws," she says. "We did not interpret the flaws as fatal . . . and concluded that the studies were still valid and that mammography screening reduces deaths from breast cancer."

The USPSTF concluded that the absolute benefit among women in their 40s is smaller than it is among older women because the incidence of breast cancer is lower at the younger age. The USPSTF also concluded that the evidence is also generalizable to women aged 70 and older (who face a higher absolute risk for breast cancer) if their life expectancy is not compromised by comorbid disease. The absolute probability of benefits of regular mammography increase along a continuum with age, whereas the likelihood of harms from screening (false-positive results and unnecessary anxiety, biopsies, and cost) diminish from ages 40 to 70. The balance of benefits and potential harms, therefore, grows more favorable as women age. The precise age at which the potential benefits of mammography justify the possible harms is a subjective choice.

the availability of screening reduces mortality from breast cancer by 20 to 30 percent (reviewed by Duffy and colleagues in 2003),[19] and that in a population that actually participates in screening mammography, the reduction can be considerably greater, nearly 50 percent.[18,97] This is not to say that every woman who undergoes screening mammography will benefit. Most women will never develop breast cancer, but the lives of many of those who do will be saved even though it is not yet possible to identify them in advance.

BREAST DENSITY AFFECTS MAMMOGRAPHIC SENSITIVITY

Breast density varies widely among women, and cancer is more difficult to detect in mammograms of women with radiographically dense breasts. Mammographic density refers to the relative lightness of a mammogram, determined by the number of x-ray photons that penetrate the breast. Fat is radiographically translucent, so x-rays pass through it relatively unimpeded making it appear darker on x-ray images. Connective and epithelial tissue, which includes the mammary glands, is radiographically dense relative to fat and blocks x-rays to a greater extent, so it appears lighter. Breast cancers and microcalcifications generally appear as whiter areas on mammograms because they tend to absorb more x-ray photons; they can be difficult to detect against the relatively light background of dense breast tissue because of the lack of contrast between them and a dense breast background.

Breast density is usually measured as part of mammographic interpretation by classifying a mammogram according to the 4-point Breast Imaging Reporting and Data System™ (BI-RADS®) breast density scale established by the American College of Radiology (see Table 2-1). The scale was revised in 2003 and now asks radiologists to include the "percentage of glandular density," or the percentage of breast tissue that is mammographically dense, when characterizing breast composition. Density level 1 indicates predominantly fatty tissue; 2 indicates scattered glandular tissue; 3 indicates heterogeneous density; and 4 indicates an extremely dense breast. Categories 3 and 4 indicate the possibility of reduced mammographic sensitivity. However, there is only moderate agreement among radiologists on these density readings,[49] and several investigators have

TABLE 2-1 BI-RADS® (fourth edition) Scale for Characterizing Breast Composition

Category	Description	Glandular Density (percent of breast tissue that is mammographically dense)
1	Predominantly fatty tissue	Less than 25%
2	Scattered glandular tissue	25–50%
3	Heterogeneously dense	50–75%
4	Extremely dense tissue	More than 75%

attempted to develop a standard quantitative approach to mammographic density measurement, such as by using x-ray digitizers and quantifiable detection systems using density algorithms. These have been carefully studied, but are not yet widely available for clinical purposes.[4,79,102]

Breast density is a risk factor for missed cancers, and both false-positive and false-negative mammographic interpretations are more likely with dense breasts.[34] In a study of more than 11,000 women with no clinical symptoms of breast cancer, the sensitivity of mammography was only 48 percent for the subset of women with extremely dense breasts compared to 78 percent sensitivity for the entire sample of women in the study.[53] Technologies that are not based on x-rays, such as magnetic resonance imaging and sonography (ultrasound), are less affected by breast density.

Many factors influence breast density, such as obesity, ethnicity, age, stage of menstrual cycle, and number of live births (parity). Overall, menopausal status, weight, and parity account for 20 to 30 percent of the age-adjusted variation in the percentage of dense breast tissue.[5] Younger women tend to have more dense breasts and thus often have mammograms that are difficult to interpret. Hormone replacement therapy increases breast density, although few women show dramatic changes, and the changes depend on the particular hormone regime (reviewed by Slanetz, 2002).[93] For example, estrogen and progestin combination therapy increases breast density to a greater degree than estrogen alone.[15]

Breast density varies within individual women as well as among different women. Breasts that are mammographically dense also tend to have areas that are not dense. Women are slightly more likely to have extremely dense breasts during the last 2 weeks of the menstrual cycle (luteal phase),[103,111] although this is not generally clinically significant. Nevertheless, performing mammography during the first 2 weeks of the menstrual cycle may increase mammographic accuracy,[111] probably because women do not feel as much discomfort during breast compression. This increases the probability of obtaining an examination without noticeable patient motion, which can degrade image quality and limit the ability to find cancers.

Obesity is commonly associated with fatty breasts and accounts for more than 40 percent of the variance in breast density.[6] Native American populations typically have lower density breast tissue, and Asian populations have greater density breast tissue than African American and white populations overall. One solution to the difficulties posed by dense breasts might be to perform ultrasound on all women with particularly dense breasts. This is standard practice in Korea and is done in many facilities in the United States, but, to date, no data have been published to indicate this would improve outcomes and which women would benefit.

THE HARMS OF MAMMOGRAPHY

Mammography has been criticized not only because of questions about its effectiveness, but for fear that it might actually cause harm. Harms that have been listed by Thornton and colleagues include physical, emotional, social, financial, intergenerational, or psychological harm.[100] Although some authors suggest that these may be lifelong, the evidence collected thus far indicates that they are generally moderate and short-lived.

Financial harm refers to the cost of tests needed for definitive diagnosis following an abnormal mammogram. Retrospective studies indicate that the additional costs of evaluating false-positive results can add up to one-third of the total cost of screening for all women.[21,63]

Intergenerational harm refers to the possibility that insurance fees might be raised for daughters of women who were diagnosed with a condition that did not lead to adverse health outcomes and was detected only during a screening mammogram.[14] However, the Committee is not aware of any published cases where this is documented.

Pain and Anxiety

Mammography requires compression of the breast, and is painful for some women primarily related to the timing of the last menstrual period or the anticipation of pain (reviewed by Drossaert and colleagues in 2002).[17]

Studies conducted prior to 1999 reported highly inconsistent results, ranging from only 1 percent to as many as 85 percent of women reporting pain during mammography. Given the known difficulty in reliably measuring pain, it is important to evaluate the methodologies used in these reports.[1,85] For example, Kornguth and his colleagues found that only 2 percent of women reported pain using a 6-point pain scale, whereas 75 to 85 percent of the *same* women reported pain when using the two more complex measures of pain (McGill Pain Questionnaire and the Visual Analog Scale and Brief Pain Inventory).[55]

Recent, appropriately designed studies report that only 15 percent[17] or 28 percent[87] of women experienced moderate or severe pain. In the latter study, 200 women were asked to rate the pain associated with a screening mammogram on a 10-point scale, where 0 is "no pain at all"; 10 is "the worst pain you have ever felt"; and 5 is "about average: for example, a mild headache or shoes that are a little too tight." Seventy-two percent of the women rated the pain at or less than 4. In general, these studies found no correlation between pain and age, breast size, or body mass index. In another recent study, 77 percent of women reported moderate or severe pain (lasting 10 minutes or less); 12 percent of them said they would be deterred from future screening, although less than 5 percent said they would like to receive pain medication prior to their next mammogram.[85]

Emotional harm includes the anxiety of waiting for results, which may take days to weeks. (The Mammography Quality Standards Act requires that women receive their mammogram results within 30 days of testing.) In one survey, women who were questioned immediately following screening mammography reported that the part of the procedure they found most stressful was waiting for results.[87] Yet another study reported that 67 percent of women were unwilling to pay even a small fee of $25 for immediate results.[81] In general, anxiety associated with waiting for mammography results does not appear to be significant for most women (reviewed in 2001 by Meystre-Agustoni and colleagues).[67]

False Alarms

An abnormal finding on a mammogram is cause for concern.[b] However, resulting psychological distress is usually transient[84] and is generally resolved if a subsequent test indicates that the interpretation was, in fact, a false positive. Nevertheless, for some women, anxiety persists long after an initial false positive is resolved, although generally at moderate levels.

One study compared the anxiety levels of women who received negative results at their first screening with those who received false-positive results. The women's anxiety levels were measured on a scale of 0 (not at all anxious) to 5 (very anxious). Depending on the measurement scale used and dimension of anxiety that was measured, the anxiety levels of the women who received false positives ranged from averages of 1.5 to 2.5. Their anxiety levels were consistently about three times higher than for women whose mammograms had been negative from the start, but they were still only "moderately anxious" and not "very anxious" (level 5) as much as eight weeks after the resolution of the false positive.[67] The initial anxiety level of the women was a strong predictor of their anxiety levels after a negative result. Although this study measured anxiety levels in about 800 women, the results are based on the much smaller group of 36 women who received false-positive results. Furthermore, the study was conducted in Switzerland during the introduction of a pilot screening program and anxiety levels with mammography presumably were influenced by the unfamiliarity of these women with screening mammography.

Two studies report that the experience of a false-positive mammogram does not deter women from obtaining subsequent mammograms.[16,80] A

---

[b]Note that call backs are prompted not only by abnormal findings (positive mammograms), but also if technical problems in the quality of the mammogram prevent a clear interpretation of the findings.

third study reports the opposite—that fewer women who received false-positive results return for a screening mammogram within three years—but the difference between groups, although statistically significant was only 3 percent and of doubtful clinical relevance.[66]

Biopsies

In the event of a positive mammogram, a woman must undergo a secondary assessment phase involving needle and/or open surgical biopsy to establish a definitive diagnosis.[c] Exposure to unnecessary biopsies is a real danger. Biopsy rates for suspected cases of breast cancer vary considerably among countries, indicating that the technical limitations of mammography are only part of the reason for biopsies. The rates are influenced by multiple factors beyond screening, such as practice variation and risk assessment. For example, the physician must take into account not only a patient's risk of breast cancer, but his or her confidence in the mammographic results (which can be influenced by patient characteristics such as breast density or previous surgeries), as well as risks associated with the health care system— such as the risk of malpractice suits. In principle, improved risk stratification should result in a lower rate of biopsies for benign conditions because there would be a smaller pool of low-risk women being screened. "Unnecessary" biopsies can also be reduced by the use of supplemental technologies.

Radiation Risk

High doses of radiation (0.2.5 to 20 Gy), such as those that occurred in the 1930s to 1950s due to atomic bomb radiation, multiple chest x-rays, and radiation treatment for breast disease, were associated with increased incidence of breast cancer in women below age 35 at exposure.[29,59] However, radiation sensitivity among women drops precipitously after age 35,[59] and although some caution may be warranted for regular mammographic screening of women below age 35,[60] calculations indicate that radiation risk is extremely small compared with the benefits, even for women in their forties.[28,29,48] Moreover, since the early days of mammography, image quality has improved markedly (Figure 2-1) and radiation exposure has been greatly reduced, so that the average amount of radiation absorbed during a mammogram is now very low.[112] It is estimated that 100,000 women who were screened annually from ages 50 to 75 would lose about 13 years from

---

[c]A "suspicious" mammogram is not necessarily a "positive" mammogram (i.e., one that shows evidence of breast cancer) and normally would be followed by additional mammography views or by ultrasound.

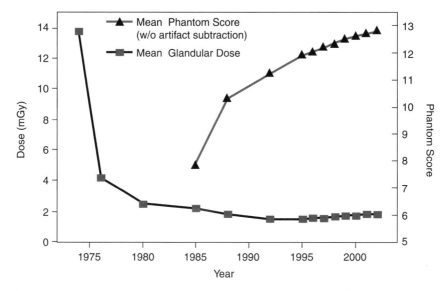

FIGURE 2-1 Trends in mammography dose and image quality. Radiation dose is shown in milliGray units. Phantom Score indicates image quality.[95]

radiation-induced cancers, but gain 12,600 years from an assumed 20 percent reduction in breast cancer mortality.[28]

Recent studies cited in the media have caused some alarm reporting greater DNA damage in human cells in cultures from low than from high x-ray doses.[8,83] Also, because BRCA1 and BRCA2 mutations are associated with deficient DNA repair,[11,56,78] it is theoretically possible that women with BRCA mutations might be more sensitive to the mutagenic effects of radiation. However, studies of mammalian cells in culture dishes have yielded inconsistent results,[37,82] and isolated cells cannot be presumed to predict comparable effects on human health. No large-scale epidemiological studies have been able to detect an increase in cancer rate due to exposure to mammography,[60] nor has a definitive correlation between BRCA1 or BRCA2 mutations and the induction of cancer (or even the induction of mutations) by the type of radiation used in mammography been demonstrated. (Other aspects of BRCA gene mutations are discussed in Chapter 4.)

THE DCIS DILEMMA

Far outstripping the current rise in all breast cancers, the diagnosis of ductal carcinoma in situ (DCIS) has increased approximately 10-fold in the

United States and other developed countries since the advent of population-based mammographic screening, raising concerns of possible overtreatment (Figure 2-2).[22,23,69]

DCIS now represents about 14 percent, or 1 in 7, of all new breast cancer diagnoses in the United States.[96,114] Among screen-detected breast cancers, 20 percent are DCIS and 1 in every 1,300 screening mammograms leads to a diagnosis of DCIS.[22,d] When younger women are diagnosed with breast cancer, it is somewhat less likely to be DCIS (Table 2-2). *All* breast cancers are more common among older women, so relatively and absolutely more of DCIS is found in older women.

Before the widespread use of screening mammography, many cases of DCIS went unrecognized; the increased numbers and proportion of DCIS cases that are now recognized do not necessarily mean that more women are developing DCIS. The reported incidence of DCIS is determined by the actual number of cases and also by the ability to detect them.

DCIS is not life-threatening *per se*, but it is a significant risk factor for invasive breast cancer. It is believed to precede the development, over time, of invasive breast cancer,[54] although the rate of development can be so slow that it never becomes life threatening.[46,77] Among women in an extensive mammography registry study who were initially diagnosed with DCIS between 1978 and 1983, 3.4 percent died of invasive breast cancer within 10 years; of those diagnosed between 1984 and 1989, the 10-year breast cancer mortality was 1.9 percent.[22] These rates, which are approximately one-tenth those for women diagnosed with localized invasive breast cancer, may reflect the effectiveness of treatment for DCIS, the mildness of the condition, or both. Deaths from breast cancer among women with DCIS are thought to result from an invasive component that was not recognized at the time of the DCIS diagnosis or because of progression to an invasive cancer.

The most important issue for DCIS is not, however, the increased detection, but rather the information, which mammography cannot provide, that would permit optimally individualized treatments. Cessation of screening mammography, or any other screening modality, would not solve the problem of overtreatment.[26] Instead, the solution lies in tailoring treatment to the biological characteristics of individual cases.

Diagnosis of DCIS

DCIS occurs when malignant epithelial cells proliferate within the breast ducts but remain confined by the basement membrane (a thin non-

---

[d]Most, but not all, cases of DCIS are detected by screening mammography; some cases are palpable and can be detected following biopsy for breast asymmetry or masses.

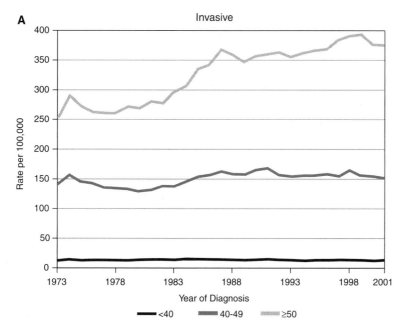

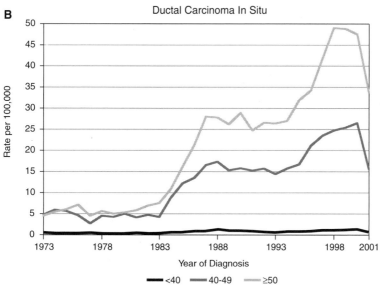

FIGURE 2-2 Female breast cancer incidence (invasive and DCIS) by age-adjusted rates from 1973 to 2001.[96]

TABLE 2-2 Age Differences in DCIS Detected by Screening Mammography[22]

Age	Approximate Number of DCIS Cases Detected per Mammogram	Approximate Incidence of DCIS Cases Detected by Mammography
40-49	1 in 1800	0.06%
50-59	1 in 1500	0.07%
60-69	1 in 1000	0.1%
70-84	1 in 900	0.1%

cellular tissue underlying epithelial cells).[40] The resulting disease ranges from low-grade lesions resembling atypical hyperplasia, to high-grade or anaplastic lesions. (Anaplastic lesions are made up of cells that have reverted to an immature or less differentiated form that is often indicative of invasive cancer.) The classification of different types of DCIS is described in Box 2-3.

The proliferation of epithelial cells in the lobules of the mammary ducts traditionally has been referred to as lobular carcinoma in situ (LCIS), but the current preferred term is lobular intraepithelial neoplasia (LIN), which includes both LCIS and atypical lobular hyperplasia.[7] LIN and DCIS are neither invasive nor metastatic. In time, however, many DCIS lesions will become both invasive and metastatic.[92] LIN, while an indicator of high risk for developing breast cancer, is not considered to be a pre-invasive cancer.[106] It has no characteristic mammographic features and is typically detected by a biopsy performed for another reason,[61] whereas the microcalcifications typical of many cases of DCIS are usually apparent on mammograms.

Only about 10 percent of mammographically detected DCIS will appear as a mass or asymmetry without calcifications; most DCIS is suspected on the basis of mammographic microcalcifications.[22,71,109] This contrasts with invasive cancer, which usually appears as a mass or density on a mammogram. Mammograms frequently underestimate the extent of DCIS, particularly for larger lesions.[41,42,43,71] Calcifications associated with DCIS vary in size, form and density, although they tend to be grouped in clusters, lines, or segmental arrangements that follow the morphology of the duct. Calcifications may also reflect the presence of benign conditions such as proliferative or nonproliferative fibrocystic change, although calcifications that result from these conditions are usually more rounded, more uniform in density, and more scattered in distribution than DCIS calcifications.[71,88]

A definitive diagnosis of DCIS requires pathologic evaluation of a biopsy specimen. To ensure complete accuracy of grading, a core or excisional biopsy must be performed.[51] Stereotactic core biopsy is recommended and

---

BOX 2-3
Classification of DCIS

Traditionally, the microscopic classification of DCIS has been based on the architecture of the lesion. Most simply, lesions are classified as either comedo or noncomedo, based on the presence or absence of plug-like necrotic material (dead tissue) filling the lumen of the affected ducts. This necrotic debris produces the typical fine, linear branching pattern of calcifications seen on mammography and is associated with more aggressive disease.[20] DCIS is graded according to the Van Nuys classification, which combines nuclear grade and the presence or absence of necrosis to predict prognosis[50,51,98] (see table below).[90] Although the Van Nuys classification is used in clinical practice, it has never been validated in a prospective clinical trial.

Comedo carcinoma or high-grade lesions are more aggressive and likely to progress to invasive disease. Studies of local recurrence rates (following local excision without subsequent radiotherapy) indicate that poorly differentiated, comedo-type tumors tend to recur earlier despite excision and radiotherapy (for excellent review, see Kessar et al., 2002).[46,46,51,57,58,94]

Van Nuys Prognostic Index

Parameter	Parameter Score		
	1	2	3
Tumor Size (mm)	15	>15-40	>40
Margins (mm)	10	2-9	<1
Pathology	Non-high-grade, no necrosis	Non-high-grade with necrosis	High-grade with necrosis

The Van Nuys Prognostic Index (VNPI). The first horizontal row represents VNPI scores and the index is calculated by adding the scores of the three parameters (VNPI varies between 3 and 9). For example, a 20-mm tumor would have a score of 2. If the margins were >10 mm (score =1) and there was no sign of necrosis or high-grade pathology in the nucleus (score =1), the total would give a VNPI of 4.

The percent of women who had no recurrence after 8 years of the initial DCIS diagnosis was highest for low VNPI scores (97 percent for VNPI = 3-4; 77 percent for VNPI = 5-7; and 20 percent for VNPI = 8-9).

---

preferred for diagnosis of DCIS, but some patients with microcalcifications are poor candidates for this procedure due to the small size and/or thickness of their breasts, the location of the calcifications, or other factors that interfere with probe function.[71] In these cases, image-directed open surgical biopsy is the preferred approach. Some facilities use vacuum-assisted biopsy to obtain more tissue for analysis. Ultrasound-guided biopsy is useful for nonpalpable masses, but usually cannot be relied on for biopsy of microcalcifications.[71]

Although it was previously believed there was a general progression of genetic abnormalities from atypical ductal hyperplasia, to low-grade DCIS, to high-grade DCIS, and finally to invasive ductal carcinoma, this is no longer believed to be true.[62,71]

Is DCIS Overtreated?

Some researchers contend that the routine biopsy and follow-up of mammographically detected DCIS constitutes overtreatment, because many such tumors would not progress to invasive disease.[33,44,51,99] This argument is based on (1) autopsy studies that indicate a significant prevalence of undetected DCIS in women who died of other causes, and (2) the observation that most women with DCIS do not experience invasive recurrence within 10 to 15 years following treatment (reviewed in Ernster et al., 2002).[22,24,108,110] However, neither of these arguments is conclusive. First, the series of studies that estimated a 30 to 50 percent risk of developing invasive cancer within 10 years of a DCIS diagnosis (and in the absence of any treatment besides surgical biopsy)[2,86] was based on cases that occurred before the widespread use of mammography and were detected by other means.[76] Second, many more cases are detected, presumably at earlier stages, and few go untreated. As a result, there are no definitive estimates of the natural course of DCIS (see Box 2-4). Moreover, later review of the earlier autopsy studies revealed that many of the DCIS cases had been overdiagnosed and failed to meet current criteria for DCIS diagnosis.[91]

Other lines of evidence suggest that DCIS is not overtreated. A small series of untreated women with DCIS, who were diagnosed before mammographic screening became widespread, were found to have more than the expected number of invasive breast cancers when compared to the general population.[2,22,25,75] Similarly, increased risk for both DCIS and invasive breast cancer also has been reported in larger, more recent studies of women treated for DCIS.[22,35,36,68,104] Findings from randomized trials indicate that the addition of radiotherapy and tamoxifen to breast-conserving surgery (BCS) reduces the chance of future invasive disease recurrence compared with BCS alone.[22,31,32,47] Finally, recent molecular genetic studies suggest that most invasive ductal breast cancers arise from DCIS (reviewed by Feig, 2000).[9,10,26,64,65,70,107] Overall, most cases of DCIS are high grade, regardless of how they were detected. Fifty-four percent of screen-detected cases and 62 percent of non-screen-detected cases were high grade.[51] High-grade tumors have a greater potential to progress to invasive disease than low-

---

BOX 2-4
Treatment for DCIS

Women with biopsy-proven DCIS are typically treated surgically with either mastectomy or BCS (also known as lumpectomy). Along with BCS, treatment often includes adjuvant radiotherapy (RT) and in some cases, hormone therapy (tamoxifen).[22,24] Although BCS is recommended for the majority of DCIS cases, mastectomy remains the treatment of choice for many women in the United States. Mastectomy is specifically indicated for women with two or more primary tumors in the breast or with diffuse malignant-appearing microcalcifications, and also when persistent positive tumor margins remain after reasonable surgical attempts.[26,71,114] Mastectomy may also be more appropriate in cases of extensive DCIS that can be removed with only a small negative margin, particularly in small-breasted patients. Total mastectomy is associated with very low rates of local recurrence (1.4 percent) and breast cancer-specific mortality (0.6 percent).[69]

Treatment guidelines recommend BCS plus RT for localized DCIS (that is, for single, nondiffuse loci) less than or equal to 4 cm, meanwhile acknowledging the inherent difficulty of accurately measuring DCIS lesions.[71] Younger women tend to have a greater risk of local recurrence after BCS plus RT, which results at least in part from the biological characteristics of disease in younger women.[105]

Although no randomized trials have yet been published, retrospective studies indicate that total mastectomy improves disease-free survival of DCIS as compared with *BCS plus RT*, but there is no evidence to suggest the superiority of mastectomy over BCS plus RT in terms of overall and breast-cancer-specific survival.[3,69,89]

There have been some reports of low recurrence rates following *BCS alone* for small-volume lesions with clear margins, but the maximum size of DCIS for which RT could be safely omitted is unknown.[69,71] Three recent randomized controlled trials demonstrated that *BCS plus RT* significantly reduces the incidence of local recurrence of DCIS.[30,31,38,47,69] Most nonrandomized trials reported findings consistent with these randomized trials and showed that adjuvant RT after BCS significantly decreased the incidence of ipsilateral (same side) breast tumor recurrence.[13,52,69,89,101] Randomized trials show that recurrence with lumpectomy alone is approximately 30 percent at 10 years and reduced by half with radiotherapy. Despite the higher rates of recurrence, there is no difference in the mortality rates for lumpectomy alone versus lumpectomy with RT; rates for both are in the range of mortality for mastectomy, which is about 2 percent. Fifty percent of recurrences are DCIS and the other 50 percent are invasive breast cancer. Although not considered a mandatory part of treatment for DCIS, tamoxifen therapy appears to benefit some patients.[32,69,114]

---

grade tumors. DCIS is now recognized to be very heterogeneous is its clinical behavior.[46]

Although there is an element of overdiagnosis of DCIS in breast cancer screening, this appears to be relatively small. For example, a recent study reported that the average incidence of nonprogressive DCIS is about 1 in

100,000 per year and estimated that only 4 percent of DCIS cases detected during incidence screening represent overdiagnosis that would *not* progress if left untreated.[113,e]

Thus, although most experts accept that a significant fraction of DCIS will remain noninvasive, many agree that until clinicians can distinguish among the heterogeneous types of DCIS and recognize those that are likely to progress to invasive, metastatic breast cancer, mammography-detected DCIS requires full diagnostic workup and treatment.[51] A critically important focus of future research will be to identify those cases of DCIS that are unlikely to progress, as well as more effective ways to arrest the development of more dangerous lesions.[45]

REFERENCES

1. Andrews FJ. 2001. Pain during mammography: implications for breast screening programmes. *Australas Radiol* 45(2):113-117.
2. Betsill WL Jr, Rosen PP, Lieberman PH, Robbins GF. 1978. Intraductal carcinoma. Long-term follow-up after treatment by biopsy alone. *JAMA* 239(18):1863-1867.
3. Boyages J, Delaney G, Taylor R. 1999. Predictors of local recurrence after treatment of ductal carcinoma in situ: a meta-analysis. *Cancer* 85(3):616-628.
4. Boyd NF, Byng JW, Jong RA, Fishell EK, Little LE, Miller AB, Lockwood GA, Tritchler DL, Yaffe MJ. 1995. Quantitative classification of mammographic densities and breast cancer risk: results from the Canadian National Breast Screening Study. *J Natl Cancer Inst* 87(9):670-675.
5. Boyd NF, Dite GS, Stone J, Gunasekara A, English DR, McCredie MR, Giles GG, Tritchler D, Chiarelli A, Yaffe MJ, Hopper JL. 2002. Heritability of mammographic density, a risk factor for breast cancer. *N Engl J Med* 347(12):886-894.
6. Boyd NF, Lockwood GA, Byng JW, Little LE, Yaffe MJ, Tritchler DL. 1998. The relationship of anthropometric measures to radiological features of the breast in premenopausal women. *Br J Cancer* 78(9):1233-1238.
7. Bratthauer GL, Tavassoli FA. 2002. Lobular intraepithelial neoplasia: previously unexplored aspects assessed in 775 cases and their clinical implications. *Virchows Arch* 440(2):134-138.
8. Brenner DJ, Sawant SG, Hande MP, Miller RC, Elliston CD, Fu Z, Randers-Pehrson G, Marino SA. 2002. Routine screening mammography: how important is the radiation-risk side of the benefit-risk equation? *Int J Radiat Biol* 78(12):1065-1067.
9. Buerger H, Otterbach F, Simon R, Poremba C, Diallo R, Decker T, Riethdorf L, Brinkschmidt C, Dockhorn-Dworniczak B, Boecker W. 1999. Comparative genomic hybridization of ductal carcinoma in situ of the breast-evidence of multiple genetic pathways. *J Pathol* 187(4):396-402.
10. Bur ME, Zimarowski MJ, Schnitt SJ, Baker S, Lew R. 1992. Estrogen receptor immunohistochemistry in carcinoma in situ of the breast. *Cancer* 69(5):1174-1181.

---

[e]Diseases can be screened for either prevalence or incidence. *Prevalence screening* represents the patient's baseline scan, and *incidence screening* represents subsequent, follow-up screening that looks for changes in the original condition.

11. Chen JJ, Silver D, Cantor S, Livingston DM, Scully R. 1999. BRCA1, BRCA2, and Rad51 operate in a common DNA damage response pathway. *Cancer Res* 59(7 Suppl):1752s-1756s.

12. Christiansen CL, Wang F, Barton MB, Kreuter W, Elmore JG, Gelfand AE, Fletcher SW. 2000. Predicting the cumulative risk of false-positive mammograms. *J Natl Cancer Inst* 92(20):1657-1666.

13. Cutuli B, Cohen-Solal-Le Nir C, De Lafontan B, Mignotte H, Fichet V, Fay R, Servent V, Giard S, Charra-Brunaud C, Auvray H, Penault-Llorca F, Charpentier JC. 2001. Ductal carcinoma in situ of the breast results of conservative and radical treatments in 716 patients. *Eur J Cancer* 37(18):2365-2372.

14. Davey C, White V, Ward JE. 2002. Insurance repercussions of mammographic screening: what do women think? *Med Sci Monit* 8(12):LE54-LE55.

15. Dixon JM. 2003. Hormone replacement therapy and the breast. *Surg Oncol* 12(4):251-263.

16. Drossaert CH, Boer H, Seydel ER. 2001. Does mammographic screening and a negative result affect attitudes towards future breast screening? *J Med Screen* 8(4):204-212.

17. Drossaert CH, Boer H, Seydel ER. 2002. Monitoring women's experiences during three rounds of breast cancer screening: results from a longitudinal study. *J Med Screen* 9(4):168-175.

18. Duffy SW, Tabar L, Chen HH, Holmqvist M, Yen MF, Abdsalah S, Epstein B, Frodis E, Ljungberg E, Hedborg-Melander C, Sundbom A, Tholin M, Wiege M, Akerlund A, Wu HM, Tung TS, Chiu YH, Chiu CP, Huang CC, Smith RA, Rosen M, Stenbeck M, Holmberg L. 2002. The impact of organized mammography service screening on breast carcinoma mortality in seven Swedish counties. *Cancer* 95(3):458-469.

19. Duffy SW, Tabar L, Vitak B, Day NE, Smith RA, Chen HH, Yen MF. 2003. The relative contributions of screen-detected in situ and invasive breast carcinomas in reducing mortality from the disease. *Eur J Cancer* 39(12):1755-1760.

20. Dummin L. Pathology Seen in Breast Imaging: DCIS. Web Page. Available at: http://medrad.city.unisa.edu.au/Breast/DCIS.html.

21. Elmore JG, Barton MB, Moceri VM, Polk S, Arena PJ, Fletcher SW. 1998. Ten-year risk of false positive screening mammograms and clinical breast examinations. *N Engl J Med* 338(16):1089-1096.

22. Ernster VL, Ballard-Barbash R, Barlow WE, Zheng Y, Weaver DL, Cutter G, Yankaskas BC, Rosenberg R, Carney PA, Kerlikowske K, Taplin SH, Urban N, Geller BM. 2002. Detection of ductal carcinoma in situ in women undergoing screening mammography. *J Natl Cancer Inst* 94(20):1546-1554.

23. Ernster VL, Barclay J, Kerlikowske K, Grady D, Henderson C. 1996. Incidence of and treatment for ductal carcinoma in situ of the breast. *JAMA* 275(12):913-918.

24. Ernster VL, Barclay J, Kerlikowske K, Wilkie H, Ballard-Barbash R. 2000. Mortality among women with ductal carcinoma in situ of the breast in the population-based surveillance, epidemiology and end results program. *Arch Intern Med* 160(7):953-958.

25. Eusebi V, Foschini MP, Cook MG, Berrino F, Azzopardi JG. 1989. Long-term follow-up of in situ carcinoma of the breast with special emphasis on clinging carcinoma. *Semin Diagn Pathol* 6(2):165-173.

26. Feig SA. 2000. Ductal carcinoma in situ. Implications for screening mammography. *Radiol Clin North Am* 38(4):653-668, vii.

27. Feig SA. 2002. Effect of service screening mammography on population mortality from breast carcinoma. *Cancer* 95(3):451-457.

28. Feig SA, Ehrlich SM. 1990. Estimation of radiation risk from screening mammography: recent trends and comparison with expected benefits. *Radiology* 174(3 Pt 1):638-647.

29. Feig SA, Hendrick RE. 1997. Radiation risk from screening mammography of women aged 40-49 years. *J Natl Cancer Inst Monogr* (22):119-124.

30. Fisher B, Constantino J, Redmond C, et al. 1993. Lumpectomy compared with lumpectomy and radiation therapy for the treatment of intraductal breast cancer. *N Engl J Med* 328:1581-1586.

31. Fisher B, Dignam J, Wolmark N, Mamounas E, Costantino J, Poller W, Fisher ER, Wickerham DL, Deutsch M, Margolese R, Dimitrov N, Kavanah M. 1998. Lumpectomy and radiation therapy for the treatment of intraductal breast cancer: findings from National Surgical Adjuvant Breast and Bowel Project B-17. *J Clin Oncol* 16(2):441-452.

32. Fisher B, Dignam J, Wolmark N, Wickerham DL, Fisher ER, Mamounas E, Smith R, Begovic M, Dimitrov NV, Margolese RG, Kardinal CG, Kavanah MT, Fehrenbacher L, Oishi RH. 1999. Tamoxifen in treatment of intraductal breast cancer: National Surgical Adjuvant Breast and Bowel Project B-24 randomised controlled trial. *Lancet* 353(9169):1993-2000.

33. Fletcher SW. 1995. Why question screening mammography for women in their forties? *Radiol Clin North Am* 33(6):1259-1271.

34. Fletcher SW, Elmore JG. 2003. Clinical practice. Mammographic screening for breast cancer. *N Engl J Med* 348(17):1672-1680.

35. Fonseca R, Hartmann LC, Petersen IA, Donohue JH, Crotty TB, Gisvold JJ. 1997. Ductal carcinoma in situ of the breast. *Ann Intern Med* 127(11):1013-1022.

36. Franceschi S, Levi F, La Vecchia C, Randimbison L, Te VC. 1998. Second cancers following in situ carcinoma of the breast. *Int J Cancer* 77(3):392-395.

37. Frankenberg-Schwager M, Garg I, Fran-Kenberg D, Greve B, Severin E, Uthe D, Gohde W. 2002. Mutagenicity of low-filtered 30 kVp X-rays, mammography X-rays and conventional X-rays in cultured mammalian cells. *Int J Radiat Biol* 78(9):781-789.

38. George WD, Houghton J, Cuzick J, et al. 2000. Radiotherapy and tamoxifen following complete local excision in the management of ductal carcinoma *in situ*: preliminary results from the UK DCIS trial. *Proc Am Soc Clin Oncol* Abstract 270.

39. Gotzsche PCOO. 2000. Is screening for breast cancer with mammography justifiable? *Lancet* 355:129-133.

40. Harris JR, Lippman ME, Veronesi U, Willett W. 1992. Breast cancer (2). *N Engl J Med* 327(6):390-398.

41. Holland R, Hendricks JH, Verbeek AL, et al. 1990. Extent, distribution, and mammographic/histological correlations of breast ductal carcinoma in situ. *Lancet* 335:519-522.

42. Holland R, Hendriks JH. 1994. Microcalcifications associated with ductal carcinoma-in-situ: mammographic-pathological correlation. *Semin Diag Pathol* 11:181-192.

43. Institute of Medicine. 2003. *Fulfilling the Potential of Cancer Prevention and Early Detection*. Washington DC: The National Academies Press.

44. Jatoi I, Baum M. 1995. Mammographically detected ductal carcinoma in situ: are we overdiagnosing breast cancer? *Surgery* 118(1):118-120.

45. Jeffrey SS, Pollack JR. 2003. The diagnosis and management of pre-invasive breast disease: promise of new technologies in understanding pre-invasive breast lesions. *Breast Cancer Res* 5(6):320-328.

46. Jensen RA, Page DL. 2003. Ductal carcinoma in situ of the breast: impact of pathology on therapeutic decisions. *Am J Surg Pathol* 27(6):828-831.

47. Julien JP, Bijker N, Fentiman IS, Peterse JL, Delledonne V, Rouanet P, Avril A, Sylvester R, Mignolet F, Bartelink H, Van Dongen JA. 2000. Radiotherapy in breast-conserving treatment for ductal carcinoma in situ: first results of the EORTC randomised phase III trial 10853. EORTC Breast Cancer Cooperative Group and EORTC Radiotherapy Group. *Lancet* 355(9203):528-533.

48. Jung H. 2001. Is there a real risk of radiation-induced breast cancer for postmenopausal women? *Radiat Environ Biophys* 40(2):169-174.

49. Kerlikowske K, Grady D, Barclay J, Frankel SD, Ominsky SH, Sickles EA, Ernster V. 1998. Variability and accuracy in mammographic interpretation using the American College of Radiology Breast Imaging Reporting and Data System. *J Natl Cancer Inst* 90(23):1801-1809.

50. Kerlikowske K, Molinaro A, Cha I, Ljung B-M, Ernster VL, Stewart K, Chew K, Moore D2, Waldman F. 2003. Characteristics associated with recurrence among women with ductal carcinoma in situ treated by lumpectomy. *J Natl Cancer Inst* 95(22):1692-1702.

51. Kessar P, Perry N, Vinnicombe SJ, Hussain HK, Carpenter R, Wells CA. 2002. How significant is detection of ductal carcinoma in situ in a breast screening programme? *Clin Radiol* 57(9):807-814.

52. Kestin LL, Goldstein NS, Martinez AA, Rebner M, Balasubramaniam M, Frazier RC, Register JT, Pettinga J, Vicini FA. 2000. Mammographically detected ductal carcinoma in situ treated with conservative surgery with or without radiation therapy: patterns of failure and 10-year results. *Ann Surg* 231(2):235-245.

53. Kolb TM, Lichy J, Newhouse JH. 2002. Comparison of the performance of screening mammography, physical examination, and breast US and evaluation of factors that influence them: an analysis of 27,825 patient evaluations. *Radiology* 225(1):165-175.

54. Kopans DB. 2003. Re: Detection of ductal carcinoma in situ in women undergoing screening mammography. *J Natl Cancer Inst* 95(6):487; author reply 487-488.

55. Kornguth PJ, Keefe FJ, Conaway MR. 1996. Pain during mammography: characteristics and relationship to demographic and medical variables. *Pain* 66(2-3):187-194.

56. Kote-Jarai Z, Eeles RA. 1999. BRCA1, BRCA2 and their possible function in DNA damage response. *Br J Cancer* 81(7):1099-1102.

57. Lagios MD. 1990. Duct carcinoma in situ. Pathology and treatment. *Surg Clin North Am* 70(4):853-871.

58. Lagios MD, Margolin FR, Westdahl PR, Rose MR. 1989. Mammographically detected duct carcinoma in situ. Frequency of local recurrence following tylectomy and prognostic effect of nuclear grade on local recurrence. *Cancer* 63(4):618-624.

59. Land CE, Tokunaga M, Koyama K, Soda M, Preston DL, Nishimori I, Tokuoka S. 2003. Incidence of female breast cancer among atomic bomb survivors, Hiroshima and Nagasaki, 1950-1990. *Radiat Res* 160(6):707-717.

60. Law J, Faulkner K. 2001. Cancers detected and induced, and associated risk and benefit, in a breast screening programme. *Br J Radiol* 74(888):1121-1127.

61. Li CI, Anderson BO, Daling JR, Moe RE. 2003. Trends in incidence rates of invasive lobular and ductal breast carcinoma. *JAMA* 289(11):1421-1424.

62. Liberman L. 2000. Ductal carcinoma in situ: Percutaneous biopsy considerations. *Semin Breast Dis* 3:14-25.

63. Lidbrink E, Elfving J, Frisell J, Jonsson E. 1996. Neglected aspects of false positive findings of mammography in breast cancer screening: analysis of false positive cases from the Stockholm trial. *BMJ* 312(7026):273-276.

64. Liu E, Thor A, He M, Barcos M, Ljung BM, Benz C. 1992. The HER2 (c-erbB-2) oncogene is frequently amplified in in situ carcinomas of the breast. *Oncogene* 7(5):1027-1032.

65. Maguire HC Jr, Hellman ME, Greene MI, Yeh I. 1992. Expression of c-erbB-2 in in situ and in adjacent invasive ductal adenocarcinomas of the female breast. *Pathobiology* 60(3):117-121.

66. McCann J, Stockton D, Godward S. 2002. Impact of false-positive mammography on subsequent screening attendance and risk of cancer. *Breast Cancer Res* 4(5):R11.

67. Meystre-Agustoni G, Paccaud F, Jeannin A, Dubois-Arber F. 2001. Anxiety in a cohort of Swiss women participating in a mammographic screening programme. *J Med Screen* 8(4):213-219.

68. Mirza NQ, Vlastos G, Meric F, Sahin AA, Singletary SE, Newman LA, Kuerer HM, Ames FC, Ross MI, Feig BW, Pollock RE, Buchholz TA, McNeese MD, Strom EA, Hortobagyi GN, Hunt KK. 2000. Ductal carcinoma-in-situ: long-term results of breast-conserving therapy. *Ann Surg Oncol* 7(9):656-664.

69. Mokbel K. 2003. Towards optimal management of ductal carcinoma in situ of the breast. *Eur J Surg Oncol* 29(2):191-197.

70. Moore E, Magee H, Coyne J, Gorey T, Dervan PA. 1999. Widespread chromosomal abnormalities in high-grade ductal carcinoma in situ of the breast. Comparative genomic hybridization study of pure high-grade DCIS. *J Pathol* 187(4):403-409.

71. Morrow M, Strom EA, Bassett LW, Dershaw DD, Fowble B, Harris JR, O'Malley F, Schnitt SJ, Singletary SE, Winchester DP. 2002. Standard for the management of ductal carcinoma in situ of the breast (DCIS). *CA Cancer J Clin* 52(5):256-276.

72. Mushlin AI, Kouides RW, Shapiro DE. 1998. Estimating the accuracy of screening mammography: a meta-analysis. *Am J Prev Med* 14(2):143-153.

73. Nystrom L, Andersson I, Bjurstam N, Frisell J, Nordenskjold B, Rutqvist LE. 2002. Long-term effects of mammography screening: updated overview of the Swedish randomised trials. *Lancet* 359(9310):909-919.

74. Olsen O, Gotzsche PC. 2001. Cochrane review on screening for breast cancer with mammography. *Lancet* 358(9290):1340-1342.

75. Page DL, Dupont WD, Rogers LW, Jensen RA, Schuyler PA. 1995. Continued local recurrence of carcinoma 15-25 years after a diagnosis of low grade ductal carcinoma in situ of the breast treated only by biopsy. *Cancer* 76(7):1197-1200.

76. Page DL, Dupont WD, Rogers LW, Landenberger M. 1982. Intraductal carcinoma of the breast: follow-up after biopsy only. *Cancer* 49(4):751-758.

77. Page DL, Gray R, Allred DC, Dressler LG, Hatfield AK, Martino S, Robert NJ, Wood WC. 2001. Prediction of node-negative breast cancer outcome by histologic grading and S-phase analysis by flow cytometry: an Eastern Cooperative Oncology Group Study (2192). *Am J Clin Oncol* 24(1):10-18.

78. Patel KJ, Yu VP, Lee H, Corcoran A, Thistlethwaite FC, Evans MJ, Colledge WH, Friedman LS, Ponder BA, Venkitaraman AR. 1998. Involvement of Brca2 in DNA repair. *Mol Cell* 1(3):347-357.

79. Pawluczyk O, Augustine BJ, Yaffe MJ, Rico D, Yang J, Mawdsley GE, Boyd NF. 2003. A volumetric method for estimation of breast density on digitized screen-film mammograms. *Med Phys* 30(3):352-364.

80. Pinckney RG, Geller BM, Burman M, Littenberg B. 2003. Effect of false-positive mammograms on return for subsequent screening mammography. *Am J Med* 114(2):120-125.

81. Raza S, Rosen MP, Chorny K, Mehta TS, Hulka CA, Baum JK. 2001. Patient expectations and costs of immediate reporting of screening mammography: talk isn't cheap. *Am J Roentgenol* 177(3):579-583.

82. Rothfuss A, Schutz P, Bochum S, Volm T, Eberhardt E, Kreienberg R, Vogel W, Speit G. 2000. Induced micronucleus frequencies in peripheral lymphocytes as a screening test for carriers of a BRCA1 mutation in breast cancer families. *Cancer Res* 60(2):390-394.

83. Rothkamm K, Lobrich M. 2003. Evidence for a lack of DNA double-strand break repair in human cells exposed to very low x-ray doses. *Proc Natl Acad Sci USA* 100(9):5057-5062.

84. Sandin B, Chorot P, Valiente RM, Lostao L, Santed MA. 2002. Adverse psychological effects in women attending a second-stage breast cancer screening. *J Psychosom Res* 52(5):303-309.

85. Sapir R, Patlas M, Strano SD, Hadas-Halpern I, Cherny NI. 2003. Does mammography hurt? *J Pain Symptom Manage* 25(1):53-63.

86. Schwartz GF, Patchefsky AS, Finkelstein SD, et al. 1989. Non-palpable in situ ductal carcinoma of the breast: predictors of multicentricity and microinvasion and implication for treatment. *Arch Surg* 124:29-32.

87. Sharp PC, Michielutte R, Freimanis R, Cunningham L, Spangler J, Burnette V. 2003. Reported pain following mammography screening. *Arch Intern Med* 163(7):833-836.

88. Sigfusson BF, Andersson I, Aspegren K, Janzon L, Linell F, Ljungberg O. 1983. Clustered breast calcifications. *Acta Radiol Diagn (Stockh)* 24(4):273-281.

89. Silverstein MJ, Barth A, Poller DN, Gierson ED, Colburn WJ, Waisman JR, Gamagami P. 1995. Ten-year results comparing mastectomy to excision and radiation therapy for ductal carcinoma in situ of the breast. *Eur J Cancer* 31A(9):1425-1427.

90. Silverstein MJ, Lagios MD, Craig PH, Waisman JR, Lewinsky BS, Colburn WJ, Poller DN. 1996. A prognostic index for ductal carcinoma in situ of the breast. *Cancer* 77(11):2267-2274.

91. Silverstein MJ, Recht A, Lagios MD. 2002. *Ductal Carcinoma in Situ of the Breast.* second ed. Philadelphia: Lippincott Williams and Wilkins.

92. Skinner KA, Silverstein MJ. 2001. The management of ductal carcinoma in situ of the breast. *Endocr Relat Cancer* 8(1):33-45.

93. Slanetz PJ. 2002. Hormone replacement therapy and breast tissue density on mammography. *Menopause* 9(2):82-83.

94. Solin LJ, Yeh IT, Kurtz J, Fourquet A, Recht A, Kuske R, McCormick B, Cross MA, Schultz DJ, Amalric R, et al. 1993. Ductal carcinoma in situ (intraductal carcinoma) of the breast treated with breast-conserving surgery and definitive irradiation. Correlation of pathologic parameters with outcome of treatment. *Cancer* 71(8):2532-2542.

95. Spelic DC. Dose and Image Quality in Mammography: Trends During the First Decade of MQSA. Accessed December 3, 2003. Web Page. Available at: http://www.fda.gov/cdrh/mammography/scorecard-article5.html.

96. Surveillance Epidemiology and End Results (SEER) Program (www.seer.cancer.gov). 2003. *SEER*Stat Database: Incidence—SEER 9 Registry Public-Use, Nov. 2002 Submission (1973-2000),* National Cancer Institute, DCCPS, Surveillance Research Program, Cancer Statistics Branch.

97. Tabar L, Vitak B, Chen HH, Yen MF, Duffy SW, Smith RA. 2001. Beyond randomized controlled trials: organized mammographic screening substantially reduces breast carcinoma mortality. *Cancer* 91(9):1724-1731.

98. The Consensus Conference Committee. 1997. Consensus Conference on the classification of ductal carcinoma in situ. *Cancer* 80(9):1798-1802.

99. Thornton H. 2000. Consequences of breast screening. *Lancet* 356(9234):1033.

100. Thornton H, Edwards A, Baum M. 2003. Women need better information about routine mammography. *BMJ* 327(7406):101-103.

101. Tunon-de-Lara C, de-Mascarel I, Mac-Grogan G, Stockle E, Jourdain O, Acharian V, Guegan C, Faucher A, Bussieres E, Trojani M, Bonichon F, Barreau B, Dilhuydy MH, Dilhuydy JM, Mauriac L, Durand M, Avril A. 2001. Analysis of 676 cases of ductal carcinoma in situ of the breast from 1971 to 1995: diagnosis and treatment—the experience of one institute. *Am J Clin Oncol* 24(6):531-536.

102. Ursin G, Astrahan MA, Salane M, Parisky YR, Pearce JG, Daniels JR, Pike MC, Spicer DV. 1998. The detection of changes in mammographic densities. *Cancer Epidemiol Biomarkers Prev* 7(1):43-47.

103. Ursin G, Parisky YR, Pike MC, Spicer DV. 2001. Mammographic density changes during the menstrual cycle. *Cancer Epidemiol Biomarkers Prev* 10(2):141-142.

104. Van Zee KJ, Liberman L, Samli B, Tran KN, McCormick B, Petrek JA, Rosen PP, Borgen PI. 1999. Long term follow-up of women with ductal carcinoma in situ treated with breast-conserving surgery: the effect of age. *Cancer* 86(9):1757-1767.

105. Vicini FA, Recht A. 2002. Age at diagnosis and outcome for women with ductal carcinoma-in-situ of the breast: a critical review of the literature. *J Clin Oncol* 20(11):2736-2744.

106. Viehweg P, Lampe D, Buchmann J, Heywang-Kobrunner SH. 2000. In situ and minimally invasive breast cancer: morphologic and kinetic features on contrast-enhanced MR imaging. *MAGMA* 11(3):129-137.

107. Walker RA, Dearing SJ, Lane DP, Varley JM. 1991. Expression of p53 protein in infiltrating and in-situ breast carcinomas. *J Pathol* 165(3):203-211.

108. Warnberg F, Bergh J, Holmberg L. 1999. Prognosis in women with a carcinoma in situ of the breast: a population-based study in Sweden. *Cancer Epidemiol Biomarkers Prev* 8(9):769-774.

109. Wazer DE, Gage I, Homer MJ, Krosnick SH, Schmid C. 1996. Age-related differences in patients with nonpalpable breast carcinomas. *Cancer* 78(7):1432-1437.

110. Welch HG, Black WC. 1997. Using autopsy series to estimate the disease "reservoir" for ductal carcinoma in situ of the breast: how much more breast cancer can we find? *Ann Intern Med* 127(11):1023-1028.

111. White E, Velentgas P, Mandelson MT, Lehman CD, Elmore JG, Porter P, Yasui Y, Taplin SH. 1998. Variation in mammographic breast density by time in menstrual cycle among women aged 40-49 years. *J Natl Cancer Inst* 90(12):906-910.

112. White SC. 1992. 1992 assessment of radiation risk from dental radiography. *Dentomaxillofac Radiol* 21(3):118-126.

113. Yen MF, Tabar L, Vitak B, Smith RA, Chen HH, Duffy SW. 2003. Quantifying the potential problem of overdiagnosis of ductal carcinoma in situ in breast cancer screening. *Eur J Cancer* 39(12):1746-1754.

114. Zellars R, Wolff AC. 2003. Local failure and prognostic factors in ductal carcinoma in situ: concentration on recent publications. *Curr Opin Obstet Gynecol* 15(1):9-12.

3

Improving Breast Cancer
Screening Services

*The controversy over mammography is often focused on whether
or not it should be used as a screening tool. But another equally
important issue, given its widespread use, is the optimization of
mammography. . . . Considerable effort should, therefore, be devoted to determining how to make mammography as effective as it
can be and to reduce the tremendous variation in interpretation
and biopsy rates.*[38]

Laura Esserman and colleagues

T|his chapter examines critical issues in providing high-quality breast
screening services. The fundamental criterion for implementing a
screening program for all women in a particular target group is that
the screening tests should have an acceptable level of accuracy, cost effectiveness, and a favorable balance of benefits to harms. Although different
programs might place relatively greater emphasis on detecting small tumors
or on reducing the false-positive rate, there is little disagreement that achieving the highest practical balance between sensitivity and specificity is central to ongoing efforts to improve the quality of mammography services.
This chapter reviews alternative approaches to the organization of breast
screening services, ways that mammography could be improved, technologies that might augment or replace mammography in breast cancer screening, and the challenges in supporting and developing a well-trained
workforce.

SCREENING OUTCOMES VARY BY COUNTRY

Nearly a dozen countries have national or regional screening programs
in which personal invitations for regular mammograms are sent to all
women over age 40 or 50, depending on the country (Table 3-1).[74] There
are international differences in breast cancer detection patterns and mortality. Examination of how these patterns are influenced by the organization
of breast cancer screening should indicate ways to improve quality.

TABLE 3-1 Breast Screening Programs in Different Countries*

	United States	Canada
Year screening program started	1988 (Medicare)	1988 (British Columbia was the 1st province)
Age of women screened (target population)	40 and older, generally until 75	50 to 69
Screening interval (years)	1-2	2[ii]
Percent of target population screened	55-63%[iv]	54%[v]
Referral type	Doctor or self-referral	Doctor or self-referral
Double reading[x]	Some[xi]	No
Number of views	2	2
Quality enforcement	National law (MQSA)[xiv]	Voluntary accreditation[xv]
Quality assurance site visits	Yes	No
Level of organization	Medicare is national; otherwise based on state and private insurance provider policies[xx]	Province[xxi]

*Finland, Luxembourg, and Japan also have national mammography screening programs; Italy, Spain, and Norway have regional programs.

[i]Swedish governments makes guidelines, but standards and practices are organized at the county level.

[ii]The Canadian Province of British Columbia offers annual mammograms.

[iii]Screening interval established individually by county.

[iv]Based on year 2000 data from Behavioral Risk Factor Surveillance System Public Use Data Tape (CDC, 2001). Also National Health Interview Survey, 2000 (CDC 2002); women over 40, and mammograms in last year; ACS Breast Cancer Facts and Figures 2003-2004.

[v]Based on 1996 data; Paquette et al. (2000); mammogram in past 2 years.

[vi]Based on 2001-2002 data; NHS Breast Screening Programme Annual Review 2003.

[vii]Based on WE trial 1977-1979; attendance after first invitation; Lynge et al.

[viii]Should be range b/c age policies differ; WE trial data is old (1977) and small sample size, but all studies go back to this same ref.

[ix]Based on 1990-1995 data; Facheboud et al., 1998, *Int. J. Cancer*.

[x]ISBN http://appliedresearch.cancer.gov/ibsn/data/double.html. Accessed February 4, 2004.

[xi]The United States does not require double reading of mammograms, but the practice is common. However, overall, double reading of screening mammograms is less common in the United States than other countries.

United Kingdom	Sweden[i]	The Netherlands	Australia
1988	1986	1989	1994
50 to 70	Beginning at 40; ending at 64 or 74	50 to 75	40 to 79
3	$1^1/_2$-2, depending on age[iii]	2	2
76%[vi]	89%[vii, viii]	78%[16]	54
Invite	Invite	Invite	Invite or self-referral
No	Yes	Yes	Yes
2[xii]	2	2[xiii]	2
Voluntary[xvi]	National law[xvii]	National law[xvooo]	National accreditation requirements[xix]
Yes	Yes	Yes	Yes
National	County (Swedish counties are comparable to stated in the U.S.)	National	National

[xii]Initial mammogram only; NHS reports as of December 2003 86% of local screening services are doing two-view mammographies.

[xiii]Initial only.

[xiv]The Mammography Quality Standards Act ensures x-ray technical quality but does not review quality of interpretation.

[xv]Canadian Association of Radiologists.

[xvi]Radiographic Quality Control Manual for Mammography.

[xvii]National Swedish law based on European Guidelines for Quality Assurance in Screening Mammography.

[xviii]Dutch Technical Protocol for Quality Control.

[xix]External quality assurance program must be established to receive funding.

[xx]No national policy. Contains aspects of both national centralized care (Medicare) and decentralized regional care (private).

[xxi]Canadian government sets has national guidelines, but standards and service organization are set at the provincial level.

Most women who undergo biopsies will not have breast cancer. Although some might describe these biopsies as "needless," in reality they reflect the lack of precision of current detection methods. Some of the imprecision is likely due to the quality of the mammographic interpretation, and some is due to the inherent limitations of the technology. Some solutions to the problem lie in organizational changes, such as adopting different procedures for interpreting mammograms, different standards, and different ways of organizing mammography services. Other solutions might lie in technological improvements.

Screening for breast cancer is organized differently in different countries. A close comparison between the different countries and the results offers some useful insights into strategies for reducing breast cancer mortality in the United States. Mortality is influenced by screening patterns, as well as patterns of care.

Screening programs can be compared according to a variety of measures, such as differences in breast cancer survival rates, rates of abnormal mammograms, or rates of false positives. But there are caveats to each of these measures.

A 2003 study reported that 5-year survival rates for all breast cancers are higher in the United States (89 percent) than in Europe (79 percent), but this was based on data from a heterogeneous group of countries including those with national or regional screening programs (Italy, Spain, The Netherlands, and the United Kingdom) and those without (Estonia and France).[101] The study, which compared the United States Surveillance Epidemiology and End Results (SEER) data set with the comparable EUROCARE data set, revealed that breast cancer survival was higher for women in the United States than in Europe, at least for breast cancers diagnosed between 1990 and 1992.[a] (During the first decade of a service screening program, most breast cancer deaths will occur in women who were diagnosed before the program started which means that a reduction in breast cancer mortality will only emerge when most of the breast cancers in the target population have been screen detected.[74]) Five-year survival was 89 percent for women in the United States and 79 percent for women in Europe.[101] Most of the difference in survival rates was due to the stage at which women were diagnosed. Forty percent of tumors in the SEER data set were early stage (T1N0M0) compared with only 30 percent in the EUROCARE set.[b] The authors attribute these differences to the availability

---

[a]Analyses of breast cancer survival outcomes do not reflect recent practice changes, either in detection or treatment, because of the need to use a study period that is at least as long as the natural course of the disease, which is about 10 years.

[b]T1 indicates a tumor less than 2 cm, N0 indicates that the cancer has not spread to the lymph nodes, and M0 indicates the absence of metastasis to other organs.

THE NATIONAL ACADEMIES PRESS

Publisher for the National Academies

National Academy of Sciences • National Academy of Engineering • Institute of Medicine • National Research Council

Visit our web site at

www.nap.edu

THE NATIONAL ACADEMIES
Advisers to the Nation on Science, Engineering, and Medicine

Use the form on the reverse of this card to order additional copies, or order online and receive a 10% discount.

ORDER CARD
(Customers in North America Only)

Saving Women's Lives: Strategies for Improving Breast Cancer Detection and Diagnosis

Use this card to order additional copies of **Saving Women's Lives: Strategies for Improving Breast Cancer Detection and Diagnosis.** All orders must be prepaid. Please add $4.50 for shipping and handling for the first copy ordered and $0.95 for each additional copy. If you live in CA, DC, FL, MD, MO, TX, or Canada, add applicable sales tax or GST. Prices apply only in the United States, Canada, and Mexico and are subject to change without notice.

___ I am enclosing a U.S. check or money order.

___ Please charge my VISA/MasterCard/American Express account.

Number: _____

Expiration date: _____

Signature: _____

FOUR EASY WAYS TO ORDER

- **Electronically:** Order from our secure website at: www.nap.edu
- **By phone:** Call toll-free 1-888-624-8422 or (202) 334-3313 or call your favorite bookstore.
- **By fax:** Copy the order card and fax to (202) 334-2451.
- **By mail:** Return this card with your payment to NATIONAL ACADEMIES PRESS, 500 Fifth Street NW, Washington, DC 20001.

All international customers please contact National Academies Press for export prices and ordering information.

PLEASE SEND ME:

Qty.	Code	Title	Price
___	SAVWOM	Saving Lives, Buying Time	$47.95

Subtotal	_____
Shipping	_____
Tax	_____
Total	_____

Please print.

Name _____

Address _____

City _____ State ____ Zip Code _____

9213

of diagnostic and treatment facilities and to the effectiveness of the different health care systems.[102] The frequency with which different breast cancer treatments were used, such as the frequency of axillary node dissection, breast-conserving surgery, and the modified radical Halstead mastectomy, varied two- to three-fold among countries.[100] Although the relative contributions of earlier detection and state-of-the-art therapy are difficult to quantify, a recent study concluded that early detection through screening had probably contributed more to the reduction of mortality rates than had improvements in therapy.[115] The study, which was conducted in Sweden, compared the results of women who participated in screening with those who did not. Cancers detected in the women who participated in screening were detected at an earlier stage and were less likely to have invaded the lymph nodes, which gained them a prognostic advantage over women whose cancer was not screen-detected but was presumably detected through physical exam or development of symptoms.

There is substantial variation between countries, as well as within the United States, in the frequency that mammograms are identified as abnormal (Figure 3-1). A review of 32 studies showed that the screening programs with high rates of abnormal mammograms also tended to be those with lower positive predictive values for biopsies, suggesting that many of those biopsies could have been safely avoided.[36]

The data collected in the screening studies reviewed do not permit determination of the underlying causes of the variation in the percentage of mammograms that are judged to be abnormal and the predictive value of biopsies. Possible sources of variation include:

- Characteristics of the population that was screened, including the age distribution, and the proportion of women being screened for the first time (prevalence screens) versus those who have been screened before (incidence screens).
- Features of the mammography examinations (such as screening interval, number of views per breast, use of single versus double readings, and availability of prior films for comparison).
- Features of physicians interpreting the mammogram (such as experience or comfort with ambiguity).
- Features of the health care system (such as malpractice concerns, financial incentives, or national policies).

Finally, although this review emphasizes international variation, the considerable variation in performance within the United States is also worth noting, suggesting that international differences such as universal access to health care, more centralized health care systems, and high cost of malpractice litigation account for only part of the differences in screening program

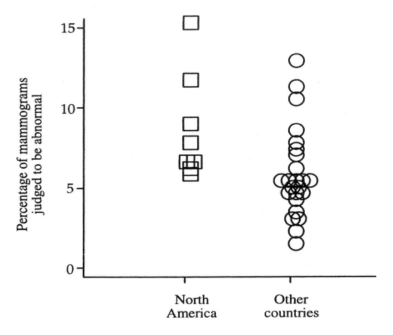

FIGURE 3-1 Frequency of abnormal mammograms in North America compared to other countries. These data are based on a review of 32 screening mammography studies.[36] With the exception of one point that indicates a study from British Columbia, Canada, all points listed for North America are from studies conducted in the United States.

performance. Although on average there are fewer "excess" biopsies in European screening programs than in the United States (at least those programs that were reviewed in the study, which was conducted in the late 1980s and 1990s), there are also European programs that appear to be worse, at least by this measure.

In 1988, the United Kingdom had the highest breast cancer mortality rate in Europe. That same year, the national breast screening program was established, and it is now one of the most well-established, well-analyzed, and extensive screening programs in the world. Since then, the United Kingdom has had the greatest reduction in breast cancer mortality for Europe.[19]

There are several important differences in the delivery of breast screening services in the United States and other countries (Table 3-2). The main programmatic differences between the United States and Britain are:

• All women in Britain receive invitations for screening mammograms at regular intervals, whereas the large majority of women in the United States are referred by a health care provider or by themselves.

- The British National Health Service pays for all screening mammograms in the United Kingdom, whereas mammograms in the United States are covered through a complex patchwork of medical payment systems that exclude millions of women.
- The volume of mammographic interpretations required of radiologists to be eligible to read mammograms in the United States is about one-tenth that required in Britain.
- The recommended interval for screening mammography is 12 months in the United States and 36 months in Britain.
- Quality assurance standards concerning mammographic interpretation for the National Health Service Breast Screening Program are set nationally and are regularly monitored through a quality assurance network.

Although the threat of malpractice is frequently cited as an important reason for the difference in screening practices between the two countries, this is part of the larger context of the health care and can not be regulated through breast cancer screening programs. (Problems of malpractice in the United States are discussed later in this chapter in the section Breast Imagers Needed.)

Table 3-2 summarizes the different outcomes of the breast screening programs in the United States and Britain. The results in Table 3-2 are only valid for comparison within the same study which directly compares the two countries because of the similar methodology used in collecting the data; other studies with different methodology may result in different statistics. Overall, women in the United States are called back after screening mammograms about twice as often as women in Britain and significantly more of the surgical biopsies they undergo turn out to be negative. But this does not translate into improved rates of cancer detection, which are not significantly different between the countries. It could be argued that women in the United States are excessively subjected to unnecessary medical procedures.

Yet, the fact that breast cancer mortality rates in the United States are lower than they are in Britain must be considered. Although differences in treatment quality cannot be ruled out, there is a more immediate reason to expect higher breast cancer mortality in Britain. Breast cancers are detected at a later stage in Britain, and stage of detection is well established as a factor in survival. The three-fold difference in screening intervals between Britain and the United States is highly likely to be a significant contributor to the differences in mortality between the two countries. Longer screening intervals are associated with more false positives, as well as in increase in

TABLE 3-2 Comparison of Screening Mammography Outcomes in the United States and Britain

	United States	Britain	Source	Comments
Sensitivity	77% (>300/month) 70% (≤300/month)	79% (>300/month)	Esserman et al., 2002 JNCI[i]	Used enriched test set; U.S. figures are for high-volume radiologists
Specificity	88% (>300/month)	88%		Volume was not significantly correlated with specificity for any of the groups.
Mammograms judged to be abnormal at 1st screen	12.0%	7.4%	Smith-Bindman, 2003 JAMA	U.S. value = median of estimates from two data sets (11.2-13.1)
Mammograms judged to be abnormal at later screens	7.4%	3.6%		U.S. value = median of estimates from two data sets (6.8-8.0)
Mammograms judged to be abnormal	6.9%	4.9%	Elmore et al., 2003 JNCI	Values are medians of estimates for three or more studies; included both 1st and subsequent screening mammograms
Women with abnormal mammograms later diagnosed with breast cancer	7.6%	12.3%		Values are medians of estimates for three or more studies
Negative biopsies	73%	40%		Included all types of biopsy
Biopsy rates/100 screening mammograms for later screens	0.33	0.28	Smith-Bindman, 2003 JAMA	Differences are *not* significant

Negative open surgical biopsies at 1st screen	82%	36%	
% Negative open surgical biopsies at later screen	22%	10%	
% Cancers detected	78.6% (>300/month) 70% (≤300/month)	83.5%	Esserman et al., 2002
# Cancers detected at 1st screen/1,000	6.8	8.4	Smith-Bindman, 2003 *JAMA*; Median of estimates from two data sets (6.3-7.2)
# Cancers detected at later screens/1,000	2.6	4.3	U.S. value = Median of estimates from two data sets (2.3-2.8)
% Invasive cancers detected at early stage (T1N0M0)	41%	26%	Sant, 2003 *Int J Cancer*; Sant, 2004 *Int J Cancer*; U.S. data from SEER; UK based on median of two counties (18-34%); for cases diagnosed in 1990s
Five-year survival rate for invasive breast cancers	89%	78%	U.S. data from SEER; U.K. data based on median of two counties (73-83%) for cases diagnosed in 1990s
Mortality rate for all breast cancers/100,000	21.2	26.8	Cancer Facts & Figures 2003, ACS

[1]This reference is from a specific study examining a relatively small group of radiologists that interpreted a specific set of mammograms; therefore, these figures are for internal comparison only and cannot be appropriately compared to the sensitivity and specificity of population-based studies.

the frequency of late-stage cancers. Although there are many aspects of the British national screening program that should be considered for adoption in the United States, the 3-year screening interval is not one of them. Mammography services in both Sweden and several Canadian provinces also have high performance standards, but there are fewer published data and direct comparisons with services in the United States, so they are not reviewed here. The British Health Service monitors and tracks the outcomes of their breast cancer screening programs more thoroughly than do other countries.[74]

QUALITY ASSURANCE IMPROVES OUTCOMES

The National Health Service Breast Screening Programme (NHSBSP) in the United Kingdom has integrated quality assurance into all clinical aspects of its programs (Box 3-1).[107] Ranges of acceptable performance for

---

BOX 3-1
Quality Assurance for Breast Screening in the United Kingdom

The United Kingdom is divided into 11 National Health Service regions, each of which is supported by a quality assurance reference center that collects and collates data about the performance and outcomes of the breast screening program, organizes quality assurance visits, and provides support for the regional director of quality assurance and the professional coordinators.

Each region has a quality assurance director for breast screening and a quality assurance reference center. Each regional quality assurance director is supported by a regional quality assurance team, which includes a professional coordinator from each of the professions that contribute to the breast screening program (radiology, radiography, pathology, surgery, breast care nursing, administration, and medical physics). Each professional coordinator meets regularly with colleagues in the region to review the performance and outcomes of the breast screening program, to share good practice, and to encourage continued improvements in the program. There is also a program of regular quality assurance visits to breast screening units.

Regional quality assurance directors and professional coordinators meet regularly in a series of national coordinating committees. The committees produce guidance on good practice and set standards and targets for staff working in the breast screening program and for the technical performance of equipment. National standards and targets for the performance and outcomes of the program are also published.

SOURCE: See http://www.cancerscreening.nhs.uk/breastscreen/quality-assurance.html. Accessed March 4, 2004.

BOX 3-2
PERFORMS: A Self-Assessment Program to
Improve Performance

PERFORMS (PERsonal perFORmance in Mammographic Screening) is an integral part of quality assurance for breast cancer screening in the United Kingdom. It is a self-assessment program for mammogram interpretation, developed in 1991 and funded by the NHSBSP. As of 2003, it is the only system of its kind in the world.[89]

The PERFORMS program film set is released early each year. It contains 2 film sets, each with 60 two-view cases (mediolateral oblique and cranio-caudal). Up to 90 percent of U.K. radiologists use the PERFORMS system to assess their mammogram interpretation skills.[124]

PERFORMS results indicate the number of malignant cases a radiologist missed in the testing film set and whether they showed any patterns in the types of cases they missed, such as dense mammograms or mammograms with many microcalcifications. Pathology information is also provided where appropriate. Particular film sets allow the individual to see a large number of examples of one particular abnormality and have been shown to improve radiologists' detection of these specific features.[124] Additional advanced training sets are also available that concentrate on the types of cases that the radiologists were most likely to misinterpret. Analysis of the PERFORMS data can provide the participating radiologist with insight into how they perform in comparison with their anonymous colleagues.

In addition, the program also can provide details concerning the specific cases that a radiologist incorrectly recalled for further assessment (false positives) or incorrectly identified as normal (false negative). Targeted training with the cases producing disagreement may achieve a higher level of consensus and reduce clinically important inconsistencies.[10] An individual's results are anonymous and are made available only to the radiologist who takes the test—although, for quality assurance purposes, the results can also be collated to provide anonymous regional or national results.

---

recall, biopsy, and cancer detections rates have been established and an organized program operates at the local and national levels to monitor and achieve these targets. All screening programs in the United Kingdom receive data that enable a comparison of their recall and cancer detection rates with other programs. Both programs and individual radiologists below a minimum standard are subject to quality assurance. In contrast, the United States has only voluntary guidelines and there is no national organization to collect or monitor data to promote high levels of performance. Finally, an organized program of professional development in the United Kingdom specifically provides instruction related to mammography interpretation (Box 3-2). Although, a self-testing program exists in the United States, it is not widely used.

Strategies for skills improvement have been much discussed among breast imagers, advocates, and policymakers. The American College of Radiology (ACR) began offering a self-assessment program called Mammography Interpretive Skills Assessment in 1999, but there is no requirement for radiologists to use this voluntary program, and—as was the case with the voluntary Mammography Accreditation Program that preceded the Mammography Quality Standards Act (MQSA)—many do not use it. (The effectiveness of the ACR self-testing program has not been tested or compared with the PERFORMS program used in the United Kingdom.)

Experience with the MQSA demonstrates that a national quality assurance program could be successful in the United States. The MQSA led to nationwide improvements in the technical quality of mammography and it is reasonable to predict that a quality assurance program could be designed to improve the delivery of mammography services in the United States. This would include, but not be limited to, efforts to improve the quality of mammographic interpretation. Organization of services that are integrated and efficient—possibly through regionalization of certain tasks—are equally important and are discussed further in Chapter 7.

However, the MQSA is not without its critics. Even though there is little debate that the technical quality of mammography and consistency among practices has improved since its inception, compliance with MQSA regulations imposes a heavy tax on mammography facilities. In fact, the reauthorization of the MQSA in February 2004 included a mandates for the Institute of Medicine (IOM) to study ways that the MQSA could be improved both to improve the quality of mammographic interpretation and to ensure an adequate workforce.

Adopting Best Practices from Other Countries Can Save Lives

Mammographic screening services in the United States are typically separated from treatment, counseling, and other support services. Screening is poorly integrated into routine health care and tends to be more opportunistic than organized.[108] In contrast, the European Code Against Cancer stresses that breast screening should be organized as part of integrated breast care centers.[18]

Another option, which has been shown to reduce the frequency of false positives, is to mandate second opinions by experts before biopsy is performed.[81] Screening could take place in outlying centers with diagnosis and workup in centralized facilities. The Netherlands and Sweden have organized their service in this way, and they have thereby achieved very low rates of false positives.

Many features of European screening programs, if adopted in the United States, could improve screening. These features include invitations to screening, double reading of mammograms, and the organization of services in centralized high-volume facilities. Such services would include centralized facilities for interpreting mammograms and other screening data, whether it would be ultrasound, magnetic resonance imaging (MRI), or other new technologies once they are developed and validated. Centralization should not, however, involve reducing access to screening services. Consolidation of interpretation facilities does not need to coincide with consolidation of facilities that women attend for mammograms. In cases where traveling long distances might limit attendance at screening facilities, image acquisition and image interpretation could be conducted at separate locations.

Callback rates in mammography screening can be reduced when mammograms are read by breast imaging specialists at a central location, as opposed to having them dispersed among the sites where the mammography is done. By centralizing the reading, the mammography service reduced the overall callback rate by 2 percent, from 11 to 9 percent, which was statistically significant.[76]

On the other hand, the quality of a breast cancer screening program cannot be measured solely by the recall rate or the cancer detection rate, although these are important considerations. It is the rate of detection of small early stage, node-negative tumors that provides the greatest opportunity to save lives. Larger tumors are less often confused with normal breast structures and are less likely to be missed or to be false positives, and thus fewer women undergo unnecessary follow-up. [109]

Improving Screening Practices Can Reduce Health Care Costs

Aggregate costs of screening mammography in the United States are more than $3 billion, and cost savings in screening practices could have a significant impact.[22] The average cost of a diagnostic workup following a false-positive mammogram is about $500 per case.[29] About 40 million women in the United States are screened each year for breast cancer, which means that if the percentage of mammograms judged to be abnormal were reduced from 10 to 5 percent, 200,000 fewer women would be called back for follow-up work every year, which would translate into an annual savings of $100 million.

Equal Access Is a Component of Quality

In addition to considering how mammography should be organized to deliver optimal quality, it is essential to optimize access to services. Because access to health care in the United States is so uneven, it is important to consider not only the internal organization of a screening service, but also how well it accommodates the financial, cultural, and educational situations of those it needs to serve.

Breast cancer mortality rates in the United States vary by race and ethnicity, and the gap between white and African American women is striking (Figure 3-2). Although the incidence of breast cancer among white females is higher than among other racial or ethnic groups, African-American women—particularly those older than age 64—have the highest risk for mortality from breast cancer.[99] (The racial and ethnic categories included in this database were white, African American, Asian/Pacific Islander, American Indian/Alaskan Native, and Hispanic.) Similarly, 88 percent of white women survive at least 5 years after diagnosis, as compared with 73 percent of African-American women. Stage-specific survival rates do not differ significantly between the two groups.[28]

Group disparities in mammography rates may result from a broad combination of socioeconomic and cultural influences. Low socioeconomic status is characterized by low income, higher rates of poverty, lower levels of education, lack of private health insurance, lack of transportation, and lack of access to health care. Together, these factors are associated with lower rates of cancer screening, higher probability for later stage diagnosis, lack of breast health awareness, and mistrust and misunderstanding of the health care system.[28,60,61,71,91,95] Higher poverty rates among African Americans are reflected in disproportionate numbers of women lacking adequate insurance, or any insurance at all.[47,90] Insurance coverage is a significant predictor of whether or not a woman will receive a mammogram.[57] Uninsured women and women with Medicaid are more likely to receive a breast cancer diagnosis at a late stage of disease, and are 30 to 50 percent more likely to die of their disease than women with private insurance.[57]

Yet when white, African-American, and Hispanic women were provided equal access to high-quality mammographic screening, all groups had similar rates of breast cancer survival regardless of age, stage of diagnosis, and socioeconomic status.[123] These circumstances are, however, far from typical (Figure 3-3).

Social factors that restrict access to health care appear to contribute to racial and ethnic differences in breast cancer mortality. Biology may also play a role; even among women who have equal access to health care, fewer African Americans than whites are diagnosed with early stage breast disease, and more African Americans are diagnosed with advanced stage cancer.[123] The peak age for incidence of breast cancer among African American women is 40 to 49, while among white women it is 50 to 59.[90,91] The incidence of estrogen receptor-negative and progesterone receptor-negative tumors, which tend to be aggressive, is also significantly higher among African American women than among whites.[61,77,90]

Social injustice, in the form of social or institutional discrimination, can

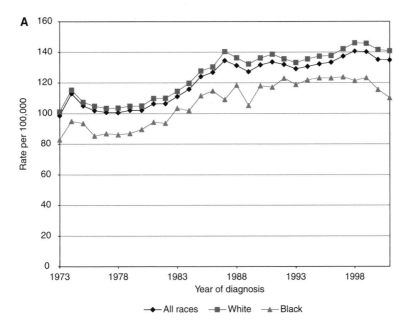

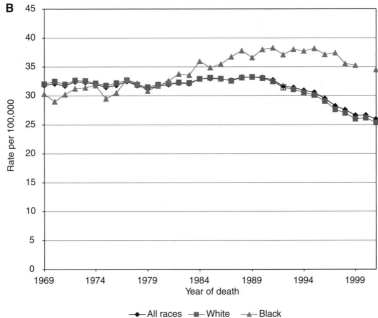

FIGURE 3-2 Breast cancer incidence (A) and mortality (B) in white and black women.[114] Statistics were generated from malignant cases only.

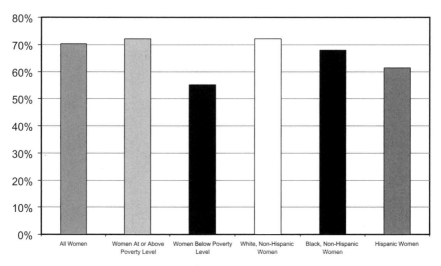

FIGURE 3-3 Poverty is a greater barrier to mammography than race or ethnicity.
SOURCE: National Center for Health Statistics, 2003.

frustrate screening attempts and create barriers for women seeking preventive screenings.[45,50] African American women may also face cultural barriers to obtaining a mammogram, including false beliefs about cancer, traditions that discourage seeking medical care, and difficulties in communicating with their physicians.[8,58,61,72,82,83]

A number of programs have been initiated since 1990 to reduce the financial barriers to mammography rates in all groups. In 1991, Medicare began to cover part of the cost of screening mammograms, but screening rates failed to increase. In 1998, the co-payment and deductibles for the Medicare screening services were eliminated. All women aged 65 and older are eligible for Medicare and 94 percent of them choose the option. Yet, as noted earlier, these are the African-American women who suffer the greatest racial disparity in breast cancer mortality, suggesting that the lack of health insurance is not the predominant cause.

The Centers for Disease Control and Prevention's (CDC's) National Breast and Cervical Cancer Detection Program was launched in 1990 to provide screening services for uninsured women who were not eligible for Medicaid. Since then it has provided nearly 4 million screenings to 1.6 million women. In principle, this program should reduce the disparities in mortality that arise from lack of health insurance, although it has never been funded well enough to cover all, or even most, eligible women. For example, in 2002 approximately 400,000 women received at least one Pap test, mammogram, or clinical breast exam through the CDC program.[26] By comparison, approximately 9 million women between the ages of 40 and 65 lacked health insurance that year. (Women over 65 are eligible for Medicare and so would have little need for this program.)

Community-based programs, such as the North Carolina Breast Cancer Screening Program, also disseminate information about prevention and guide women to mammographic services.[32]

Equal access is a prerequisite for reducing the unequal burden of breast cancer, but other factors that contribute to equal use of health care services are also critical and must be taken into account.

IMPROVING MAMMOGRAPHY

Quality Assurance by Law

Mammography is possibly the most heavily legislated medical procedure in history. Between 1980 and 1994 alone, 43 state laws were passed concerning different aspects of screening for breast cancer.[44] As a rule, state laws regulating mammography have been enacted before federal mammography laws. For example, 33 states had already passed laws supporting treatment and care following the detection of a breast malignancy when a similar federal law, the Breast and Cervical Cancer Prevention and Treatment Act (BCCPTA), was passed in 2000. Currently, more than 10 federal laws specifically address breast cancer screening, including laws governing quality and access (Box 3-3).

When Congress enacted the Medicare program as part of the Social Security Amendments in 1965, preventive services were explicitly excluded. (Although breast screening does not prevent the occurrence of breast cancer, it is considered *secondary prevention* because early detection can prevent deaths from breast cancer and, thus, mammography is considered a preventive service.) Since 1965, many preventive services have been added, but each addition requires a specific Act of Congress. Not every benefit recommended by experts has been added, and some have been added that were not recommended (such as bone density and prostate serum antigen [PSA] screening). Mammography benefits were initially included in the Medicare Catastrophic Act of 1988, which was repealed the following year, but subsequently included in the 1990 Budget Reconciliation Act. Women's health and breast cancer advocacy groups were instrumental in the inclusion of mammography benefits.[43]

A Sweeping Act for Technical Quality

The MQSA was enacted in 1992 to ensure that all women have access to quality mammography for the detection of breast cancer in its earliest,

BOX 3-3
Breast Cancer Legislation

2003 Reauthorization of MQSA

Legislation reauthorized for two years awaiting the findings of two Congressionally mandated reports. The first by the General Accounting Office to assess the States as Certifiers program and mammography access issues. The second by the Institute of Medicine on ways to improve physician recruitment, mammography interpretation, and mammography services.

2003 Medicare Prescription Drug and Modernization Act

Created a prescription drug benefit for Medicare beneficiaries. The legislation also increased payments for mammography and provided an additional $10 million in funding for the National Breast and Cervical Cancer Early Detection Program, bringing the total to $220 million. The program is intended to provide 32,000 diagnostic and screening services to additional women who are hard to reach and have never been screened for these cancers.

2001 Native American Breast and Cervical Cancer Treatment Technical Amendment Act

Amended Title XIX of the Social Security Act to clarify that Indian women with breast or cervical cancer who are eligible for health services provided under a medical care program of the Indian Health Service or of a tribal organization are included in the optional Medicaid eligibility category of breast or cervical cancer patients added by the BCCPTA of 2000.

2000 BCCPTA

Gave States the option of providing medical assistance (Medicaid) for breast and cervical cancer-related treatment services to certain low-income women without creditable coverage who have already been screened for such cancers under the CDC breast and cervical cancer early detection program, and who need treatment.

1998 Reauthorization of MQSA

- Required a summary of the written report concerning a mammogram to be provided directly to the patient in terms easily understood by a lay person.
- Empowered the Secretary to require a facility to notify patients who received mammograms inconsistent with standards so as to present a significant risk to the individual or public health.

1997 Veterans' Benefits Act

Directed the Under Secretary for Health to develop a national policy for the Veterans Health Administration on mammography screening for veterans.

1997 Stamp Out Breast Cancer Act

Authorized the U.S. Postal Service to issue a first-class breast cancer stamp. Seventy percent of the net amount raised is given to the National Institutes of Health and 30 percent is given to the Breast Cancer Research Program at the Department of Defense.

1993 Preventive Health Amendments

Revised and authorized FY94-FY98 appropriations for a CDC program providing grants to states for breast and cervical cancer prevention programs, including mammography and Pap smear screening services.

1992 Indian Health Amendments

- Amended the Indian Health Care Improvement Act to authorize appropriations for Indian health programs, and for other purposes
- Provided for screening mammography for rural and urban American Indian women.

1992 MQSA

- To amend the Public Health Service Act to establish the authority for the regulation of mammography services and radiological equipment, and for other purposes.
- Required Department of Health and Human Services (HHS) certification of facilities providing mammography services.
- Authorized HHS to approve state agencies or private nonprofit organizations as mammography facility accreditation bodies.
- Directed HHS to develop and enforce quality standards for mammography facilities, equipment, and medical personnel.
- Mandated annual HHS or state inspections of mammography facilities.
- Provided for civil penalties, or suspension or revocation of a certificate, for certain violations by mammography facilities.
- Authorized HHS grants for research on the effectiveness of breast cancer screening programs.

1990 Omnibus Budget Reconciliation Act

Reauthorized Medicare payment and certification standards for screening mammography for women.

1990 Breast and Cervical Cancer Mortality Prevention Act

Authorized FY91-FY93 appropriations for HHS grants to states for breast and cervical cancer screening, medical treatment referrals, and information development and dissemination; training of health professionals in breast and cervical cancer prevention and control; and mammography and cytological procedure quality assurance activities.

1988 Medicare Catastrophic Coverage Act

Established Medicare payment and certification standards for screening mammography for women (repealed in 1989).

BOX 3-4
Bodies Approved to Certify and Accredit the Quality of Mammography Facilities

Certification Bodies
(issue approval to provide mammography services)

- Food and Drug Administration (FDA)
- State of Illinois
- State of Iowa

Accreditation Bodies
(review quality of mammography facility)

- American College of Radiology (ACR)
- Arkansas Department of Health
- Iowa Department of Health
- Texas Department of Health

Any state can apply to the FDA to become a mammography certification body and any state or nonprofit organization can apply to become an accreditation body; however, as of June 2004, only those listed above are currently approved by the FDA. In May of 2004 the State of California voluntarily withdrew its application seeking status as a mammography facility accreditation body. Most states have relied upon the ACR to set standards for mammography facilities.

---

most treatable stages by establishing baseline quality standards for facilities performing mammography.[118] It is the single most sweeping legislation affecting the early detection of breast cancer. The MQSA is responsible for the stringent set of regulations that govern clinical image quality, equipment, medical records, consumer complaint mechanisms, and personnel qualifications. As a result, mammography is unique among radiologic procedures for the requirements that outline every aspect of daily practice.

The initial push for MQSA legislation was sparked by public concern about the inconsistent quality of mammography and was spearheaded in a national effort led by women's health organizations and breast cancer advocates. It was shepherded through the legislative process by Senator Barbara Mikulski.

The MQSA includes requirements that breast imaging facilities performing mammography must be certified by the Secretary of Health and Human Services and be accredited by an approved body (see Box 3-4). The basic requirements that breast imaging facilities must meet for accreditation are established by the law which, in turn, directs the Food and Drug Administration (FDA) to set the standards for accreditation and to oversee enforcement of the MQSA.

In 1998, the first reauthorization of the MQSA added the requirement that women receive direct notification of their mammography results. Another reauthorization of the MQSA was passed by the Senate for reauthorization in February 2004, but to date the House has taken no action. Senate sponsors predict a major reauthorization of the MQSA in 2005. In the meantime, the Consolidated Appropriations Act for FY 2004, which was passed in January 2003 (Pub. L. No. 108-199), included a mandate for studies to be conducted by the U.S. General Accounting Office (GAO) and the IOM on how to further improve mammography quality and make appropriate adjustments to the MQSA. Included is a request for those studies to be completed in time for Congress to consider the studies' results in the debate in the spring of 2005 for the MQSA reauthorization.

For the most part, the MQSA regulations are based on standards established by the ACR Mammography Accreditation Program. That program was set up as a voluntary means of technical quality improvement, and only about half of the mammography screening facilities participated. The ACR lacked the funds to conduct on-site visits and the legal authority to enforce compliance among imaging facilities.

After the federal enforcement of quality standards, the percentage of facilities with acceptable image quality increased significantly and site-to-site variations in radiation doses decreased.[16] Along with the positive results of the legislation, considerable costs are associated with adherence to the standards. These costs include staff time, inspection fees, and the maintenance of paperwork for performance documentation.

The MQSA regulations set standards primarily for the technical quality of mammography, whereas quality standards for the interpretation of mammography are almost nonexistent. The only regulation relating to quality of interpretation requires that physicians who interpret mammograms must interpret a minimum of 960 mammograms every two years, an average of 480 per year (see following discussion under Variation in Mammographic Interpretation).

The MQSA requires every mammographic facility to keep track of all positive mammograms (BI-RADS® 4 and 5; Box 3-5), including follow-up correlation of pathology results with the interpreting physician's mammography report. Facilities are audited every year to be sure the data have been collected and that each radiologist has seen his or her own results, but there is no further requirement for the use of the data, such as for skills improvement.

BOX 3-5
ACR BI-RADS®: Breast Imaging Reporting and Data System

BI-RADS® was introduced by the ACR to provide a uniform system of assessing mammography results. Besides the categories shown in this box, BI-RADS® includes a detailed lexicon for standardized descriptions of lesions and other breast abnormalities. It is intended to guide radiologists and referring physicians in a decision-making process that facilitates the management of patients based on breast imaging.

BI-RADS® is a useful and widely used tool for standardizing the interpretation of mammograms and for quantitative analysis. However, a serious limitation of quantitative analysis based on BI-RADS® is that the 6-point scale is not continuous and does not provide enough gradations of positive mammograms. It is also important to note that there inevitably will be some variability in how different readers assign mammograms to different categories. Although invaluable in communicating and quantifying results, it has not yet been demonstrated that use of BI-RADS® reduces variability among radiologists (reviewed by Elmore and colleagues, 2002).[27,35]

BI-RADS® system for standardization of mammogram interpretation and reporting. (Fourth Edition, 2003)

BI-RADS® Category	Assessment	Recommendations
0	Incomplete	Other mammographic views and techniques or ultrasound needed
1	Negative, no findings	Routine screening
2	Benign finding	Routine screening
3	Probably benign abnormality	Short-term follow-up to establish stability
4	Suspicious abnormality	Biopsy should be considered
5	Highly suggestive of malignancy malignancy	Appropriate action should be taken
6	Known biopsy-proven malignancy	Appropriate action should be taken

Variation in Mammographic Interpretation

Mammograms consist of shadowy outlines of fat and soft tissue in varying shades of gray. Interpreting them requires skill and experience, and, as for every type of imaging test, different radiologists may interpret the same mammograms differently. Many factors influence the accuracy of individual radiologists in recognizing clinically important abnormalities during screening mammography, but many other factors influence the consistency of mammographic interpretation (reviewed by Beam, Elmore, Sickles, and colleagues [7,15,35,41,105]).

The accuracy of radiologists in interpreting mammograms depends on many factors, including case variation, practice variation, training and experience, and the type of screening program in which they practice. Box 3-4 summarizes those factors that have been reported in the peer-reviewed literature to be correlated with the interpretation of screening mammograms. It is important to keep in mind that estimates of performance are different for screening and diagnostic mammography. In screening, the central decision is whether or not to conduct additional workup (i.e., the callback decision). The goal of screening mammography is not to provide a definitive diagnosis or to recommend biopsy without further consideration. A true positive in screening occurs whenever a woman with breast cancer is given a recommendation for additional workups, whereas a true positive in diagnosis would be whenever breast cancer is detected.

Case Variation Influences Performance Measures

Individual characteristics such as breast density or history of breast cancer are known to increase the likelihood of both false-positive and false-negative results (Table 3-3).[8,24,27] In addition, ambiguous mammograms such as those revealing possible microcalcifications—which are often difficult to interpret—increase the likelihood of disagreement among radiologists. A mammography practice that serves younger women is likely to have an overall lower sensitivity rating than an otherwise identical practice that serves older women. This is reflected in the observation by Beam and his colleagues that case-related differences accounted for more variation than individual differences among radiologists.[10] For example, mammographic sensitivity increases with a woman's age (Figure 3-4).

Also, approximately twice as many breast cancers are detected at first screens as compared to subsequent screens. This is because a cancer detected at a subsequent screen generally would have developed to the point where it can be seen on a mammogram only since the previous screen, whereas a cancer detected at a woman's first screen could have been present for years. The result is not only a higher rate of cancers detected at first

TABLE 3-3 Factors That Affect the Quality of Screening Mammography

Primary Source of Variation	Underlying Sources of Variation
Case Variation	
Breast density	Breasts that are mammographically dense are associated with more false positives and false negatives[42,65]
	• Hormone replacement therapy generally increases breast density.
	• Menopause generally lowers breast density.
	• Overweight women usually have less dense breasts.
	• Breast density usually decreases with age.
Breast cancer history	Family history of breast cancer[63]
	Previous biopsy
Practice Variation	
Individual radiologists	Subspecialty training in breast imaging
	Volume of mammograms read (but see text)
	Years since training
Organization of mammography services	• High volume centers tend to have higher accuracy, above and beyond the increase attributable to reading volume of individual radiologists
	• Number of diagnostic exams performed
	• Number of image-guided breast interventional procedures (biopsies?) performed
	Double-reading of mammograms by two radiologists improves accuracy[51]
	Use of computer-assisted detection (CAD) by nonspecialists (but see text)
	Center designated as breast diagnostic and/or screening center or freestanding mammography center
	Availability of prior mammograms for comparison increases specificity
Health care cystem	False-positive rates have increased over time in the United States and are higher than in other countries.

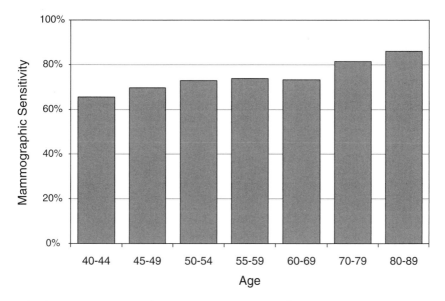

FIGURE 3-4 Mammographic sensitivity increases with a woman's age.

screens, but a higher percentage of abnormal mammograms, biopsies, and false-positive findings. Therefore—if judged by rates of false positives—the apparent performance of a mammography service or individual radiologist would be influenced by the proportion of how many women are receiving their first mammogram.

Performance and Volume

A relationship between the volume of procedures performed and the outcome of those procedures has been established for many complex medical procedures, particularly in surgery and oncology.[55] Many studies have suggested that the volume of mammograms read by a radiologist is correlated with accuracy, and mammography volume standards are mandated by federal law. However, relatively few studies have directly compared the number of mammograms read by a radiologist and the accuracy of their interpretations. The results of these are variable, and are shown in Table 3-4. The most comprehensive study to date was the analysis by Beam and his colleagues in 2003,[12] which indicated that the volume of mammograms interpreted by a radiologist accounts for less than 2.5 percent of the variation. This means that more than 97 percent of inconsistency in interpretation is due to *other* factors.

TABLE 3-4 Relationship Between Volume of Mammograms Read and Accuracy of Interpretation Is Inconsistent

Comparison Groups (Average numbers of mammograms read per year for comparison groups)	Outcome Measured	Results
Volume does not affect performance.		
U.S. radiologists (n = 110)	Analyzed on the basis of the total number of mammograms read in the past year (average number = 1,900; range =1-12,000)	The number of mammograms read in the past year was not significantly associated with interpretive accuracy[11]
High-volume readers perform better.		
U.S. radiologists (n = 59) < 1201 1201-3600 > 3600	Accuracy at reading PERFORMS2, which is a teaching set of mammograms enriched for cancer cases	High-volume readers perform better Average sensitivity was equal for both low and medium volume groups (70%), but higher for the high volume group (77%)** [37]
High-volume readers do not perform better.		
Canadian radiologists with >3 years experience (n = 35) < 2,000 2,000-2,999 3,000-3,999 4,000-5,199	Percent of screening mammograms interpreted as abnormal and cancer detection rate*	The midvolume readers (2,000-3,999) detect fewer abnormal mammograms than the low- and high-volume groups. No significant difference in detection rates[61]

* This figure includes both true positives and false positives, but because the great majority of women screened do not have breast cancer, the percent of mammograms judged to be abnormal will depend more on the false-positive rate than on the true-positive rate.

** This reference is from a single study examining a group of radiologists that interpreted a common set of mammograms. Therefore, these sensitivity values should be compared only within this study and do not necessarily apply to population-based studies.

The volume of mammograms read by individual breast imagers is likely to be important—if not directly, perhaps as a proxy for other characteristics such as advanced training, specialization in breast imaging, or working in an organization with a mammography quality improvement program.

Specialists Are More Accurate Than Generalists

One study reported that compared to general radiologists, breast imaging specialists detect more cancers, recommend more biopsies, and have lower recall rates. In general, the specialists, who interpreted more than 5,000 mammograms per year, found two to three more cancers than general radiologists for every 1,000 mammograms.[11]

However, only 12 percent of radiologists interpreting mammograms are specialists,[23] and most women do not see specialists. The false positive rates of community radiologists (those who work outside academic research centers) are quite variable. One study reported rates of false positives that ranged from 3 to 16 percent.[35]

Error Rates Depend on Context and Organizational Factors

Accuracy depends on context. Rates of false positives in the United States have increased over the years, and they vary among countries and health care systems. Defensive medicine is widely presumed to be prevalent in the United States, especially in mammography. Leonard Berlin testified on behalf of the ACR in Congress that malpractice suits in the United States are decided in favor of plaintiffs so often that many radiologists do not attempt to contest even seemingly frivolous cases.[14]

Rates of false positives in the Unites States nearly doubled from 1985 to 1993, from roughly 5 to 10 percent.[35] This increase parallels the steadily increasing rates of malpractice suits related to failures to detect breast cancer through mammography, which is often proposed as a driving force in rates of false positives. Radiologists in the United States may be practicing more defensive medicine because they fear malpractice suits, which their counterparts in the United Kingdom face to a much lesser degree.[34] Although British radiologists also report that they worry about malpractice, the scope of the problem is considerably less than it is in the United States. Only about 25 percent of British practices admitted to being sued over breast cancer, with nearly all cases being dropped.[89] Many believe that concern over malpractice is an important factor in the relatively high rate of false-positive results in the United States, and anecdotal evidence supports this view. However, there are no reliable data to measure the extent of this problem, and such sensitive data would be difficult to obtain.

Options for Improving Mammographic Interpretation

As a rule, health care quality is less often improved by weeding out individual, low-performing "bad apples" than it is by organizational improvements. Health care depends more on the development of organizational structures and processes that support high-quality performance and that have built-in systems for continuous improvement and feedback about performance.[54] The various options that have been proposed for improving the quality of mammographic interpretation in the United States are discussed below. They include increasing the required volume of mammograms, restricting the number of radiologists permitted to interpret mammograms, greater standardization of assessment categories, public reporting of performance, and better training for radiologists in mammographic interpretation.

Increase Volume Requirements

The MQSA standards for the minimum number of mammograms to be interpreted by certified radiologists are lower in the United States than for other countries with breast screening programs (Table 3-5). When the MQSA standards for mammography volume were established, the volume standards were designed to balance the perceived benefits of high volume against the need to avoid discouraging the already limited workforce from interpreting mammograms at all. Beam and his colleagues concluded that a 1 percent increase in accuracy would require 3,000 more mammograms to be read per radiologist per year.[11] The Society of Breast Imaging "strongly disagrees with the implication that American radiologists recommend excessive workups and should be required to read 5,000 mammograms annually, as is required of British radiologists."

TABLE 3-5 Mammography Volume Standards[12]

	Required Number of Mammograms	Average per Month
United States	960 over a 2-year period	40
British Columbia, Canada	2,500 per year	>200
Sweden	No target set, but only specialists interpret mammograms	>1,000
United Kingdom	5,000 per year	>400

Restricting the Number of Radiologists Permitted to Interpret Mammograms

Beam and his colleagues predicted that health policy recommendations based on improving mammographic interpretations based solely on radiologist volume will be "misleading and ineffectual."[11]

Beam and his colleagues estimated the effects of increasing median accuracy by prohibiting low-performing radiologists from interpreting mammograms.[12] They calculated that, to achieve a 5 percent increase in the median accuracy among radiologists, the 2,200 radiologists at the bottom of the performance spectrum would need to be prohibited from interpreting mammograms. This would translate into a reduction in national service capacity of about 25 percent. The net effect of such a policy would be more likely to increase rather than decrease the number of women whose breast cancer escapes early detection. Further reducing a workforce that is already in short supply is deemed not the best option.

Greater Standardization

Use of ACR BI-RADS® could, in principle, lead to less variability among radiologists (see Box 3-5). However, recommendations for BI-RADS® categories have been shown to be applied inconsistently for mammographic abnormalities, suggesting that use of BI-RADS® by itself is not enough to reduce variability in mammography.[116] For most BI-RADS® assessments, community radiologists make consistent recommendations, with an overall concordance of 97 percent. However, agreement is substantially lower when the assessments are "probably benign finding" (BI-RADS®), with a concordance of only 47 percent.[69] This is the assessment most commonly associated with errors of interpretation, as well as malpractice cases. Agreement among radiologists is also lower for mammograms of women with dense breasts.[69]

Public Reporting of Performance

Publicly reporting mammogram interpretation performance results of radiologists has been resisted by radiologists. Quality conclusions based on performance might be misleading in view of differing risks, ages, or other characteristics of caseload among radiologists and facilities that could legitimately lead to differing results, as noted earlier. Although radiologists review nondiscoverable outcomes data for their positive cases on an annual basis, follow-up on negative mammograms is not possible. Also, it is feared that public reporting would provide targets for litigation and major professional and economic disincentives to radiologists entering or remaining in the field of mammography, already a relatively unattractive and risky service with low reimbursement. In the United Kingdom, for example, individual performance results are provided only to the radiologist. Finally, in practice, publicly released health care performance data are rarely used by consumers even when available. In contrast, health care providers do use performance data results to improve the quality of their health care services. Marshall and colleagues reviewed studies on the public disclosure of health care performance data and concluded that[78]

> . . . the use of public performance data by consumers and purchasers or for regulation purposes will remain relatively less important for the foreseeable future than use of the data as a catalyst to stimulate and promote *internal* [italics added] quality improvement mechanisms at the level of the organizational provider.

Better Training

Continuing medical education is required for radiologists in the United States, but the content is not uniformly organized and almost never targets recall or cancer detection rates. There is a view that continuing quality assurance through feedback of results could improve performance. In contrast, the United Kingdom has established a program that is voluntary but is used by more than 90 percent of radiologists who practice mammography.

OTHER TECHNOLOGY OPTIONS

As noted earlier, no breast cancer screening tool has better sensitivity and specificity than screen-film mammography, although it could be better. However, even with similar sensitivity and specificity, there may be ways to improve storage, transmission, cost, ease of use, and other characteristics of mammography that would add value. Certainly, any new technology or refinement should have equal success in accurately detecting abnormalities and an equal or better effect on health outcomes compared to current screening mammography. Reviewed briefly below are some leading technologies that are FDA approved and are being examined for their roles in breast cancer detection and diagnosis. Digital mammography and CAD have been proposed for use in screening of average risk women, whereas MRI is not expected to improve outcomes for average risk women but is being tested for use in certain groups of high-risk women.

Digital Mammography

For more than 10 years, researchers have been developing digital mammography devices in the hope that digitizing radiographic data will improve on conventional imaging methods by allowing the different tasks of image acquisition, processing, and display to be separated and therefore refined, as well as allowing adjunct technologies such as CAD to be used more easily.[59] But despite the introduction of full-field digital mammography units into the market, the question of whether digital actually improves cancer detection rates or workflow remains open.

Digital mammography systems offer better contrast and lower spatial resolution at a lower radiation dose than traditional screen film mammography.[59] The relative diagnostic accuracy of digital mammography compared to traditional mammography is still undergoing study through the large Digital Mammographic Imaging Screening Trial (DMIST). As of this writing, digital mammography appears to improve specificity—possibly due to the flexibility of image display available to the interpreting radiologists.[31] Digital units probably also improve workflow, allowing radiologists to view images in less than a minute, compared to the 8 to 10 minutes required from screen film systems.

Because digital mammography devices are more expensive than conventional devices, they will have to offer substantial advantages over film-screen mammography in order to be widely used. Research to date has not shown a dramatic difference between the two techniques. In a 2001 study, 4,945 women had both conventional and digital screening mammography exams. The conventional mammography device found a few more cancers than the digital unit; both devices missed cancers the other found. Overall, there were no major differences in cancer detection rates between the two techniques, although if the digital technique had been used alone, recall rates would have been lower.[70] Similar results were reported in 2003 from a Norwegian study of 3,683 women.[106] Each woman in the study had both digital and screen film mammography exams and they were independently interpreted. The cancer detection rates for the two imaging modalities were not significantly different, although the recall rate was slightly higher for digital mammography and the positive predictive value based on needle biopsy was slightly higher for screen film mammography.

In 2001, the National Cancer Institute (NCI) and the American College of Radiology Imaging Network (ACRIN) launched the multicenter DMIST study to compare digital mammography with standard mammography for the detection of breast cancer. The 49,520 women enrolled in the study will be followed for one year after receiving both digital and conventional mammograms. For further discussion of ACRIN and DMIST, see Chapter 6.

Computer-Aided Detection

Since 1989, technology developers have conducted experiments on the use of computer capability to aid in reading radiological images. Because using mammography to detect cancer in normal breast tissue is fundamentally a signal-to-noise exercise, it is particularly suited to CAD technology.[30] Because factors such as radiologist fatigue and distraction, the complexity of breast structure, and the subtle characteristics of early stage disease make interpreting mammograms challenging and contribute to both false-positive and false-negative results, the use of CAD with mammography becomes particularly attractive, offering experienced radiologists the option of a "double read."

Basic CAD systems consist of a workstation with display and signal processing software. The CAD unit reads either manually digitized mammography films or directly digitized images and highlights areas of concern such· as masses, calcifications, or architectural distortions, for the radiologist's review. Images can be printed or displayed in soft copy on a monitor. CAD for mammography was formally introduced in 1998 when the FDA approved the first CAD device, ImageChecker M1000®, made by R2 Technology of Sunnyvale, California. In addition to ImageChecker, two other CAD devices cleared for use in the United States: (1) Second Look® by Nashua, New Jersey-based iCAD® and (2) MammoReader® by Intelligent Systems Software of Clearwater, Florida. ImageChecker and Second Look are also approved by the FDA for use with full-field digital mammography devices.

In a 2001 study, radiologists who interpreted mammograms, using both conventional mammography reading techniques as well as CAD technology, found nearly 20 percent more cancers with CAD than they did without, and the proportion of early stage malignancies detected increased from 73 to 77 percent. But they also found that the recall rate increased, from 6.5 percent when the radiologist interpreted the mammogram without CAD to 7.7 percent when CAD was used.[46] This study analyzed only the ImageChecker M1000® system produced by R2 Technology and the results cannot be assumed to apply to every CAD system.

The reproducibility of CAD results has improved as the technology has been advanced. Bin Zheng and colleagues used 100 mammographic cases with four views each from a database of more than 1,000 digitized images and diagnostic results. The cases included 25 with microcalcification clusters and 75 with masses. Two-thirds of the cases had been confirmed malignant. Using ImageChecker®, Zheng scanned the images three times over a period of 3 weeks, checking for sensitivity, false-positive rates, and reproducibility of the results. The researchers found identical results in 213 of 400 images, for a reproducibility rate of 53 percent, an improvement from 38 percent found in a 2000 study based on an earlier version of the CAD system.[125]

The greatest clinical value in CAD probably does not lie in its ability to raise the performance level of *all* breast imagers, but rather in its potential to bring the performance level of general radiologists to that of breast imaging specialists.[88] As noted earlier, the great majority of screening mammography is done by general radiologists who tend to have lower sensitivity rates and higher false-positive rates than breast imaging specialists. In fact, a 2004 study reported that the use of CAD was not associated with statistically significant changes in recall or breast cancer detection rates.[49] However, all radiologists in that study were considered breast imaging specialists, and the results of this study should not be extrapolated to use by community radiologists who vary widely in their proficiency.

An often overlooked challenge in establishing the value of CAD systems is that they are not all the same. There has been a series of peer-reviewed papers documenting the efficacy of the CAD systems produced by R2 Technology, but, to date, there are no peer-reviewed reports on the efficacy of any other commercially available CAD systems for breast imaging. Even for systems that have been analyzed in the peer-reviewed literature, when a manufacturer produces an "upgraded" system, the changes should be assessed in terms of diagnostic accuracy—as opposed to subjective evaluations of clarity of image, or other aspects of image processing that might appeal to the eye but not improve interpretation.

Reimbursement for this technology may be a key factor in the adoption of CAD, helping offset the cost of acquiring the technology and integrating the process into the existing organization of breast care services. The Center for Medicare & Medicaid Services (CMS) provides some support for the adoption of this new technology. In 2003, its reimbursement rate for CAD was $19.13 per exam. Also, in 2002 the agency expanded its coverage to include diagnostic exams and the use of CAD with digital mammography. CAD is treated as an add-on procedure to screening or diagnostic mammography. Ironically, although CAD offers a "second look" at a mammogram and is reimbursed by CMS (although not by all health care insurers and providers), actual double reading done by two radiologists is not reimbursed, even though the practice reportedly increases cancer detection by 5 to 15 percent.[51]

Whether the use of CAD technology affects a center's workflow remains open to debate. In a facility that uses screen-film mammography devices, CAD can slow down workflow because of the extra time needed to digitize films. For many, CAD makes more sense in a digital environment, where the images can go directly from the mammography unit to the CAD device; yet even with direct digital images, image processing can be affected by the different algorithms used for image detection, digitization techniques, and methods of display each CAD system employs.

However, for those who do decide to incorporate CAD into their facility, the technology may provide an additional benefit beyond clinical ones. Because radiologists are the targets of litigation—especially for missed breast cancer diagnoses—more than any other specialist, it may be worth the additional workflow impact or fiscal cost if the use of CAD reduces the likelihood of capricious judgments. If a radiologist and a CAD system both fail to detect an abnormal mammographic finding, then it becomes less likely that the missed cancer can be successfully argued to be due to negligence on the part of the interpreting radiologist.

Magnetic Resonance Imaging (MRI)

[In its current state,] MRI has nothing to do with the average woman undergoing screening for breast cancer. It's a promising technology, but right now it's overreaching to say it's useful for the average woman.[84]

William J. Gradishar, M.D.
Northwestern University

Researchers have been exploring the use of MRI in breast cancer detection for more than 15 years.[104] In 1991, the FDA cleared MRI for use as a diagnostic tool to evaluate breast tissue abnormalities found in other exams—but not as a screening tool. It has been suggested that MRI is useful in a number of clinical indications such as finding small breast lesions that are sometimes missed in mammograms, generating better images of dense or augmented breast tissue, revealing multifocality of breast cancer, and aiding in treatment staging and follow-up.[103] There is also growing agreement in the clinical community that MRI could be a valuable tool in screening protocols for women at higher risk for breast cancer.

Results of the largest prospective, multicenter study of MRI screening to date were presented at the 2003 meeting of the American Society of Clinical Oncology. The study compared the findings of yearly x-ray mammography and MRI breast exams in more than 1,000 women at higher than average breast cancer risk. Over 2 years, 40 breast cancers were found. Sixteen percent of the cancers were identified by clinical exam, 36 percent by mammography exams, and 71 percent by MRI.[67] However, MRI was less specific than mammography (88 versus 95 percent). In another 2003 study, researchers found that, for use as a tool in screening women with breast cancer gene mutations and helping diagnose disease earlier, MRI appeared to be superior to mammography and sonography (ultrasound).[92]

Likewise, mammography is also the primary technique for detecting ductal carcinoma in situ (DCIS). Recent research indicates that contrast-enhanced MRI might help detect otherwise occult foci (such as those that occur in DCIS), or in patients with small or dense breasts for whom mammography can be less reliable (Figure 3-5).[53,121] A gadolinium-based con-

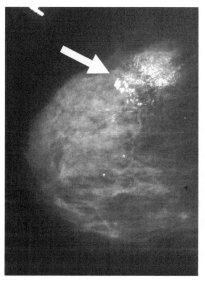
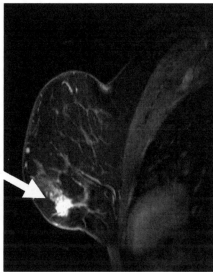

FIGURE 3-5 Examples of MRI and x-ray images of two different cases of DCIS. The case on the left is an x-ray mammogram of a breast showing DCIS in the upper portion of the breast. The case on the right is an MRI mammogram showing DCIS in the lower portion.
SOURCE: X-ray; UHrad.com. Women's Imaging Teaching Files. http://www.uhrad. com/mamarc/mam016.htm [Accessed August 21, 2003]. MRI; Magnetic Resonance Science Center at University of California San Francisco. Breast MRI Website. http://www.mrsc.ucsf.edu/breast/dcis.html [Accessed August 21, 2003].

trast agent is administered intravenously to provide better soft-tissue contrast, and this helps differentiate cancer from benign surrounding tissue. The principle behind contrast-enhanced MRI relies, in part, on the assumption that cancerous lesions will have characteristic features. For example, compared to benign breast lesions, cancerous lesions tend to absorb the contrast agent faster and the gadolinium-based agents are washed out faster.

A prospective study of 51 patients with biopsy-proven DCIS who underwent contrast-enhanced MRI before surgical treatment indicated that contrast-enhanced MRI had significantly higher sensitivities and negative predictive values than mammography in the detection of residual disease, occult invasive cancer, and multicentric DCIS.[53] Although contrast-enhanced MRI was statistically significantly more accurate than mammography for detecting multicentric DCIS, it was significantly less specific than mammography for detecting associated invasive disease.[53]

It is important to keep in mind that results for MRI based on high-risk populations should not be extrapolated to the general screening population, because the positive predictive value of a screening testing depends on the prevalence of the condition being screened. By definition, breast cancer will be more prevalent in high-risk women. In addition, the lower specificity of MRI compared to mammography would translate into a substantially higher rate of false positives. According to Daniel Sullivan, Associate Director for the Cancer Imaging Program at the NCI, determining the value of MRI screening for the general population would require a study of more than 40,000 patients, a minimum of 3 years, and tens of millions of dollars.[84] Unfortunately, the lack of evidence in support of MRI for breast cancer screening and the lack of FDA approval do not necessarily protect the public from misleading marketing (see Box 1-3 in Chapter 1).

The techniques for performing and interpreting breast MRI are not standardized. As a result, breast MRI performance has been variable, and it has been challenging to determine its clinical efficacy. The results of the 5-year International Breast MRI Consortium (Trial #6883), a study funded by the NCI and the National Institutes of Health (NIH) Office on Women's Health, will soon be reported and will be a major step forward in clarifying and optimizing the clinical value of MRI. This multicenter study, conducted at 14 institutions, evaluated the diagnostic performance of breast MRI in women with suspicious mammographic or clinical findings. It is expected to yield definitive results about the diagnostic accuracy of breast MRI and should lead to recommendations for performing and interpreting breast MRI images. In addition, as of early 2004, an ongoing ACRIN trial testing the use of MRI to screen the contralateral, or noncancerous breast, in women with breast cancer is attempting to further define the role of MRI in detecting breast cancer in a high-risk population (Trial #6667).

Ultimately, more research on how MRI performs as a screening modality and exactly how high-risk women would benefit remains to be done.[104] MRI is expensive, about 10 times the cost of conventional mammography, and because it will generate more false-positive results, it will become even more expensive with the added costs of additional biopsies and/or other diagnostic follow-up.

Ultrasound

Also known as sonography, ultrasound gained FDA approval in 1977 as a means to evaluate suspicious mammographic findings (see Appendix A). Ultrasound is especially useful in determining whether such findings depict benign cysts or solid lesions. When rigorous criteria are applied, the accuracy of ultrasound for diagnosing fluid-filled "simple" cysts—which are always benign and therefore require no further evaluation—has been found to be 98 to 100 percent.[64] Ultrasound is also used to investigate palpable abnormalities, of which 20 to 25 percent are simple cysts.[6] It is often used instead of mammography to investigate palpable breast abnormalities in women who are pregnant, to avoid exposing the fetus to x-rays, and in women under age 30, for whom mammography is not as effective due to breast density (see Chapter 2).[80] Unlike mammography, ultrasound is not affected by breast density.

Ultrasound can also determine whether a lesion located near the surface of the breast occurs within the skin, where it is unlikely to be malignant, or in the underlying breast tissue, necessitating further investigation.[80] Because it can reveal various characteristics of suspicious lesions such as the likelihood of invasiveness, and spread within the ducts, ultrasound may in some cases inform the staging of breast cancer.[68,80] Ultrasound can also contribute to attempts to distinguish between benign and malignant solid lesions, but criteria for assessing malignant features have yet to be established and validated in controlled multicenter clinical studies.[6,80]

The combination of screening mammography and ultrasound is highly sensitive for breast cancer in non-symptomatic women. For example, in the largest screening series of bilateral whole-breast ultrasound, which encompassed more than 13,000 examinations in women with dense breasts and previously negative mammograms, a "double screen" of mammography plus ultrasound detected 97 percent of breast cancers; other, smaller studies have produced similar results.[6] As a competing technology, as opposed to a complementary technology, ultrasound falls short of mammography due to its relatively poor sensitivity for microcalcifications, the hallmark of DCIS.[6] When ultrasound depicts microcalcifications, they are usually associated with a mass, and therefore indicative of invasive cancer (reviewed by Mehta, 2003).[80] This raises the possibility that ultrasound actually finds the majority of DCIS that has become invasive[6] (see also Chapter 2).

Some researchers have claimed, and published studies strongly suggest, that ultrasound can detect breast cancers that both mammography and clinical breast exams would miss (reviewed by Kopans, 2004).[66] However, because breast screenings were not conducted independently in any of these studies, their results were potentially biased (for example, by researchers' knowledge of a participant's mammography findings prior to conducting ultrasound).[66] Better information on the potential role of ultrasound in breast cancer screening should be forthcoming from a multicenter clinical trial that is currently being conducted by ACRIN with support from the Avon Foundation (see Chapter 6).[6] The protocol, which includes blinded sonographic screening, aims to compare the sensitivity, specificity, and positive and negative predictive values of ultrasound and mammography combined with that of mammography alone. In order to make obvious any disparities that may exist among mammography, clinical breast examination, and ultrasound, the trial is limited to women with dense breasts who are at high risk for breast cancer.

Because the ACRIN trial will not measure death rates, but will rely on surrogate endpoints such as lesion size, nodal status, and diagnostic yield, it cannot directly determine whether the combination of ultrasound and mammographic screening has any effect on mortality from breast cancer (reviewed in Kopans 2004).[66] Rather, it is intended as a preliminary, best-case scenario of ultrasound screening for breast cancer which, given promising results, would justify broader study.[6] Moreover, even if the efficacy of screening ultrasound were established, several technical and practical limitations could hinder its adoption. Chief among these is the variability of results obtained in current clinical practice.[6,68,80] Ultrasound tends to be more difficult in larger and fatty breasted women. However, a systematic study of factors that influence the performance of breast ultrasound—which may include breast size and shape, as well as lesion location—has yet to be conducted.[6] Finally, as it is currently performed, ultrasound demands too much physician time to be a cost-effective screening method.[6]

BREAST IMAGERS NEEDED

Demand for breast imaging is rising as the U.S. population ages and as increasing numbers of women require routine screening.[56,119] Improved screening methods and new technologies may help keep pace with these trends, but greater capacity in both personnel and imaging facilities will also be needed to ensure patient access. These resources are also crucial to the improvement of breast cancer detection, because a robust process of assessment, adoption, and dissemination of innovative technology and techniques by practitioners requires an equally robust workforce.

Despite these mounting demands, many in the breast imaging field point to stagnant growth, if not decline, in the availability of the services they provide. Over the long term, such a trend could threaten the advancement of breast cancer detection, which is already limited by the scarcity of radiologists conducting research in this area. The development of new technology also has the potential to solve some of the problems of demand by focusing mammographic services on populations who are most at risk, although these applications are probably at least 5 to 10 years in the future. The need for and difficulty in developing a large and well-trained workforce will likely help to push for research and adoption of technology that improves our ability to target mammographic screening to those who will benefit most. This section describes key factors influencing supply and demand for breast imaging and recommended measures to ensure the accessibility and advancement of breast cancer screening.

Access to Breast Cancer Screening Is Endangered

Recent increases in average waiting times for mammograms indicate that breast cancer screening facilities are operating at or near full capacity.[56] In New York City, patients waited an average of more than 40 days in 2003 for first-time screening mammograms, as compared with 14 days in 1998; in parts of Florida, waiting times of three months are common.[75] Such delays are likely to occur in locations where facilities have closed or where radiologic technologists (the individuals who actually perform mammograms) or radiologists who interpret mammograms—or both—are in short supply. Although no published studies document this trend, there is widespread consensus among breast imagers that workforce issues limit access to mammography and this problem is becoming more acute.

A 2002 report by the GAO found that women in some locations have problems obtaining timely mammography services and raised the prospect of future staff shortfalls, but concluded that the nation's capacity was "generally adequate to meet the growing demand for these services."[119] Impressions of current capacity within the field of breast imaging are far less sanguine, and that community has criticized the GAO report on several counts.[85] For example, they note that it does not distinguish among those radiologists who read some mammograms and those who are breast imaging subspecialists,[c] and therefore may have overestimated capacity for mammogram interpretation. Although approximately 20,000 radiologists interpret mammograms in the United States,[12] only 2,000 of them are members of the subspecialty society, the Society of Breast Imaging. (There are also a small number of nonradiologists who meet the requirements for interpreting mammograms, but the great majority are radiologists, so for simplicity, this report refers simply to radiologists.)

In addition, the GAO may have underestimated the number of radiologic technologists required to meet national mammography needs. A 2000 GAO report found an 18 percent job vacancy rate for radiologic technologists, and a majority of participating hospitals reported greater difficulty in hiring technologists than in the previous year.[119] Among radiologic technologists, the number of first-time examinees for mammography certificates has declined substantially each year from 1996 to 2000.[85] Moreover, the most recent GAO projections do not take into account the time spent by technologists on activities other than screening, such as performing diagnostic mammograms, breast interventional procedures, and quality assur-

---

[c]A radiologist can interpret mammograms and other breast imaging examinations (such as breast MRI and breast ultrasound) but not all do. Even fewer radiologists perform breast interventional procedures, such as needle biopsies. A radiologist who identified him/herself as a subspecialist in breast imaging (a breast imager) is either a radiologist who is self-trained and experienced in the specialty, or one who has completed a fellowship in breast imaging.

ance activities mandated by the MQSA.[86] Finally, many radiologic techni-
cians are involved in other radiology work and are not available to work
full-time on mammography tasks.

Financial Woes Close Screening Facilities

A decline in the number of mammography screening facilities was reported by the ACR, which found that facility closures (979) outpaced
openings (401) by more than two to one between April 2001 and February
2003 (Figure 3-6). Financial factors were the most frequently cited main
reason for these closures. Although some facility closures probably reflect
consolidation of services with more efficient service delivery, the scale of
the closures suggests a serious decline in access.

For years, radiologists and health care administrators have asserted
that reimbursement for mammography does not cover procedure costs,
which include the soaring expense of malpractice liability insurance (see
below) and the cost of compliance with MQSA regulations.[56] Medicare
now pays slightly more than $82 per mammogram; the ACR estimates that
a screening mammogram costs about $87 to perform in a freestanding

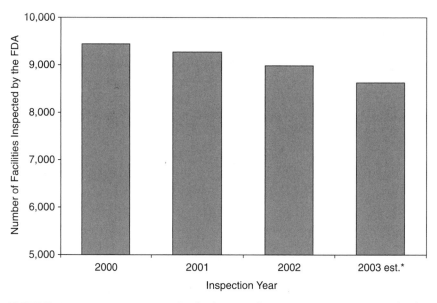

FIGURE 3-6 Fewer mammography facilities each year. Fewer mammography facilities are being inspected by the FDA each year.[87] Under the MQSA, which is
enforced by the FDA, yearly inspections are required for accreditation. The year
2003 data were estimated from the initial result of the inspections in the first half
of 2003 extrapolated using the trend from the previous 3 years.

clinic and more than $105 in a hospital.[d] For high volume settings, even relatively small shortfalls for a particular procedure can add up to large operating deficits. This is compounded in settings that are dedicated to providing a single procedure because there are no opportunities for cost recovery on other, profitable procedures.

A financial analysis of seven university-based breast programs reported that they all incurred losses in the professional component of mammography services.[4] The driver of the loss was diagnostic mammograms.[37] However, it should be noted that because women often seek out university-based programs for second opinions or difficult diagnoses, such programs are likely to conduct a larger proportion of diagnostic mammograms as compared with community facilities (Dieter Enzmann, personal communication).

Increasing Demand for Breast Imagers

The term "crisis" is routinely used in the radiology community to describe the shortage of breast imagers. Based on U.S. population estimates, 1.25 million additional women become age eligible for recommended mammography screening each year, while only about one to three dozen breast imaging subspecialists enter the profession each year (Priscilla Butler, ACR, personal communication). Although only about 12 percent of all mammograms are interpreted by breast imaging subspecialists (Barbara Monsees, personal communication), they spend more of their time doing breast imaging than other radiologists and tend to be more proficient. Thus increasing their ranks may not only help meet the growing demand for screening mammograms, but also improve the quality of breast image interpretation.

Mammography here is pretty awful. Five centers closed in 18 months and we're working very hard, too hard. Two technologists put in their notice and the three of us part-time mammographers may have to leave because the insurance company is putting an extra charge to read mammography —i.e., my premium and hence, tail coverage will cost more than my husband, who is full time. Pretty crazy. It will take all of us leaving Florida mammography to make a change.

Anonymous Florida radiologist
January 2004

---

[d]Medicare reimbursement for mammography services comprises a *professional component*, the amount paid for the physician's interpretation of the results of the examination, and a *technical component*, the amount paid for all other services (including technician and equipment costs).

This is unlikely to happen soon, however, given the relative dearth of medical students entering radiology and, in particular, breast imaging. While the number of radiologists is growing by an estimated 2 percent per year, their workload is increasing by about 6 percent annually, and is likely to continue to outpace workforce expansion.[2,112,113] Even more scarce than radiologists are those who choose to specialize in breast imaging. In a 2001 survey of radiology residents in accredited U.S. programs, 64 percent said they would not consider doing a fellowship in breast imaging. [9] The same proportion of respondents said they did not want to spend more than 25 percent of their work time interpreting mammograms, due to reasons such as lack of interest, fear of lawsuits, high stress, low pay, and the fact that breast imaging is perceived as a female-dominated field. Even without a general shortage of radiologists for procedures other than mammography, there is great concern over the shortage of breast imagers.

Malpractice litigation is a particular concern for breast imagers due to the disproportionate number of claims against radiologists who interpret mammograms (see Box 3-6) and the comparatively high price they pay for malpractice insurance (Barbara Monsees, personal communication). Recent, precipitous increases in malpractice insurance premiums for all physicians reportedly have led significant numbers of physicians in high-risk specialties and/or locations to retire, relocate, or restrict their practices in order to avoid lawsuits.[33,93] Such claims were only partially substantiated in a GAO assessment of the effects of rising malpractice premiums on access to health care, however.[120] The ensuing report included an analysis of access to mammograms in five states that were cited by the American Medical Association (AMA) and other national health care provider organizations as facing "full blown liability crises." The GAO concluded that access to mammograms had not been subject to "major reductions" in these states (unlike access to emergency surgery and newborn deliveries, which were found to be restricted in several, mostly rural, locations). The AMA disputed the GAO's findings, claiming that the scope of the agency's investigation was insufficient to support its conclusions.

To ensure adequate capacity over the long term for radiological services (and, more specifically, for breast imaging) the causes of the decline in workforce must be identified, prioritized, and addressed. Possible solutions to these larger issues include incentives to increase the number of breast imagers and radiologic technologists (such as by enriching the professional opportunities and resources for research), more efficient technology, better reimbursement for mammography, efforts to increase breast imagers' productivity, and mechanisms to reduce the burden of malpractice insurance, such as tort reform.[110]

Problems relevant to tort reform are particularly intense in, but by no means limited to, mammography—or even, for that matter, limited to health

BOX 3-6
Mammograms and Malpractice

The threat of malpractice litigation disturbs breast imagers and radiology residents, and perhaps for good reason. Breast cancer in women leads to more malpractice claims than any other medical condition and is second only to the neurological impairment of newborns in the expense of paid claims, according to a 2002 report by the Physicians Insurers Association of America (PIAA) based on claims paid between January 1995 and June 2001.[97]

The latest PIAA study also found that an increasing percentage of claims regarding breast cancer are being filed against radiologists who interpret mammograms. Radiologists accounted for the largest proportion (33 percent) of paid claims involving breast cancer, up from 24 percent during the previous PIAA study based on claims paid between 1990 and 1995.[96] Surprisingly, among breast cancer claims, obstetricians and gynecologists were the second largest group (23 percent). Other claims for missed breast cancer diagnosis, in descending order of percentage, named insurance corporations, surgical specialists, family and general practitioners, and internal medicine practitioners.

The PIAA represents about 60 percent of physicians in private practice. Over the more than 16 years that the PIAA has collected data on medical malpractice claims related to breast cancer, an average of about 200 such claims per year have been reported by its member companies. Forty-one percent of these claims were successful and, by 2001, paid an average indemnity of more than $290,000.

Focusing on the 450 paid claims involving the delayed diagnosis of breast cancer during the 2002 study period, the PIAA found that 74 percent of those claims involved pre- or peri-menopausal women. More than one-third of these claims involved women under age 40, who compose less than 5 percent of invasive breast cancer cases.[3] This group accounted for 43 percent of the total cost of claims, and nearly half of all deaths, in malpractice cases involving delay of diagnosis of breast cancer.

Successful malpractice claims for delayed diagnosis among younger women may be due to a combination of factors. Younger women tend to have more dense breasts, resulting in mammograms that are difficult to interpret (see Chapter 2) and thereby increasing the likelihood of a missed diagnosis. Yet because people tend to overestimate the benefits of mammography (see Chapter 4), particularly for younger women, jurors may not appreciate its limitations. As for the relatively high indemnities paid in such cases, awards to injured patients tend to reflect the severity of the damage sustained (an early death, in many of these cases), less than they reflect the degree of negligence attributed to the injury.[13,20]

Just as there are no simple cures for the malpractice liability crisis facing physicians across the United States[110] (see Box 3-7), there is no straightforward solution to the particular legal vulnerability of radiologists who interpret mammograms. Instead of exploring risk management strategies that might reduce a radiologist's exposure to lawsuits, this report recommends a variety of measures aimed at reducing the likelihood of a missed diagnosis. These could include the reorganization of breast cancer screening services to better serve young women at higher-than-average risk for breast cancer, improving the quality of mammographic interpretation, and developing more effective technologies to detect and diagnose breast cancer.

BOX 3-7
The IOM on Tort Reform

For the first time in nearly 20 years, the United States is facing a broad-based crisis in the availability and affordability of malpractice liability insurance for physicians, hospitals, and other health care providers. Although liability is intended to provide a system of accountability, there is widespread agreement that the current system of tort liability is a poor way to prevent and redress injury resulting from medical error.[17]

The randomness and delay associated with the present pattern of accountability not only prevents severely injured patients from receiving prompt and fair compensation, but destabilizes liability insurance markets and attenuates the signal that liability is supposed to send health care providers regarding the need for quality improvement. The shortcomings of the current malpractice system come from three directions, all of which have contributed to the present crisis: inefficient and inequitable legal processes for resolving disputes, problematic responses by clinicians to the threat and cost of liability, and volatile markets for liability insurance.

The best way to create a legal environment that fosters both high-quality patient care and relieves financial strain and administrative burden for health care providers is to replace tort liability with a system of patient-centered and safety-focused nonjudicial compensation—linking claims resolution to organization-based error disclosure and safety improvement processes.

SOURCE: Committee on Rapid Advances Demonstration Projects: Health Care Finance and Delivery Systems, *Fostering Rapid Advances in Health Care,* IOM, 2003.

---

care.[79] The problem of malpractice is unlikely to be solved by individual medical specialties. The American College of Obstetrics and Gynecology worked hard to encourage the passage of federal legislation to regulate lawsuits for health care liability related to ob/gyn care, but in both 2003 and 2004 the bills they supported were defeated. It is not clear that the mammography field would have any more success. Moreover, this Committee was not comprised of experts in medical law and did not address the issue in depth, although a previous IOM Committee discussed medical malpractice and tort reform in its 2003 report on *Fostering Rapid Advances in Health Care* (see Box 3-7).[52]

More Radiologists Needed in Research

The erosion of access to mammography is not the only potential consequence of a shortage in radiologists who interpret mammograms. Radiologists, and particularly breast imaging subspecialists, are needed to refine, test, and disseminate new technologies. Anticipated advances could enhance, redirect, or replace current breast imaging technologies used to detect and evaluate abnormalities, or they could take the form of new methods for the diagnosis, biopsy, treatment, and surveillance of treated patients. However, a decline in the number of breast imaging professionals, especially at academic institutions, is likely to limit scientific advancement in the field.

University clinicians play key roles in medical innovation—including the refinement, standardization, and evaluation of novel devices—and they make important contributions to the design of clinical trials, providing expertise in methodology and the measurement of outcomes such as quality of life, quality-adjusted survival, and cost-effectiveness.[48] Radiologists appear to be in high demand in academia; a recent survey of radiology department chairs by the Radiological Society of North America found about 600 such job openings per year.[1]

Academic vacancies in radiology leave remaining radiology faculty with less time to engage in research. This is especially troubling given that radiologists' research presence is relatively minor compared to most other medical specialists. Overall, about 3 percent of physicians in nonsurgical specialties cite research as their primary activity, whereas only 0.6 percent of radiologists do (Figure 3-7).[94] In 2000, there were roughly 21,000 diagnostic radiologists in the United States, of whom only 127 cited research as their major professional activity. By comparison there were a similar number cardiologists, of whom 748 identified themselves primarily as researchers—nearly six times as many as their counterparts in radiology. The high service workload for breast imagers also takes a toll on research involvement. Many breast imagers who previously volunteered their time to serve as grant reviewers can no longer afford to take the time from their clinical practices (Barbara Monsees, personal communication). This is a loss not only because breast imagers are less available to contribute their perspectives to research on improving breast cancer detection, but they are also deprived of an opportunity to learn about new directions in research.

Radiology equipment is expensive and ever changing. Clinicians with research expertise play an important role in evaluating the impact of new technologies on health outcomes, but few radiologists who interpret mammograms receive any research training. While some radiologists serve as alpha or beta testers for commercial products, few undertake the sort of carefully designed clinical trials needed to demonstrate the medical value of new procedures or technologies. Better training of radiologists would enable more critical evaluation of equipment and techniques.

As C. Douglas Maynard, co-chair of the ACR's Task Force on Human Resources commented, "We really need to be producing more research to take advantage of opportunities at the NIH, (but) in fact we are producing

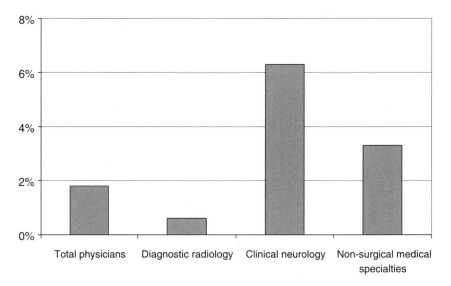

FIGURE 3-7 The ranks of academic radiologists are thin compared to other specialties.

less."[1] In principle, research participation by radiologists could get a boost from the newest institute at NIH, the National Institute of Biomedical Imaging and Bioengineering (NIBIB). However, the NIBIB budget is small. At approximately $280 million, the 2003 budget for NIBIB was the second smallest of the NIH institutes and a mere 6 percent of the NCI budget. (The smallest budget was that of the National Institute of Nursing Research.) In addition, at least for the first round, fewer than one in 5 grant applications were from physician researchers; over 80 percent were from Ph.D. researchers (Barbara McNeil, NIBIB Council Member, personal communication).

Practitioners Drive Technology Adoption

The pending (or worsening) shortage in mammography personnel at all levels—from radiologist to technologist, in academia and in private practice—presents both barrier and impetus to innovation. Development may be driven by the need to improve process and efficiency to meet the growing demand for screening, but it may also be impeded by a lack of professionals who can assess and appropriately apply new technologies. The latter situation may occur if recruitment into the field of breast imaging fails to keep pace with the demand for screening, but it may also result from technical and regulatory demands that increase workload.

In today's cost-conscious medical environment, even novel technologies that improve patient outcome present problems if they necessitate new investments in training and equipment.[73] If such technologies expand—rather than replace—current methods for breast cancer detection and diagnosis, then innovation may further burden an overtaxed workforce.[73] For example, as noted in *Mammography and Beyond*, current practice guidelines and standards of care for breast cancer detection, which are already complex, may be made more complicated with the incorporation of new technologies.

Breast imagers are essential not only in preserving access to breast cancer screening, but also in the evaluation of new technologies and the adoption of technological advances in breast cancer detection that will improve health outcomes in the future. The speed of adoption for new technologies and evidence-based practice guidelines for breast cancer detection is likely to vary according to region (urban versus rural) and clinical setting (community clinic versus academic health center). However, the rate of innovation ultimately is determined by the actions of individual physicians, who must be persuaded of the potential value of a new technique or technology if it is to become widely available. Appropriate research also has the potential to reduce the spread of inappropriate technologies such as those that increase costs but do not improve outcomes.

Righting the Balance of Supply and Demand

Where radiological services are in short supply, institutions have adopted a variety of short-term measures to meet their needs. They have used offsite "moonlighters" to take the place of attending physicians; called in retired radiologists; established cross-coverage agreements to share specialists among (sometimes competing) hospitals; and offered flexible schedules and the opportunity to work at home as a way to make a comparatively low-paying job more attractive.[1] Many radiology facilities are increasingly relying on foreign radiologists.

Teleradiology has also been used in a variety of settings with limited local imaging capacity. The Air Force, anticipating the loss of half of its radiology staff between 2002 and 2005, developed a network that links radiologists at eight stateside hospitals operated by the U.S. Army, Air Force, or Navy with eight overseas hospitals (as of April 2003).[21] According to an Air Force spokesperson, teleradiology "will not fix the shortage, but it will make maximum use of the radiologists we currently have."[117] Some U.S. hospitals have used similar arrangements to outsource interpretation—such as the reading of emergency scans performed during the night—to radiologists overseas.[98] Although this scenario raises concerns about maintaining the quality of services, it presents a model that could be adapted to establish centralized domestic facilities for mammographic interpretation, as described earlier in this chapter under the section Organization of Screening Services.

The supply of radiologists (and therefore of breast imagers) is unlikely to grow as quickly as demand for their expertise. Significant barriers exist to expanding training programs, and to permitting well-trained radiologists to immigrate to the United States.[5] A freeze—at 1996 levels—on the number of house officers at institutions supported by CMS effectively limits the growth of residency programs, even for fields in such high demand as radiology. Visa restrictions, in addition to the burden of state and hospital licensure and ACR certification requirements, inhibit the immigration of highly qualified foreign radiologists. Given these circumstances, the committee focused on optimizing the productivity of the limited and increasingly precious supply of radiologists who interpret mammograms.

Expanding Capacity with Physician Extenders

Physician extenders such as physician assistants (PAs) and nurse practitioners have long been employed to increase capacity in a variety of medical specialties and settings, and their numbers are growing rapidly. Until recently, hospitals with residency training programs tended to rely on residents, whose costs were paid by CMS and who worked comparatively long hours, to perform duties that could have been performed by non-physicians.[5] Today, with the number of residents capped and residents' hours limited by new work rules, hospitals are hiring more physician extenders. Nonphysician provider training programs produced twice as many graduates in 1997 as they did in 1992, and several state legislatures have passed laws enabling them to practice.[5] Until now, however, this trend has largely bypassed radiology, which employs less than 0.5 percent of all PAs.[5]

The position of radiology PA was introduced in the 1970s. At that time, candidates trained in baccalaureate programs at the University of Kentucky and at Duke and Brown Universities, but they have since closed due to lack of interest.[5] In 1996, responding to a shortage of radiologists in the armed services, the Department of Defense (DoD) supported the launch of a baccalaureate training program at Weber State University in Utah for a distinct position known as the Radiology Practitioner Assistant. Although the DoD no longer funds this program, it continues to produce graduates, who are eligible for certification by their own board.

Most recently, the ACR and the American Society of Radiological Technologists (ASRT) have jointly defined a new physician extender with expertise in medical imaging, the radiological associate (RA).[2] The RA offers a partial solution to the continuing chronic shortage of personnel in the field of radiology by simultaneously reducing radiologists' workload and establishing a career path by which to attract and retain radiation technologists (RTs), who are also in short supply, to the field. The RA's duties are proposed to include patient management, certain routine procedures under direct supervision of a radiologist, and the communication of results to referring physicians; image interpretation, even on a preliminary basis, is expressly excluded. However, because individual states control licensing and regulation of nonphysician practitioners, an RA's role and responsibilities may depend on his or her location.[5,111] With ASRT funding, RA training programs catering to experienced RTs have been initiated at Loma Linda University, Midwestern State University, the University of North Carolina, and the University of Medicine and Dentistry in New Jersey, and are being developed at eight additional institutions.[5]

Should Nonphysicians Interpret Mammograms?

While RAs would enable breast imagers to focus on image interpretation and biopsies, physician extenders who interpret screening mammograms under the supervision of breast imaging specialists can further extend capacity. Evidence suggests that RTs could be specially trained to prescreen mammograms for the presence or absence of abnormalities[25,111] or to double-read mammograms along with a radiologist.[122] A series of studies supports the prospect for training and evaluation of physician extenders in mammographic interpretation.

Some of the most relevant experience of nonphysicians interpreting screening mammograms has occurred in the United Kingdom, where—despite a less burdensome malpractice environment and a different reimbursement structure—there is also a long-standing shortage of radiologists who interpret mammograms.[40,122] One English "rapid access" breast clinic faced with unacceptably long wait times due to increased demand for mammograms coped with this problem by allowing mammograms of patients meeting specific criteria for concern to be interpreted initially by two specially trained RTs.[25] [e] (Candidate patients were not pregnant or lactating and were over 35, without clinically obvious cancer or axillary problems, but with worrisome symptoms such as breast pain, palpable masses, Paget's disease, or nipple discharge.) Their findings were later reviewed by two radiologists, who decided whether the women should be recalled for additional studies. In 511 women thus screened and tracked for approximately two years, the sensitivity, specificity, and accuracy obtained by the RTs was comparable to that of radiologists. The women reportedly did not object when informed that an RT would provide the initial read on their exams.

---

[e]RTs are referred to as radiographers in the United Kingdom.

In another study conducted in the United Kingdom, three RTs in a hospital that was otherwise unable to maintain double reading requirements for mammograms were trained to meet national certification standards.[122] The trained radiographers performed well and were comparable in both accuracy and speed to that of the four participating radiologists.

A 6-week study of 33 experienced RTs conducted in a U.S. hospital found that even without training, the technologists could classify screening mammograms as to their need for additional workup (such as additional views, sonography, or biopsy) with "reasonable" accuracy.[111] The technologists assigned each of the more than 3,000 women whose mammograms they reviewed to one of two categories: either she needed additional workup to explore possible abnormalities, or no workup was required. The RTs' classification of more than 80 percent of these cases matched those of the hospital's nine radiologists, and the RTs identified most of the cases that later proved to be malignant.

Each of the studies described above involved the interpretation of screening mammograms by RTs working under the supervision of a board-certified radiologist, and do not apply to diagnostic mammograms. The Committee does not suggest that RTs should interpret diagnostic mammograms or that screening mammograms should be interpreted solely by an RT; rather, they would work to expand the capacity of radiologists. RTs could also take on other tasks commonly performed by radiologists such as filling out forms, dictating, and hanging and taking down films. Having a physician extender support the work of breast imagers would add the cost of an extra salary, but this could result in overall reduced costs if they could take on other tasks commonly done by radiologists.

The most important requirement that would have to be met if nonphysicians were to interpret mammograms would be that the quality of the mammography service was shown to improve, or at least, did not decline. In fact, the use of physician extenders for double-reading has the potential to increase quality. Because double-reading by a second radiologist is not reimbursed by Medicare, few mammography facilities can afford to have two radiologists interpret each mammogram, even though this practice is known to improve sensitivity. Another requirement would be that mammograms interpreted by physician extenders should also be viewed by an interpreting radiologist.

Challenges to this proposal include the acceptance of the radiology profession and malpractice coverage. In May 2004 the ACR leadership council recently voted against a proposal to allow the interpretation of *any* imaging examination by nonphysicians. However, resistance to expanding professional boundaries has been overcome by other medical specialties, for example, the use of nurse practitioners and midwives in obstetrics and gynecology; these professionals have also dealt with similar malpractice issues. Indeed, it is even conceivable that malpractice rates for radiologists could be *lowered* if they adopted the practice of double-reading made possible by supportive assistance from nonphysicians with specialized training in mammography.

The MQSA stipulates that mammograms are to be interpreted only by a physician specifically certified in mammography (Box 3-8). The Act does not, however, preclude other personnel from examining the mammograms that are *also* interpreted by certified physicians. Although not widely appreciated and rarely practiced, it would in fact be permissible within the provisions of the MQSA to have nonphysician personnel examine mammograms—as long as a certified physician signed the mammogram report indicating that he or she had interpreted it. This suggestion that physician

---

BOX 3-8
Who Does What in Mammography

This includes only the initial requirements established by law in the MQSA. Further requirements are set by the FDA in the Code of Federal Regulations for Mammography, 21 CFR 900.12.

Interpreting Physician—Interprets mammograms

- Must have state license to practice medicine
- Must be certified in an appropriate specialty area by an FDA-approved accreditation body or have 3 months of training in mammographic interpretation
- Must complete 60 hours of category I medical education in mammography
- Must interpret a minimum of 240 mammograms every six months

Radiologic Technologist—Performs mammograms

- Must be licensed to perform radiographic procedures by FDA-approved accreditation body (See Box 3-4).
- Must complete 40 hours of training specific to mammography
- Must perform 200 mammograms every 2 years

Medical Physicist—Surveys mammography equipment and oversees quality assurance practices

- Must be state licensed to perform physics survey
- Must have a Master's degree or higher in physical science
- Must complete 20 hours of specialized training in conducting surveys of mammography facilities
- Must conduct surveys of at least 1 mammography facility and a total of 10 mammography units

extenders could be enlisted to help read mammograms would thus offer women a more thorough examination than is currently typical of most mammography facilities where mammograms are viewed only by a single breast imager. Physician extenders could potentially improve the overall accuracy of mammographic interpretation through double reading, as well as alleviate the burden on the breast imaging physicians by prescreening the mammograms to allow the interpreting physician to spend more time on the more problematic mammograms.

SUMMARY

Mammography is not a perfect screening technology, but it can reduce mortality from breast cancer. However, there is wide variation in performance among breast imaging facilities and individual breast imagers. Organizing breast screening services to increase the utilization of services as well as their quality and efficiency should thus be priority for health care payers and providers.

Approaches to improving mammography that need to be examined include organizational changes such as those implemented in some European countries including limiting interpretation to more expert and experienced breast imagers, and regionalization and reading at a central location. Although the evidence for how such changes might improve mammography in the United States is mixed, they have led to improvements in some European countries. Certainly, better accuracy and lower rates of callbacks and false positives should result in more cost-effective care.

Even without the single-payer, universal access health care system common to all other developed countries, screening services in the United States could adapt many features of those systems to regionally based programs. As pointedly noted by Harmon Eyre and his colleagues at the American Cancer Society:[39]

> Screening under opportunistic condition rather than through a system is inefficient at both the individual level and population level; moreover, without a system, there is no readiness to implement any new early detection technology that could improve disease control.

> A comprehensive system of early-detection potentially not only leads to high levels of participation but also insures that all the elements of a program of early detection an intervention are highly competent, interrelated, and inter-dependent. A system has the potential not only to increase quality but also to reduce the volume of small errors that contribute to incremental erosions of efficiency . . . .

> While there are many practical barriers that must be overcome to establish true population-based screening programs, a system of organized

screening holds the greatest potential to realize the benefits of reducing the incidence rate of advanced cancers.

Harmon J. Eyre, Robert A. Smith, Curtis J. Mettlin
Cancer Screening and Early Detection, 2003

State and federal legislators have taken an active role in exploring ways to improve breast cancer detection. The federal Mammography Quality Standards Act represents an unusual governmental intervention aimed at, and successful in, improving the technical quality of mammography. In the future, the MQSA may address the vexing problem of variation in radiologist interpretation of breast images. In spite of the impression left by widespread coverage in the national media,[f] differences among radiologists are not the largest component of the problem of inconsistency in interpretation. Other factors, notably organizational factors, have received much less attention, and are more difficult to control than individual factors, such as volume or training requirements.

New technologies, such as digital mammography, CAD, and MRI are being examined. Although they have advantages in some situations that may justify their use, they can add significant costs, and their value as improvements in sensitivity and specificity over screen-film mammography has not been established.

Organizational factors such as double reading by two radiologists improves accuracy; high volume centers on average have higher accuracy, above and beyond the increase attributable to reading volume of individual radiologists; and use of CAD can reduce the variability in mammographic interpretation among different readers.

As the U.S. population ages, demand for mammography will rise at a time when supply of personnel and facilities appears to be falling, increasingly threatening access. Among other things, low reimbursement and the unattractiveness of breast imaging as a subspecialty due to stress and malpractice litigation seem to be driving the impending shortages. Other problems include a dearth of radiologist researchers to conduct trials and investigate new approaches to breast cancer detection. To address the shortage of mammographers, expansion of responsibilities by nonphysicians to include preliminary interpretation of images should be considered. A key to improving mammographic interpretation is to reduce known and controllable sources of variability in quality, but at the same time to avoid adding to the burden of an already overextended workforce.

---

[f]See, for example, series of articles by Michael Moss in the *New York Times* (October 24, 2002).

REFERENCES

1. The radiology shortage: will it continue? 2003. *Radiological Society of North America News* 13(2):10-11.
2. Radiology assistants will share workload in diagnostic imaging. 2004. *Radiological Society of North America News* 14(2):5-6.
3. American Cancer Society. 2003. *Breast Cancer Facts and Figures 2003-2004*. Atlanta, GA: American Cancer Society.
4. American College of Radiology. ACR Mammography Practice Cost Survey Executive Summary. Unpublished as of March 9, 2004.
5. American College of Radiology. Intersociety Conference 2003 Summary. Unpublished as of March 9, 2004.
6. American College of Radiology Imaging Network (ACRIN). Current Protocols: Screening Breast Ultrasound in High-Risk Women (ACRIN Protocol A6666-Open). Accessed May 12, 2004. Web Page. Available at: http://www.acrin.org/current_protocols.html#A6666.
7. Andrews FJ. 2001. Pain during mammography: implications for breast screening programmes. *Australas Radiol* 45(2):113-117.
8. Barroso J, McMillan S, Casey L, Gibson W, Kaminski G, Meyer J. 2000. Comparison between African-American and white women in their beliefs about breast cancer and their health locus of control. *Cancer Nurs* 23(4):268-276.
9. Bassett LW, Monsees BS, Smith RA, Wang L, Hooshi P, Farria DM, Sayre JW, Feig SA, Jackson VP. 2003. Survey of radiology residents: breast imaging training and attitudes. *Radiology* 227(3):862-869.
10. Beam CA, Conant EF, Sickles EA. 2002. Factors affecting radiologist inconsistency in screening mammography. *Acad Radiol* 9(5):531-540.
11. Beam CA, Conant EF, Sickles EA. 2003. Association of volume and volume-independent factors with accuracy in screening mammogram interpretation. *J Natl Cancer Inst* 95(4):282-290.
12. Beam CA, Conant EF, Sickles EA, Weinstein SP. 2003. Evaluation of proscriptive health care policy implementation in screening mammography. *Radiology* 229(2):534-540.
13. Berlin L. 2003. Missed mammographic abnormalities, malpractice, and expert witnesses: does majority rule in the courtroom? *Radiology* 229(1):288; author reply 289.
14. Berlin L. 2003. Testimony of Leonard Berlin, M.D. Regarding the Mammography Quality Standards Act Reauthorization. Senate Committee on Health, Education, Labor, and Pensions.
15. Betsill WL Jr, Rosen PP, Lieberman PH, Robbins GF. 1978. Intraductal carcinoma. Long-term follow-up after treatment by biopsy alone. *JAMA* 239(18):1863-1867.
16. Birdwell RL, Wilcox PA. 2001. The Mammography Quality Standards Act: Benefits and Burdens. Pisano ED, Editor. *Breast Imaging*. Amsterdam, Oxford: IOS Press.
17. Bovbjerg RR, Miller RH, Shapiro DW. 2001. Paths to reducing medical injury: professional liability and discipline vs. patient safety—and the need for a third way. *J Law Med Ethics* 29(3-4):369-380.
18. Boyle P, Autier P, Bartelink H, Baselga J, Boffetta P, Burn J, Burns HJ, Christensen L, Denis L, Dicato M, Diehl V, Doll R, Franceschi S, Gillis CR, Gray N, Griciute L, Hackshaw A, Kasler M, Kogevinas M, Kvinnsland S, La Vecchia C, Levi F, McVie JG, Maisonneuve P, Martin-Moreno JM, Bishop JN, Oleari F, Perrin P, Quinn M, Richards M, Ringborg U, Scully C, Siracka E, Storm H, Tubiana M, Tursz T, Veronesi U, Wald N, Weber W, Zaridze DG, Zatonski W, zur Hausen H. 2003. European Code Against Cancer and scientific justification: third version (2003). *Ann Oncol* 14(7):973-1005.

19. Boyle P, d'Onofrio A, Maisonneuve P, Severi G, Robertson C, Tubiana M, Veronesi U. 2003. Measuring progress against cancer in Europe: has the 15% decline targeted for 2000 come about? *Ann Oncol* 14(8):1312-1325.
20. Brennan TA, Sox CM, Burstin HR. 1996. Relation between negligent adverse events and the outcomes of medical-malpractice litigation. *N Engl J Med* 335(26):1963-1967.
21. Brewin B. 2003, February 12. DOD system brings medical expertise closer. Accessed April 11, 2003. Web Page. Available at: http://www.bio-itworld.com/news/021203_report2006.html.
22. Burnside E, Belkora J, Esserman L. 2001. The impact of alternative practices on the cost and quality of mammographic screening in the United States. *Clin Breast Cancer* 2(2):145-152.
23. Butler P (American College of Radiology). Personal communication, March 1, 2004.
24. Carney PA, Miglioretti DL, Yankaskas BC, Kerlikowske K, Rosenberg R, Rutter CM, Geller BM, Abraham LA, Taplin SH, Dignan M, Cutter G, Ballard-Barbash R. 2003. Individual and combined effects of age, breast density, and hormone replacement therapy use on the accuracy of screening mammography. *Ann Intern Med* 138(3):168-175.
25. Casey B. 2003, March 11. Breast center enlists radiographers for first look at mammograms. Accessed February 19, 2004. Web Page. Available at: http://www.auntminnie.com/default.asp?Sec=sup&Sub=wom&Pag=dis&ItemId=57614&stm=radiographers.
26. CDC (Centers for Disease Control and Prevention). 2003. *The National Breast and Cervical Cancer Early Detection Program: Reducing Mortality Through Screening*. Atlanta, GA: Centers for Disease Control and Prevention: Department of Health and Human Services.
27. Christiansen CL, Wang F, Barton MB, Kreuter W, Elmore JG, Gelfand AE, Fletcher SW. 2000. Predicting the cumulative risk of false-positive mammograms. *J Natl Cancer Inst* 92(20):1657-1666.
28. Chu KC, Lamar CA, Freeman HP. 2003. Racial disparities in breast carcinoma survival rates: separating factors that affect diagnosis from factors that affect treatment. *Cancer* 97(11):2853-2860.
29. Cyrlak D. 1988. Induced costs of low-cost screening mammography. *Radiology* 168(3):661-663.
30. D'Orsi CJ. 2001. Computer-aided detection: there is no free lunch. *Radiology* 221(3):585-586.
31. Dakins DR. 2002. Mammography debate raises digital quality bar. *Diagnostic Imaging. Com.* Accessed March 3, 2002. Web Page. Available at: http://www.dimag.com/db_area/archives/2002/.
32. Earp JA, Eng E, O'Malley MS, Altpeter M, Rauscher G, Mayne L, Mathews HF, Lynch KS, Qaqish B. 2002. Increasing use of mammography among older, rural African American women: results from a community trial. *Am J Public Health* 92(4):646-654.
33. Eisenberg D, Sieger M, Tsiantar D, Berryman A, Cuadros P, Peltier M. 2003. The doctor won't see you now. *Time* 161(23):46-56.
34. Elmore JG, Carney PA. 2002. Does practice make perfect when interpreting mammography? *J Natl Cancer Inst* 94(5):321-323.
35. Elmore JG, Miglioretti DL, Reisch LM, Barton MB, Kreuter W, Christiansen CL, Fletcher SW. 2002. Screening mammograms by community radiologists: variability in false-positive rates. *J Natl Cancer Inst* 94(18):1373-1380.

36. Elmore JG, Nakano CY, Koepsell TD, Desnick LM, D'Orsi CJ, Ransohoff DF. 2003. International variation in screening mammography interpretations in community-based programs. *J Natl Cancer Inst* 95(18):1384-1393.

37. Enzmann DAPHCVL. 2001. Providing professional mammography services: financial analysis. *Health Policy Prac* 219:467-473.

38. Esserman L, Cowley H, Eberle C, Kirkpatrick A, Chang S, Berbaum K, Gale A. 2002. Improving the accuracy of mammography: volume and outcome relationships. *J Natl Cancer Inst* 94(5):369-375.

39. Eyre HJ, Smith RA, Mettlin CJ. 2003. Cancer Screening and Early Detection. In: Holland JF, Frei E, Bast RC, Kufe DW, Pollack RE, Weichselbaum RR, Editors. *Cancer Medicine.* 6th ed. Ontario: BC Decker.

40. Field S. 1996. UK radiology workforce survey—breast imaging services. *Royal College of Radiologists Newsletter* 45:10-12.

41. Fisher B, Dignam J, Wolmark N, Mamounas E, Costantino J, Poller W, Fisher ER, Wickerham DL, Deutsch M, Margolese R, Dimitrov N, Kavanah M. 1998. Lumpectomy and radiation therapy for the treatment of intraductal breast cancer: findings from National Surgical Adjuvant Breast and Bowel Project B-17. *J Clin Oncol* 16(2):441-452.

42. Fletcher SW, Elmore JG. 2003. Clinical practice. Mammographic screening for breast cancer. *N Engl J Med* 348(17):1672-1680.

43. Foote SB, Blewett LA. 2003. Politics of prevention: expanding prevention benefits in the Medicare program. *J Public Health Policy* 24(1):26-40.

44. Fowler BA. 2000. Variability in mammography screening legislation across the states. *J Womens Health Gender-Based Med* 9(2):175-184.

45. Freeman H. 2004. Reducing Disparities in Cancer. *Fulfilling the Potential of Cancer Prevention and Early Detection: An American Cancer Society and Institute of Medicine Symposium.* Washington, DC: The National Academies Press.

46. Freer TW, Ulissey MJ. 2001. Screening mammography with computer-aided detection: prospective study of 12,860 patients in a community breast center. *Radiology* 220(3):781-786.

47. Fronstin P. 2000. *Sources of Health Insurance and Characteristics of the Uninsured: Analysis of the March 2000 Current Population Survey.* EBRI Issue Brief Number 228 ed. Washington, DC: Employee Benefits Research Institute.

48. Gelijns AC, Thier SO. 2002. Medical innovation and institutional interdependence: rethinking university-industry connections. *JAMA* 287(1):72-77.

49. Gur D, Sumkin JH, Rockette HE, Ganott M, Hakim C, Hardesty L, Poller WR, Shah R, Wallace L. 2004. Changes in breast cancer detection and mammography recall rates after the introduction of a computer-aided detection system. *J Natl Cancer Inst* 96(3):185-190.

50. Han B, Wells BL, Primas M. 2003. Comparison of mammography use by older black and white women. *J Am Geriatr Soc* 51(2):203-212.

51. Harvey SC, Geller B, Oppenheimer RG, Pinet M, Riddell L, Garra B. 2003. Increase in cancer detection and recall rates with independent double interpretation of screening mammography. *Am J Roentgenol* 180(5):1461-1467.

52. Hayes JC. 2002, December 3. Annual oration analyzes mammography controversies. Web Page. Available at: www.dimag.com/cgi-bin/webcast02/display_news.cgi?105.

53. Hwang ES, Kinkel K, Esserman LJ, Lu Y, Weidner N, Hylton NM. 2003. Magnetic resonance imaging in patients diagnosed with ductal carcinoma-in-situ: value in the diagnosis of residual disease, occult invasion, and multicentricity. *Ann Surg Oncol* 10(4):381-388.

54. Institute of Medicine. 2001. *Crossing the Quality Chasm: A New Health System for the 21st Century.* Washington, DC: National Academy Press.

55. Institute of Medicine. 2001. *Interpreting the Volume-Outcome Relationship in the Context of Cancer Care.* Washington DC: National Academy Press.

56. Institute of Medicine. 2001. *Mammography and Beyond: Developing Technologies for the Early Detection of Breast Cancer.* Washington, DC: National Academy Press.

57. Institute of Medicine. 2002. *Care Without Coverage: Too Little, Too Late.* Washington, DC: The National Academies Press.

58. Institute of Medicine. 2003. *Fulfilling the Potential of Cancer Prevention and Early Detection.* Washington DC: The National Academies Press.

59. James JJ. 2004. The current status of digital mammography. *Clin Radiol* 59(1):1-10.

60. Jones BA, Patterson EA, Calvocoressi L. 2003. Mammography screening in African American women: evaluating the research. *Cancer* 97(1 Suppl):258-272.

61. Joslyn SA, West MM. 2000. Racial differences in breast carcinoma survival. *Cancer* 88(1):1114-1123.

62. Kan L, Olivotto IA, Warren Burhenne LJ, Sickles EA, Coldman AJ. 2000. Standardized abnormal interpretation and cancer detection ratios to assess reading volume and reader performance in a breast screening program. *Radiology* 215(2):563-567.

63. Kerlikowske K, Carney PA, Geller B, Mandelson MT, Taplin SH, Malvin K, Ernster V, Urban N, Cutter G, Rosenberg R, Ballard-Barbash R. 2000. Performance of screening mammography among women with and without a first-degree relative with breast cancer. *Ann Intern Med* 133(11):855-863.

64. Kerlikowske K, Smith-Bindman R, Ljung BM, Grady D. 2003. Evaluation of abnormal mammography results and palpable breast abnormalities. *Ann Intern Med* 139(4):274-284.

65. Kolb TM, Lichy J, Newhouse JH. 2002. Comparison of the performance of screening mammography, physical examination, and breast US and evaluation of factors that influence them: an analysis of 27,825 patient evaluations. *Radiology* 225(1):165-175.

66. Kopans DB. 2004. Sonography should not be used for breast cancer screening until its efficacy has been proven scientifically. *Am J Roentgenol* 182(2):489-491.

67. Kriege M, Brekelmans CT, Boetes C, Rutgers EJ, Oosterwijk JC, Tollenaar RA, Manoliu RA, Holland R, de Koning HJ, Klijn JG. 2001. MRI screening for breast cancer in women with familial or genetic predisposition: design of the Dutch National Study (MRISC). *Fam Cancer* 1(3-4):163-168.

68. Kubota M, Inoue K, Koh S, Sato T, Sugita T. 2003. Role of ultrasonography in treatment selection. *Breast Cancer* 10(3):188-197.

69. Lehman C, Holt S, Peacock S, White E, Urban N. 2002. Use of the American College of Radiology BI-RADS guidelines by community radiologists: concordance of assessments and recommendations assigned to screening mammograms. *Am J Roentgenol* 179(1):15-20.

70. Lewin JM, Hendrick RE, D'Orsi CJ, Isaacs PK, Moss LJ, Karellas A, Sisney GA, Kuni CC, Cutter GR. 2001. Comparison of full-field digital mammography with screen-film mammography for cancer detection: results of 4,945 paired examinations. *Radiology* 218(3):873-880.

71. Li CI, Malone KE, Daling JR. 2003. Differences in breast cancer stage, treatment, and survival by race and ethnicity. *Arch Intern Med* 163(1):49-56.

72. Liang W, Burnett CB, Rowland JH, Meropol NJ, Eggert L, Hwang YT, Silliman RA, Weeks JC, Mandelblatt JS. 2002. Communication between physicians and older women with localized breast cancer: implications for treatment and patient satisfaction. *J Clin Oncol* 20(4):1008-1016.

73. Lohnberg A, van der Meulen B, Brown N, Nelis A, Rappert B, Webster A, Cabello C, Rosales M, Sanz-Menéndez L. 1999. *Studying Innovation Strategies for Future Medical Technologies: Conceptual Framework and Methodologies for the FORMAKIN Project*. European Commission Targeted Socio-Economic Research Programme.

74. Lynge E, Olsen AH, Fracheboud J, Patnick J. 2003. Reporting of performance indicators of mammography screening in Europe. *Eur J Cancer Prev* 12(3):213-222.

75. Maguire P. 2003. Is an access crisis on the horizon in mammography? *ACP Observer*.

76. Mainiero MB. 2003. Breast-Imaging Specialists Are More Efficient Than General Radiologists at Reading Mammograms. *103rd Annual American Roentgen Ray Society Meeting*. San Diego, CA.

77. Marbella AM, Layde PM. 2001. Racial trends in age-specific breast cancer mortality rates in US women. *Am J Public Health* 91(1):118-121.

78. Marshall MN, Shekelle PG, Leatherman S, Brook RH. 2000. The public release of performance data: what do we expect to gain? A review of the evidence. *JAMA* 283(14):1866-1874.

79. Meadows S, Wingert P, Rosenberg D, Carmichael M, Johnson D, Childress S, Sinderbrand R, Breslau K, Shenfeld H. 2003. Civil Wars. *Newsweek*. Pp. 43-51.

80. Mehta TS. 2003. Current uses of ultrasound in the evaluation of the breast. *Radiol Clin North Am* 41(4):841-856.

81. Meyer JE, Eberlein TJ, Stomper PC, Sonnenfeld MR. 1990. Biopsy of occult breast lesions. Analysis of 1261 abnormalities. *JAMA* 263(17):2341-2343.

82. Miller AM, Champion VL. 1997. Attitudes about breast cancer and mammography: racial, income, and educational differences. *Women Health* 26(1):41-63.

83. Mitchell J, Lannin DR, Mathews HF, Swanson MS. 2002. Religious beliefs and breast cancer screening. *J Womens Health (Larchmt)* 11(10):907-915.

84. Mitka M. 2003. Researchers seek mammography alternatives. *JAMA* 290(4):450-451.

85. Monsees B. 2002. Is the GAO report on mammography correct? *SBI News*.

86. Monsees B. 2002. The breast imaging profession: take my job, please! *SBI News*.

87. Mourad WG. 2003, May 5. Mammography equipment evaluations and the annual survey—is your equipment up to the task? Accessed March 24, 2004. Web Page. Available at: http://www.fda.gov/cdrh/mammography/scorecard-article4.html.

88. National Cancer Institute. 2004. *Fifth National Forum on Biomedical Imaging in Oncology Meeting Summary*. Bethesda, MD.

89. National Health Service. Cancer Screening Programmes. 2003. *NHS Breast Screening Programme Annual Review 2003*.

90. Newman LA, Mason J, Cote D, Vin Y, Carolin K, Bouwman D, Colditz GA. 2002. African-American ethnicity, socioeconomic status, and breast cancer survival: a meta-analysis of 14 studies involving over 10,000 African-American and 40,000 White American patients with carcinoma of the breast. *Cancer* 94(11):2844-2854.

91. Oluwole SF, Ali AO, Adu A, Blane BP, Barlow B, Oropeza R, Freeman HP. 2003. Impact of a cancer screening program on breast cancer stage at diagnosis in a medically underserved urban community. *J Am Coll Surg* 196(2):180-188.

92. Pal S. 2003, November 30. Women with genetic history of breast cancer benefit from MR screening. Accessed February 19, 2004. Web Page. Available at: http://www.auntminnie.com/default.asp?Sec=rca&Sub=rsna_2003&pag=dis&ItemId=60243&stm=November+30%2C+2003+pal.

93. Pallarito K. 2003, February 27. Spike in malpractice premiums hurting access to care—survery. Accessed February 28, 2003. Web Page. Available at: http://www.auntminnie.com/default.asp?Sec=sup&Sub=imc&Pag=dis&ItemId=57516.

94. Pasko T, Seidman B (American Medical Association). 2002. *Physician Characteristics and Distribution in the US, 2002-2003 Edition.* Chicago, IL: AMA Press.
95. Philadelphia Black Women's Health Project. 2002. Detection, Diagnosis, and Prevention of Breast Cancer. Accessed June 9, 2003. Web Page. Available at: http://www.blackwomenshealthproject.org/aabreastcancer.htm.
96. Physician Insurers Association of America. 1995. *PIAA Breast Cancer Study.* Rockville, MD: PIAA.
97. Physician Insurers Association of America. 2002. *PIAA Breast Cancer Study.* Rockville, MD: PIAA.
98. Pollack A. 2003, November 16. Who's reading your x-ray? *The New York Times.* 3. P. 1.
99. Russell A, Langlois T, Johnson G, Trentham-Dietz A, Remington P. 1999. Increasing gap in breast cancer mortality between black and white women. *WMJ* 98(8):37-39.
100. Sant M. 2001. Differences in stage and therapy for breast cancer across Europe. *Int J Cancer* 93(6):894-901.
101. Sant M, Allemani C, Berrino F, Coleman MP, Aareleid T, Chaplain G, Coebergh JW, Colonna M, Crosignani P, Danzon A, Federico M, Gafa L, Grosclaude P, Hedelin G, Mace-Lesech J, Garcia CM, Moller H, Paci E, Raverdy N, Tretarre B, Williams EM. 2004. Breast carcinoma survival in Europe and the United States. *Cancer* 100(4):715-722.
102. Sant M, Capocaccia R, Coleman MP, Berrino F, Gatta G, Micheli A, Verdecchia A, Faivre J, Hakulinen T, Coebergh JW, Martinez-Garcia C, Forman D, Zappone A. 2001. Cancer survival increases in Europe, but international differences remain wide. *Eur J Cancer* 37(13):1659-1667.
103. Schnall MD. 2001. Application of magnetic resonance imaging to early detection of breast cancer. *Breast Cancer Res* 3(1):17-21.
104. Schnall MD. 2003. Breast MR imaging. *Radiol Clin North Am* 41(1):43-50.
105. Sickles EA, Wolverton DE, Dee KE. 2002. Performance parameters for screening and diagnostic mammography: specialist and general radiologists. *Radiology* 224(3):861-869.
106. Skaane P, Young K, Skjennald A. 2003. Population-based mammography screening: comparison of screen-film and full-field digital mammography with soft-copying reading—Oslo I study. *Radiology* 229(3):877-884.
107. Smith-Bindman R, Chu PW, Miglioretti DL, Sickles EA, Blanks R, Ballard-Barbash R, Bobo JK, Lee NC, Wallis MG, Patnick J, Kerlikowske K. 2003. Comparison of screening mammography in the United States and the United Kingdom. *JAMA* 290(16):2129-2137.
108. Smith RA, Wender RC. 2004. Cancer screening and the periodic health examination. *Cancer* 100(8):1553-1557.
109. Society of Breast Imaging. 2003, October 24. SBI response to JAMA article. Web Page. Available at: http://www.sbi-online.org/JAMA_Response.htm.
110. Studdert DM, Mello MM, Brennan TA. 2004. Medical malpractice. *N Engl J Med* 350(3):283-292.
111. Sumkin JH, Klaman HM, Graham M, Ruskauff T, Gennari RC, King JL, Klym AH, Ganott MA, Gur D. 2003. Prescreening mammography by technologists: a preliminary assessment. *Am J Roentgenol* 180(1):253-256.
112. Sunshine JH, Burkhardt JH. 2000. Radiology groups' workload in relative value units and factors affecting it. *Radiology* 214(3):815-822.
113. Sunshine JH, Cypel YS, Schepps B. 2002. Diagnostic radiologists in 2000: basic characteristics, practices, and issues related to the radiologist shortage. *Am J Roentgenol* 178(2):291-301.

114. Surveillance Epidemiology and End Results (SEER) Program (www.seer.cancer.gov). 2003. *SEER*Stat Database: Incidence—SEER 9 Registry Public-Use, Nov. 2002 Submission (1973-2000)*. National Cancer Institute, DCCPS, Surveillance Research Program, Cancer Statistics Branch.

115. Tabar L, Yen MF, Vitak B, Chen HH, Smith RA, Duffy SW. 2003. Mammography service screening and mortality in breast cancer patients: 20-year follow-up before and after introduction of screening. *Lancet* 361(9367):1405-1410.

116. Taplin SH, Ichikawa LE, Kerlikowske K, Ernster VL, Rosenberg RD, Yankaskas BC, Carney PA, Geller BM, Urban N, Dignan MB, Barlow WE, Ballard-Barbash R, Sickles EA. 2002. Concordance of breast imaging reporting and data system assessments and management recommendations in screening mammography. *Radiology* 222(2):529-535.

117. Trevino M. 2003. Air Force Teleradiology Project aims to alleviate staff shortages: plan could even out workflow and improve access to subspecialty reads. Accessed May 13, 2002. Web Page. Available at: http://www.diagnosticimaging.com/pacsweb/cover/cover05090202.shtml.

118. U.S. Food and Drug Administration. 2003, June 3. About Mammography Quality Standards Act (MQSA). Web Page. Available at: http://www.fda.gov/cdrh/mammography/mqsa-rev.html.

119. United States General Accounting Office. 2002. *Mammography—Capacity Generally Exists to Deliver Services*. Washington, DC: GAO.

120. United States General Accounting Office. 2003. *Medical Malpractice: Implications of Rising Premiums on Access to Health Care*. Washington, DC: GAO.

121. Viehweg P, Lampe D, Buchmann J, Heywang-Kobrunner SH. 2000. In situ and minimally invasive breast cancer: morphologic and kinetic features on contrast-enhanced MR imaging. *MAGMA* 11(3):129-137.

122. Wivell G, Denton ER, Eve CB, Inglis JC, Harvey I. 2003. Can radiographers read screening mammograms? *Clin Radiol* 58(1):63-67.

123. Wojcik BE, Spinks MK, Stein CR. 2003. Effects of screening mammography on the comparative survival rates of African American, white, and Hispanic beneficiaries of a comprehensive health care system. *Breast J* 9(3):175-183.

124. Wooding D. 2003, July 8. PERsonal perFORmance in Mammographic Screening. Accessed May 12, 2004. Web Page. Available at: http://ibs.derby.ac.uk/performs/index.shtml.

125. Zheng B, Hardesty LA, Poller WR, Sumkin JH, Golla S. 2003. Mammography with computer-aided detection: reproducibility assessment initial experience. *Radiology* 228(1):58-62.

4

Understanding Breast Cancer Risk

Every woman is at some risk for breast cancer, but the degree of risk for individual women ranges from very low to very high. Understanding risk is important because it affects medical decisions—from whether a symptom-free woman should have a mammogram to how intensively to treat existing breast disease to how aggressively to pursue prevention strategies, such as the use of anti-estrogens or prophylactic mastectomy and removal of a woman's ovaries.

If a screening technology existed that was so simple and so inexpensive that it could be used often enough to detect even fast-growing cancers, so reliable that no supplemental screening or diagnostic tools would be needed, and so convenient and comfortable that every woman would be willing and able to undergo frequent screening, then every woman could be screened and risk assessment would not be necessary. Unfortunately, not a single one of these conditions is met by current screening options for any type of cancer. Nor are there any tools on the horizon that promise to meet these conditions in the near term. Risk assessment is and will almost certainly remain an essential component of early detection of breast cancer.

Risk factors are identified (and new ones continue to be identified) through epidemiologic research studies, which typically measure the *relative risk* of the factors being studied (see Box 4-1). If a woman has a factor that is associated with a relative risk greater than 1, then—all other things being equal—her risk will be higher than the population average. If she does not have that factor, her risk will be lower.

Risk, or *absolute risk*, is a measure of the probability of developing cancer over a specified time interval. This is sometimes expressed as the

BOX 4-1
Relative Versus Absolute Risk

A *relative risk* compares the risk of disease among people with a particular risk factor to the risk among people without that risk factor. If the relative risk is above 1.0, then risk is higher among those with the risk factor than those without. Relative risks below 1.0 indicate a protective effect, or lower risk, associated with a particular factor.

Relative risks are useful for comparisons, but they do not provide information about the *absolute* amount of additional risk experienced by the group with the risk factor in question. For example, current users of combination estrogen and progestin hormone replacement therapy (HRT) have a relative risk of 1.26, or a 26 percent increased risk. Although this increased risk may seem substantial, it proves to be less so in absolute terms because of the very low risk of breast cancer among young women in general.

Among 10,000 women who have been using HRT for 5.2 years, 38 breast cancers would be expected to be diagnosed. Among 10,000 similar women who never used HRT, 30 cases would be expected over the same period. Therefore, the 26 percent increased relative risk results in an absolute risk of only 8 additional breast cancer cases per 10,000 women over a period greater than 5.2 years.

Adapted from the American Cancer Society, *Breast Cancer Facts and Figures 2003-2004*.[1]

lifetime risk, or the risk to, say, age 70. Or the risk may be expressed as the probability that a woman of a given age will develop cancer in the next 10 years.

The statistic that one in eight women who survive to age 85 will develop some form of breast cancer in her lifetime is alarming, but this masks the important influence of age on risk (Table 4-1). Fewer than 5 percent of invasive breast cancers occur in women under age 40, whereas over three-quarters are in women over the age 50.

Numerous case-control and cohort studies over the past several decades have identified various factors, some of which have been shown to be consistently associated with risk, such as reproductive hormones, and others that are less consistent, such as dietary factors (Box 4-2, Table 4-2). Risk factors such as body mass index and dietary fat have been associated with specific types of breast cancer whose growth is stimulated by the sex hormones estrogen and progesterone.[15] Family history increases risk although not as much as some women believe. Eighty-nine percent of women who develop breast cancer have no family history among their first-degree relatives (mother, daughter, or sister).[16] The amount of increased risk depends on how close a relation the affected relative is, the age at which they developed breast cancer, and the number of relatives affected.

TABLE 4-1 Age-Specific Probabilities of Developing Breast Cancer[1]

If current age is	Then the probability of developing breast cancer in the *next 10 years* is:	or 1 in:
20	0.05%	2,152
30	0.40%	251
40	1.45%	69
50	2.78%	36
60	3.81%	26
70	4.31%	23

BOX 4-2
Epidemiological Methods for Discovering Genetic Links to Disease

Case-control studies are retrospective observational studies in which investigators identify one group of patients with a specified outcome (cases) and another group without the specified outcome (controls). Investigators then compare the histories of the cases and the controls to determine the extent to which each had the possible risk factor being investigated.

Cohort studies are observational studies in which outcomes in a group of patients who possess the possible risk factor being tested (the cohort) are compared with outcomes in a control group of patients who do not possess the possible risk factor. For example, the occurrence of breast cancer would be compared between two groups of women neither of whom have breast cancer at the beginning of the study; one of the groups would possess the possible risk factor and the other group would not. The number of new cases of breast cancer in the two groups would be compared over time.

Approximately 70 percent of women who develop breast cancer have the type of cancer called hormone receptor positive, which means that the cancerous tissue contains receptors for estrogen and/or progesterone. This association may, therefore, prove to be more relevant among women with elevated levels of these hormones, for example, premenopausal women or women using hormone replacement therapy.[17,40,46] More research into risk profiles of such subtypes of breast cancers may elucidate a clearer connection between risk factors and the development of breast cancers. Although many factors that influence risk have been identified, it is still not possible to determine which women will develop breast cancer and which will not.

TABLE 4-2 Risk Factors for Breast Cancer

Risk Factor	Relative Risk	Category at Risk	Comparison Category
Germ-line mutation	200?	Heterozygous for BRCA1, age <40	Not heterozygous for BRCA1, age <40
	15?	Heterozygous for BRCA1, ages 60-69	Not heterozygous for BRCA1, ages 60-69
Cytological findings (fine-needle aspiration; nipple aspiration fluid)	18.1	Proliferation with atypia and positive family history	No abnormality detected
	4.9-5	Proliferation with atypia	No abnormality detected
	2.5	Proliferation without atypia*	No abnormality detected
Other histologic findings	17.3	Ductal carcinoma in situ	No abnormality detected
	16.4	Lobular carcinoma in situ	No abnormality detected
Positive breast biopsy	11	Hyperplasia with atypia and positive family history	No hyperplasia, negative family history
	5.3	Hyperplasia with atypia	No hyperplasia
	1.9	Hyperplasia without atypia	No hyperplasia
Past history of breast cancer	6.8	Invasive breast carcinoma	No history of invasive breast carcinoma
Current age	5.8	65 or older	Less than 65
Radiation exposure	5.2	Radiation therapy for Hodgkin's disease	No exposure
	1.6	Repeated fluoroscopy	No exposure

TABLE 4-2 Continued

Risk Factor	Relative Risk	Category at Risk	Comparison Category
Breast density	4[7,72]	More than 75% of breast is mammo-graphically dense	Less than 25% of breast is mammo-graphically dense
Family history	3.6	Two 1st-degree relatives with breast cancer	No 1st- or 2nd-degree relative with breast cancer
	3.3	1st-degree relative with premenopausal breast cancer	No 1st- or 2nd-degree relative with breast cancer
	1.8	1st-degree relative 50 years or older with postmenopausal breast cancer	No 1st- or 2nd-degree relative with breast cancer
	1.5	2nd-degree relative with breast cancer	No 1st- or 2nd-degree relative with breast cancer
Age at first birth	1.7-1.9	Nulliparous or 1st child after 30	1st child before 20
Late menopause	1.2-1.5	Older than 55 years	Younger than 45
Hormone replacement therapy [65, ≠]	2.70	Current user of estrogen and progestin	Never used
	1.96	Current user of estrogen only	Never used
Early menarche	1.3	Younger than 12 years	Older than 15 years
Alcohol intake	1.2	2 drinks per day	Nondrinker
Body mass index	1.2	80th percentile	20th percentile

*There is controversy over whether pathologic hyperplasia detected in breast biopsy samples is directly equivalent to cytologic hyperplasia detected in samples obtained through fine-needle aspiration or nipple aspiration.

?These relative risks are subject to ascertainment bias and may overestimate the true risk associated with germline mutations in BRCA genes.[5]

≠The data for hormone replacement therapy was updated due to the release of a new study after the original risk of hormone replacement was presented by Singletary et al., 2003.[64]

SOURCE: Adapted from Singletary and colleagues.[64]

BREAST DENSITY

Mammographic breast density may be the most undervalued and underused risk factor in studies investigating breast cancer.[13,38,73] It is a heritable trait, although the contribution of breast density to increased risk is independent of the risk associated with BRCA1 and BRCA2 mutations.[7] Despite the ethnic variation in breast density, breast cancer risk rises with increasing breast density for each of the ethnic groups recently analyzed by Ursin and colleagues; the groups they analyzed included African Americans, Asian Americans, and non-Latino whites.[69] A 2002 study reported that the average relative risk of breast cancer for women in the highest category of percentage of dense tissue compared with those in the lowest category is about 4.[7] Previous studies reported relative risk estimates ranging from 2 to 6, with the majority of those studies reporting a relative risk of 4 or more (reviewed by Boyd and colleagues, 2002).[7] The genetic factors that determine breast density may also play a role in breast cancer.[73]

GENETIC RISK FACTORS

Before a cell becomes cancerous, it must accumulate a "critical mass" of molecular changes that alter key genes or their functions. The end result is a loss of the normal molecular controls on the cell's growth and differentiation. Some of the cellular changes that make a woman susceptible to developing breast cancer can be inherited. Such germ-line mutations are believed to account for the striking incidence of breast cancer in certain families, especially breast cancer that develops in both a woman's breasts and/or at a young age. But less than 10 percent of all breast cancer cases are thought to stem from inherited mutations, such as BRCA1 and BRCA2, that individually increase risk by a substantial amount.[41]

The majority of breast cancer cases are due to an accumulation of cellular (somatic) changes that occur during a patient's lifetime. This is why age is such a significant factor in most cancers—because the longer a person lives, the more time there is for mutations to accumulate. These changes are not inherited, but rather stem from factors such as exposure to carcinogens in the external environment, or from excessive or untimely exposure to breast cancer-promoting substances within the body, such as circulating hormones, or simply because of random mutations that occur during cell division. Inherited genes can also influence genetic mutations that occur during a person's lifetime if they increase the susceptibility of *other* genes to mutation. For example, the ability of a cell to correct mistakes in gene replication that occur during cell division is diminished when the genes that normally support DNA repair have mutated. As a result, mutations accumulate faster than they would otherwise.

BRCA Genes and the Shortcomings of Genetic Testing

Studies of families with an exceptionally large number of members with breast and ovarian cancer led to the discovery of the first two inherited breast cancer susceptibility genes. By searching for genetic markers shared by all affected family members (linkage analysis), researchers in the 1990s were able to pinpoint two breast cancer susceptibility genes, BRCA1 and BRCA2.[41] Both genes are rare, but they confer very high risk. Both genes code for proteins that are thought to play a role in the repair of genetic defects, and therefore mutations that decrease their ability to repair or limit the proliferation of cells with genetic defects will increase the susceptibility to breast cancer.[41]

Initial studies suggested that women who tested positive for either mutation would have nearly a 90 percent chance of developing breast cancer by age 70.[29] A recent study found that Ashkenazi Jewish women who carry one of the three BRCA1 and BRCA2 mutations associated with Ashkenazi ancestry and who reach age 80 have an 82 percent risk of developing breast cancer; those who reach age 60 have a 55 percent risk.[45]

These studies indicate that BRCA1 and BRCA2 tests would be a useful clinical tool to identify women at high risk for breast cancer, but the lifetime probability estimates for developing breast cancer among women who test positive for mutations of BRCA1 or BRCA2 (also called penetrance of the genes) is variable and often overestimated. Lifetime risks of breast cancer in women in the general population who test positive for BRCA1 (that is, women who are not preselected on the basis of a family history of breast cancer) could be as low as 45 percent, and 26 percent in such women who test positive for BRCA2 (reviewed by Begg, 2002).[5] Other studies based on women from the general population produced higher penetrance estimates, but none was as high as those seen in women from high-risk families.

Overestimates of the penetrance of BRCA1 or BRCA2 result from sampling bias. Studies of women who have breast cancer and are known to have a family history of breast cancer will generate higher estimates of penetrance than studies that start with women in the general population and assess the overall percentage of women who test positive for BRCA mutations and develop breast cancer. Women with BRCA mutations who develop breast cancer usually have several other risk factors that are likely to be shared with their relatives. These relatives could be at somewhat greater than average risk of developing breast cancer, even if they do not test positive for BRCA mutations. Consequently, the percentage of these women who test positive and develop breast cancer is likely to be greater than that of women who test positive in lower-risk populations.[5]

Evidence shows that environmental factors also play a role in determining the penetrance of BRCA genes. Some studies find that a woman's reproductive history can modify the penetrance of BRCA1 or BRCA2 (reviewed by Burke and Austin, 2002).[10] Other studies find that cancer risk is relatively greater in younger women who test positive for BRCA mutations than in older women.[10,45] Birth cohort and physical exercise also have been shown to partially mitigate the influence of BRCA1.[45] Ashkenazi Jewish women born with one of the three mutations associated with Ashkenazi ancestry who were born before 1940 have an average lower likelihood of developing breast cancer than similar women born after 1940. In the same study, women with those mutations who had been physically active as teenagers and were not obese as young adults showed an approximate risk reduction of 10 years—that is, a 60-year-old woman who was not obese at age 21 and with a history of physical activity had approximately the same average risk as a 50-year old woman with a history of obesity and no physical activity. Such a change in penetrance over time is likely due to the influence of a changing environment.

As Wylie Burke and Melissa Austin summarize in an editorial in the *Journal of the National Cancer Institute*:

> The most important implication of penetrance studies should perhaps be to temper our expectations for predictive genetic tests. Without a healthy respect for the many factors that may influence penetrance, we will continue to overestimate the risk conferred by BRCA 1 and BRCA 2 mutations alone and, thus, miss opportunities to develop truly effective prevention strategies for women who are genetically susceptible to breast cancer that are based on a broad understanding of causative factors.[10]

The wide range of penetrance estimates complicates decisions for preventive interventions like prophylactic mastectomy or tamoxifen chemoprevention, although even the lowest penetrance estimates might be high enough to suggest that women who test positive for BRCA mutations should be screened more aggressively. However, one study found that annual mammograms and biannual physical exams were less sensitive, and detected tumors at later stages in women with BRCA mutations than in women at greater than average risk for breast cancer who lack the mutations.[9] Furthermore, studies have found that BRCA2-deficient cells are hypersensitive to the effects of radiation,[54] so there is concern (but so far no evidence) that women, especially those with BRCA2 mutations, might be susceptible to radiation-induced genetic defects and cancer.

Another problem is that researchers have detected more than 2,000 mutations of BRCA1 or BRCA2,[54] but the clinical significance of these is not yet known; some may not influence breast cancer risk. Consequently, more than 1 in 10 BRCA tests yields inconclusive results because the clinical significance of the specific mutations detected by the tests is unknown.[2]

Women also may test negative for mutations in BRCA1 or BRCA2 and still harbor a BRCA mutation that increases their risk of breast cancer because this mutation falls outside the range of mutations detected by current BRCA1 or BRCA2 tests.[66] There is only one commercially available test for BRCA mutations. It costs about $450, and tests only for the three Ashkenazi mutations. A test for all of the known mutations in BRCA1 and BRCA2 genes would cost nearly $3,000 (Personal communication, W.A. Hockett III, Myriad Genetics, Inc., Vice President of Corporate Communications for Myriad Genetics, Inc., December 2, 2003). Testing negatively for BRCA mutations also does not rule out the possibility that a woman with a strong family history for breast cancer has inherited mutations in other genes that increase her breast cancer risk.[63]

Perhaps the biggest limitation is that less than one-quarter of 1 percent of women in the general population are believed to harbor BRCA mutations,[18,32,57] and mutations in either of the BRCA genes account for only 2 to 3 percent of all breast cancers (reviewed by Wooster and Weber, 2003).[71] Because more than 10 percent of women will develop breast cancer in their lifetimes, BRCA tests clearly will be a small piece in the puzzle of identifying individual risk.

Many more genetic risk factors have been published than have been verified. A literature review of epidemiological studies that assessed associations between polymorphisms and risk of cancer found that only a small proportion of the published studies were large and population-based.[35] Because studies based on small samples sizes are prone to false-positive or false-negative findings, large and well-designed studies of genetic risk are essential. Studies that analyze multiple genes or polymorphisms would be especially useful in improving our understanding of breast cancer.

Polymorphisms

The search for other genetic markers that determine breast cancer susceptibility is ongoing and has focused on subtle DNA changes, known as polymorphisms, that are shared by many people, and that may affect susceptibility to carcinogens and cancer promoters in the environment or the body, or affect the body's immune response to cancer cells. Each polymorphism probably increases or decreases breast cancer risk by only a small amount, perhaps a few percentage points. But because these polymorphisms are found in all people, their impact on breast cancer risk may be considerably greater than that of the relatively rare BRCA mutations,[22] and the combined impact of several polymorphisms on breast cancer risk could be substantial.

A compilation of various polymorphisms might enable the stratification of some women into low- or high-risk breast cancer groups. However, research on genetic polymorphisms that influence breast cancer susceptibility is in its infancy, and many more studies are needed before they are useful in stratifying women into breast cancer risk groups.[22]

Researchers seeking to discover polymorphisms that boost breast cancer risk have tended to focus their search on the most biologically plausible genes, such as those known to be involved in the metabolism of carcinogens, or the regulation of estrogen levels, or that are the normal variants (proto-oncogenes) of genes known to cause cancer (oncogenes). (Proto-oncogenes are involved in the regulation of normal cell growth and differentiation.) For the most part, reports of polymorphisms that affect susceptibility to breast cancer have been based on relatively small studies.

Table 4-3 presents the results of meta-analyses of studies on genetic polymorphisms that have been linked to breast cancer risk. Precise and validated estimations of the genetic risk associated with these polymorphisms will require large case-control studies. Of 35 polymorphisms in 19 different genes described in at least two breast cancer studies, only 13 polymorphisms in 10 genes showed an association with breast cancer. Only TNF-alpha and a variant of the HSP-70 protein show odds ratios higher than 3. Although an odds ratio of 3 or higher is a common benchmark of an important risk factor, this is still much lower than what is needed for screening tests, and would involve high false-positive or -negative rates, or both. Thus, although statistically significant at the population level, such a risk factor would not, by itself, be helpful in predicting individual risk. As of this writing, except for BRCA1 and BRCA2, no single genetic risk factor predicts the development of breast cancer well enough to be used on its own for individual risk stratification.

Relatively little research has been performed on combinations of polymorphisms which are addressed in only a few studies in breast cancer patients. Because the products of several genes interact (for example, nearly half of the genes reviewed by de Jong and colleagues play a role in estrogen metabolism), interactions between the genes are likely. Some investigators believe a whole genome screen would be the ideal method to detect new breast cancer susceptibility genes. This method, however, is still too expensive to carry out in large study populations.[22] Until this is feasible, it would be useful to collect data on appropriately sized, well-described study populations.[22] Analysis of several (or all) of the polymorphisms already known to be associated with breast cancer in the same population may increase our understanding of the etiology of breast cancer and permit better risk assessments (reviewed in 2001 by de Jong).[22]

TABLE 4-3 Genes Other Than BRCA1 and BRCA2 Involved in Breast Cancer Susceptibility[22]

Gene	Description	Effect on Breast Cancer Risk	Odds Ratio*
Rare genetic syndromes with increased breast cancer risk			
Tp53	Mutation of this gene causes Li-Fraumeni syndrome and is characterized by an increased risk of several cancers. Expressed in three different variants.	Associated with increased risk, particularly in white populations. Risk not shown in Hispanic, African-American, or Pakistani study participants.	1.08 CI 0.88-1.13
ATM	Mutation of this gene causes ataxia telangiectasia, a neurodegenerative disease characterized by lack of coordination, red lesions, and immune defects.	Few patients survive to an age at which breast cancer occurs, but a role in increased risk is plausible and has been shown in some small studies.	N/A
PTEN	Mutation of this gene causes Cowden syndrome, characterized by malformations resembling tumors composed of mature tissues, especially of the skin, mucous membranes, breast, and thyroid.	Not likely to have an effect in the sense of classical heredity. Unknown if PTEN plays a role in sporadic breast cancer susceptibility.	N/A
LKB1	Mutation of this gene causes Peutz-Jeghers syndrome and is characterized by freckle-like spots on the lips, mouth and fingers and benign polyps in the intestines.	Only likely to play a role in increased risk among those patients with Peutz-Jeghers syndrome.	N/A
Low penetrant cancer susceptibility genes: *Proto-oncogenes*			
HRAS1	Protein product is a protein kinase that transmits signals from growth factor receptors. When mutated can result in abnormal cell cycle control.	Moderately associated with increased risk.	2.04 CI 1.73-2.41

continued

TABLE 4-3 Continued

Gene	Description	Effect on Breast Cancer Risk	Odds Ratio*
L-myc	Protein product is a transcription factor that helps initiate cell division. When mutated can result in accelerated cell division and tissue growth.	No association found.	1.12 CI 0.77-1.63
TGFBR1*6a	TGFBR1*6a is a variant of one of the receptors through which Transforming Growth Factor (TGF) exerts its actions. TGF-B is the most potent naturally occurring inhibitor of cell growth.	A high-frequency, low-penetrance allele that is moderately associated with increased risk.[42]	1.48 CI 1.11-1.96[42]

Low penetrant cancer susceptibility genes: *Metabolic pathways*

Gene	Description	Effect on Breast Cancer Risk	Odds Ratio*
NAT1/NAT2	Protein product is an enzyme that can bioactivate several known carcinogens through acetylation.	No association found.	1.13 CI 0.91-1.39
GSTM1	Protein product is an enzyme responsible for the metabolism of a broad range of chemicals and carcinogens.	Marginally significant increase in risk.	1.13 CI 1.02-1.26
GSTP1	Protein product is an enzyme that plays an important role in detoxification.	Appears to play a role in increased risk in a few small studies.	1.19 CI 0.91-1.56
GSTT1	Protein product is an enzyme found in red blood cells; may detoxify some synthetic chemicals.	No association found.	1.04 CI 0.86-1.25
CYP1A1	Protein product is an enzyme responsible for metabolizing estrogens and polycyclic aromatic hydrocarbons.	m1 polymorphism: Small increase in risk in the white population. m2 polymorphism: Moderately increased risk in postmenopausal women.	0.99 CI 0.83-1.19 1.18 CI 0.94-1.48

TABLE 4-3 Continued

Gene	Description	Effect on Breast Cancer Risk	Odds Ratio*
CYP1B1	Protein product is an enzyme responsible for metabolizing polycyclic aromatic hydrocarbons (3 variants codon 119, 432, and 453).	No association found in pooled data from several studies.	1.62 CI 1.15-2.29
CYP2D6	Protein product is an enzyme involved in the metabolism of commonly prescribed drugs including codeine.	May play a role in increased risk.	1.19 CI 0.97-1.45

Low penetrant cancer susceptibility genes: *Estrogen pathway genes*

Gene	Description	Effect on Breast Cancer Risk	Odds Ratio*
CYP17	Protein product is an enzyme that mediates formation of estrogens, progesterones, and androgens.	No association found in analysis of several studies. However, because age was not accounted for, increased risk for breast cancer in young women cannot be excluded.	0.99 CI 0.88-1.11
CYP19	Protein product is an enzyme that converts androgens into estrogens and maintains the local level of estrogen.	Might play a minor role.	1.15 CI 0.72-1.85
ER	Protein product is a receptor that binds and transfers estrogen to the nucleus; regulates the production of several transcription factors.	Only five relatively small studies examined polymorphisms in the *ER* gene. Due to a small sample size, an association cannot be confirmed or excluded.	0.84 CI 0.40-1.78
PR	Protein product is a receptor that binds and transfers progesterone to the nucleus; regulates the production of several transcription factors.	Results showed a decrease in risk.	0.95 CI 0.78-1.16

continued

TABLE 4-3 Continued

Gene	Description	Effect on Breast Cancer Risk	Odds Ratio*
AR	Protein product is a receptor that binds and transfers androgen to the nucleus; regulates the production of several transcription factors.	Does not play a major role.	N/A
COMT	Protein product is an enzyme that degrades catecholamine transmitters including estrogens, dopamine, epinephrine, and norepinephrine.	No increase in risk.	0.92 CI 0.76-1.10
UGT1A1	Protein product is an enzyme that helps maintain levels of estrogens and enhances the elimination of many synthetic chemicals.	No association found.	0.99 CI 0.80-1.24

Low penetrant cancer susceptibility genes: *Immunomodulatory pathway genes*

Gene	Description	Effect on Breast Cancer Risk	Odds Ratio*
TNF-alpha	Protein product is a cytokine that stimulates inflammation and immunological response to tumor cells.	Association with increased risk shown in one small study. Additional data are required to define the precise association.	3.49 CI 1.62-7.51
HSP70	Protein product is chaperone protein that regulates structure, localization, and turnover of cellular proteins.	HSP70-hom: Increased risk associated.	3.56 CI 1.26-10.01
		HSP70-2: No association found.	1.74 CI 0.55-5.52

Low penetrant cancer susceptibility genes: *Iron metabolism genes*

Gene	Description	Effect on Breast Cancer Risk	Odds Ratio*
HFE/HH	Mutation of this gene can cause iron accumulation resulting in cirrhosis of the liver, diabetes, abnormal skin pigmentation, and heart failure.	Do not play major roles in increased risk.	N/A

TABLE 4-3 Continued

Gene	Description	Effect on Breast Cancer Risk	Odds Ratio*
Other genes			
VDR	Protein product is a receptor that acts as a transcriptional regulatory factor and can stimulate cell differentiation.	Study results are contradictory; association remains unclear.	0.95 CI 0.74-1.20
APC	Tumor suppressor gene that arrests the cell cycle and prevents further cell division and unregulated growth. When mutated the gene is associated with colorectal cancer.	Probably does not play a role in increased risk of breast cancer.	N/A

*Odds ratios for only heterozygous genotype for most common variant alleles are listed (CI= 95% confidence interval).

MANAGING RISK

Individualized Risk Prediction

Understanding that women do not have uniform risk for breast cancer suggests the possibility that they could be stratified into high- or low-risk groups. In theory, such stratification should indicate which women are most likely to benefit from more intensive screening for breast cancer (Figure 4-1). For example, most women would gain no medical benefit from screening before age 40 or from twice-yearly screening, but a small minority could. Conversely, many women could safely be screened for breast cancer only every 2 years, or perhaps even at longer intervals. And even though men can develop breast cancer, it occurs too rarely to warrant mammography screening for men in the general population (Box 4-3). The goal of improving risk assessment is to stratify breast cancer detection strategies with the aim of increasing survival in high-risk women while decreasing cost and complications in low-risk women.[23] The challenge lies in developing a more refined understanding of how to assess risk in individual women, and that depends on data from well-designed, large-scale epidemiological studies.

Mammography screening guidelines already take into account two of the most significant risk factors, gender and age. But we could do much

Breast cancer risk ranges from low to high	Different screening strategies	Outcomes

Most screening guidelines recommend annual mammograms for every woman over 50.

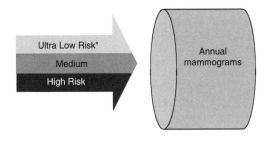

Some women will receive no medical benefit, because:

(a) they are not susceptible to breast cancer, or
(b) their breast cancers were not detected early enough for life-saving treatment

For every, 1,000 women over age 50 screened, mammograms will reveal approximately 3-5 cases of invasive or in situ breast cancer (DCIS).

Better risk assessment tools would permit a more individually-tailored, or stratified, approach to breast cancer screening.

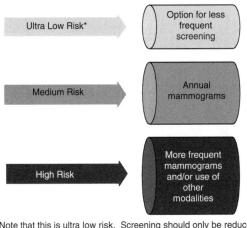

• Fewer women will undergo unnecessary procedures. Their personal concerns about breast cancer will be reduced.

• Fewer mammograms can reduce health care costs.

• Fewer mammograms would allow more resources to be devoted to improving quality and consistency of interpretations.

• More intensive screening for high-risk women should result in fewer missed cancers and more lives saved.

* Note that this is ultra low risk. Screening should only be reduced in cases where it has been demonstrated definitively that less frequent screening will not increase mortality, and it is important that women and their physicians not be misled into underestimating risk.

FIGURE 4-1 Breast cancer screening based on stratified risk assessments.

BOX 4-3
Male Breast Cancer Occurs, but
Too Rarely to Screen with Mammography

Breast cancer is not only a woman's disease. Each year about 1,300 men in the United States are diagnosed with new cases of invasive breast cancer, and about 400 will die of breast cancer.[1] The American Cancer Society reports that breast cancer is 100 times less common in men than women, and accounts for less than one-quarter of 1 percent of cancer deaths among men.

The symptoms and types of breast cancers found in men are similar to those found in women, except for lobular cancers, which men do not develop. Many breast cancers among men are found only after the late onset of cancer symptoms are identified as malignant through biopsy without performing a mammogram. The prognosis for men with breast cancer was once thought to be worse than for women, but this is not true. Stage for stage, the survival rates are equal. With the exception of BRCA1 mutations and other gender-specific factors such as menarche and childbirth, breast cancer risk factors for men are similar to those in women, with older age and history of cancer being the predominant factors. However, the absolute risk of breast cancer is so low that screening mammography is not warranted in men. It is possible, but unlikely, that a risk factor for male breast cancer would be discovered that was so informative that it would identify a group of men whose risk of breast cancer was high enough to warrant screening, but current knowledge does not support the search for such a hypothetical factor. Mammography may, however, be useful in screening for recurrence or development of a new cancer in men who have already had breast cancer. And, clearly, physicians should be aware that although it is rare, male breast cancer does occur and any single signs or symptoms of breast cancer in a man should be investigated.

---

better. Earlier attempts to base screening strategies on factors other than gender and age, such as family history or reproductive factors, have not been successful, largely because the relative risks of those factors are too low (reviewed by Smith, 1999;[16] IOM, 2001[41]). A risk factor that is used to stratify screening strategies must identify enough added risk that it is reliably linked to different outcomes.

Individualized risk prediction for breast cancer was first popularized with publication of the "Gail model."[33] In this model, five known risk factors are used to obtain risks of cancer over fixed time periods. The factors used are:

- Age,
- Age at menarche,
- Age at first live birth,
- Number of prior breast biopsies, and
- Number of first-degree relatives with breast cancer.

The model was derived by Mitchell Gail and his colleagues who used a retrospective database obtained from the Breast Cancer Detection Demonstration Project study conducted in the 1970s to evaluate a variety of potential risk factors, including some that were not significantly associated with breast cancer risk, such as cigarette smoking or the use of oral contraceptives. The sample size included more than 200,000 women, which made it large enough to allow accurate prediction and internal validation of the predicted risks. The model has subsequently been validated in other datasets, and expanded to be relevant to women of different ethnic backgrounds (reviewed by Eva Singletary in 2003).[64] The Gail model allows for simple tables that can be used to easily assess the risk for an individual woman while she is in the clinic for counseling, and has been used widely to stratify women in important ways. For example, eligibility for major breast cancer prevention trials, such as the National Surgical Adjuvant Breast and Bowel Project (NSABP) Study of Tamoxifen and Raloxifene (STAR) trial,[a] is based on the Gail risk score. Only those with a sufficiently high personal risk are eligible.

But the Gail model has some limitations. It has predictive value only for women over age 35 who have not previously been diagnosed with breast cancer,[67] and it does not incorporate specific genetic risk factors. Although it is highly accurate at predicting the aggregate number of women within various age or other risk groups who will develop breast cancer within 5 years, its ability to predict which individual women will develop breast cancer is only slightly better than chance.[60] It is, nonetheless, used to assist in determining whether individual women should engage in cancer prevention measures, because there are no better models that have been validated for individual risk prediction.

In summary, risk prediction based on easily obtained epidemiologic factors is currently accomplished widely using the Gail model. Genetic risk is predicted independently of this for women with BRCA mutations.[29,45] An integrated approach to risk prediction is desirable and, in principle, risk models should also include the likelihood of adverse events. False positives and unnecessary treatment are adverse events, but they are not identifiable because it is not possible to predict which cases of breast cancer (including ductal carcinoma in situ, or DCIS) will become life-threatening without

---

[a]The NSABP is a clinical trials cooperative group supported by the National Cancer Institute under whose auspices the STAR, one of the largest breast cancer prevention studies ever, is being conducted. This 5-year study opened in the summer of 1999 and aims to recruit 19,000 volunteers.

treatment. In any event, it is a matter of debate as to whether the harms of breast cancer screening are severe enough to be included in risk models, and they might be more appropriately considered in the context of shared decision making (see discussion in Chapter 2 on harms of mammography).

A number of hurdles still need to be overcome, including the development of more encompassing tests to predict genetically based risk that would not limit the scope of breast cancer risk prediction to the influence of just one or two genes and their narrow range of known mutations, but instead would consider the effects of a wide array of genes and environmental factors that together determine breast cancer risk. Models that integrate risk information from two or more different types of assessments, such as BRCA test results and family history, are also needed. Certainly, there is no reason why risk calculated through methods similar to those used by Gail could not also be used to inform the intensity of the screening strategy.

The Committee believes that individual screening strategies are essential to improving the early detection of breast cancer, and risk assessment is an essential step in the development of individualized screening strategies (Box 4-4). In theory, assessment of individuals' breast cancer risk could foster more accurate and less costly early breast cancer detection by determining screening strategies that are tailored to individual risks. However, the Committee emphasizes that even with individual risk assessment, at the current level of predictive accuracy, it is important to uphold the consensus guidelines for the minimum recommended use of mammography screening developed by nationally recognized organizations whose members are experts in the methodology of screening studies and who have carefully evaluated the evidence.

Caveats in Risk Stratification

The costs and benefits of *increasing* versus *decreasing* screening intensity are decidedly different. In considering a reduction in screening frequency, the benefits of lower costs and less inconvenience would be weighed against an added risk of dying from breast cancer. In contrast, a more aggressive strategy for high-risk women has the potential to save more lives. This, too, would require validation in appropriately designed clinical trials. Breast cancer is relatively rare in younger women, and the number of younger women who are at high risk would be even lower. But these relatively few high-risk women also tend to be those for whom standard mammography is less effective. Better methods of risk stratification could thus be of particular benefit to high-risk young women who would benefit from intensified screening—such as with more frequent screening or using technologies that compensate for the limitations of mammography.

Recommendations to begin mammography screening only after age 40

BOX 4-4
A Blood Test to Forego Mammography?

Imagine a blood test that could identify women whose risk of breast cancer is so low that they could safely forego regular mammogram screening. A recent study of post-menopausal women by Steven Cummings and colleagues suggests that such a test might someday be possible.[19]

Their study included more than 7,000 post-menopausal women whose average age was 66 years, and they found that the 4-year rate of breast cancer in women with undetectable serum estradiol levels was only 0.6 percent, compared to a rate of 3.0 percent for women whose estradiol levels were greater than 10 pmol/L (2.7 pg/mL), which translates into an approximately seven-fold difference between the two groups.

For comparison, the average 10-year risk for a 40-year old woman is approximately 1.5 percent, which is at or below the threshold for recommending regular mammograms. It is important to note, however, that Cummings' study reported 4-year rates, and these cannot be assumed to be the same as 10-year rates. But the comparison remains impressive—and suggests that some women over 60 might have a lower risk of breast cancer than average-risk 40-year-old women.

It has been known for some time that the risk of developing breast cancer drops with declining levels of serum estradiol, which is the most active type of estrogen,[37] but this study used a highly sensitive test to measure estradiol that allowed greater resolution of low estrogen levels than is possible in standard tests.

In fact, this is one of the caveats of the study. The minute quantities of estradiol that differentiate between high- and low-risk women required more expensive and sensitive tests than are currently available for clinical use. Assays used in daily clinical practice measure estradiol levels in the range of 10 to 20 pg/mL, and are not sensitive enough to distinguish levels between 0 and 10 pg/ml, whereas the average level of estradiol in the study was about 3 pg/mL.[48]

Another caveat is that because the study consisted of a 4-year follow-up period, breast cancer incidence might only be delayed to a later point in time in post-menopausal women with ultralow estradiol levels.

To date, there is no commercially available test. Research on the long-term accuracy and development of a clinically useful test will need to be completed before the test can be used to evaluate a woman's risk of breast cancer.

Other potential uses of highly sensitive estradiol measurements might be to identify women whose risk profiles make them candidates for preventive treatments, such as anti-estrogen. Such a test would be a welcome addition to the mix of risk assessment tools.

are largely based on the fact that cancer incidence increases with age, but also because mammography is less sensitive in women younger than 40, because they tend to have dense breasts. More frequent mammography screening in younger women also has the downside of exposing a more radiation-sensitive breast to radiation, yet breast cancers in younger women tend to be more aggressive, suggesting younger women should be screened more often.

The fact that mammography is generally less sensitive in younger women and that younger women are more sensitive to radiation alters the balance of risk and benefit. Detection technologies that do not involve radiation would thus be likely to offer a relatively greater advantage to younger women.

Risk Perception Is Often Distorted

Women fear breast cancer more than any other disease,[51,52] but their perception of risk is often distorted. In general, women in the United States and Canada tend to overestimate their risk of breast cancer, whereas women in the United Kingdom are more likely to underestimate their risk (reviewed by Hopwood in 2000).[39] Many women are also unclear about risk factors. More than three-quarters of women in one large survey recognized family history as a major determining factor for developing breast cancer, but only 13 percent correctly identified old age as a risk factor.[51] As a result, older women are more likely to underestimate their risk than younger women,[20,36] who tend to overestimate their risk. One study reported that women in their forties overestimated their probability of dying of breast cancer within 10 years by more than 20-fold.[6] The women in that study also overestimated the effectiveness of mammography. Considering the extreme bias in the media toward telling personal breast cancer stories of women in their thirties and the rarity of such stories of older women, these distorted perceptions are perhaps not surprising.[11]

The likelihood that a woman will adhere to screening recommendations depends, in part, on her perceived risk of developing breast cancer.[3,14] Despite the general validity of the Gail model in predicting risk, it does not predict risk perception or the inclination of a woman to follow mammography guidelines. A 1996 study in which more than 900 women were interviewed found a striking disparity between Gail model objective risk factors and the accuracy of women's beliefs about their own risk and adherence to mammography screening guidelines.[20] The observation that participation in screening mammography programs declines with age reflects this discordance between belief and behavior (Figure 4-2).

Reports of risk factors in the media as well as the scientific literature typically highlight relative risk rather than absolute risk which makes sense in the attempt to identify risk factors (see Box 4-1 for definitions), but it encourages exaggerated perceptions of personal risk. Most women whose mother had breast cancer are acutely aware that they are "at risk" for breast cancer, but few of them appreciate the moderate extent of their added risk. For example, the relative risk of developing breast cancer for a woman whose mother had breast cancer after age 50 is estimated to be 1.8 (see Table 4-2). If that woman is 40 years old, her underlying risk of

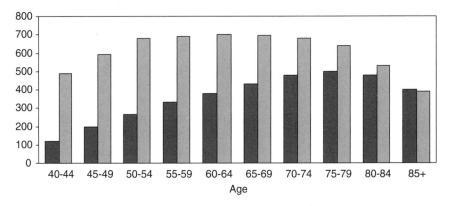

■ Breast cancer incidence (per 100,000), 1996-2000
☐ Number of women receiving mammograms in past year (per 1,000), 2003

FIGURE 4-2 Mammography use declines when breast cancer risk is greatest.
SOURCE: Data obtained from Medstat (2003)[49] and Ries et al. (2003).[59]

developing breast cancer within 10 years would be, on average, about 1.5 percent (Table 4-1). With her family history that risk is multiplied by 1.8 which gives her a 10-year breast cancer risk of 2.7 percent—higher than average, but still relatively low. Indeed, many women are surprised to learn than almost 90 percent of women who develop breast cancer have no close family history; that is, neither a mother, sister, or daughter with breast cancer.

Some women have gone to extreme measures to reduce their risk. For example, one study reported on 75 high-risk Canadian women who underwent bilateral mastectomy to avoid breast cancer, but the researchers found that on average the women had overestimated their lifetime risk of developing breast cancer before surgery three-fold.[50] The women in the study with strong or limited family histories of breast cancer estimated their lifetime risk for breast cancer as approximately 75 percent, whereas their calculated risks were only 25 percent (for strong family histories) and 18 percent (for limited family histories). In contrast, the women with BRCA gene mutations estimated their lifetime risk as 80 percent, while the model used to calculated their risk (BRCAPRO) indicated a 65 percent lifetime risk—a difference that was not statistically significant. Of course, there is no way to be sure that the models are accurate for the individual women in this study because of uncertainty about the penetrance of the BRCA mutations in each woman.

Distorted risk perception includes perceptions about prognosis as well. Although the prognosis for DCIS is excellent, the prognosis for early inva-

TABLE 4-4 Percent of Women Who Rated Certain Outcomes "Likely" Was Not Significantly Different for Diagnoses, Despite Significantly Different Prognoses

	Perceived Risk Among Women with Different Diagnoses*	
Possible Event	DCIS	Early Invasive Breast Cancer
Developing a local recurrence	53%	45%
Developing a distant recurrence	36%	39%
Dying of breast cancer	27%	27%

*None of the differences between diagnoses meet statistical significance.

sive breast cancer is not. Ten years after a diagnosis of DCIS, 2 percent of women will have died of breast cancer compared to 11 percent of women diagnosed with early invasive breast cancer.[28] Despite the different levels of risk, a study of 228 patients with either DCIS or early invasive breast cancer found no significant differences between the two groups in terms of perceived risk for recurrence or death from breast cancer (Table 4-4).[58] In addition, both groups of women expressed similar levels of anxiety and depression: 56 percent of women with DCIS and 54 percent of women with early invasive breast cancer reported anxiety; 41 percent of women with DCIS and 48 percent of women with early invasive breast cancer reported depression.

Finally, not only do many women have distorted perceptions of their risks of developing breast cancer, but most women misunderstand or overestimate the benefits of mammography.[6,24] A survey conduced in 1999 reported that a 57 percent majority of women in the United States believe that mammography affects their risk of developing breast cancer, compared to 37 percent who correctly responded that mammography does not influence breast cancer risk (Table 4-5).[24] Women in the United Kingdom and Italy who were surveyed overestimated the benefits of mammography to an even greater extent, 69 and 81 percent, respectively. Likewise, most women in all countries surveyed overestimated the extent to which mammography can reduce mortality due to breast cancer.

Decisions and Uncertainty

When information is certain, decisions are simple. A 40-year-old woman with an invasive breast tumor that will metastasize within 5 years

TABLE 4-5 Most Women in the United States Overestimate the Benefits
of Mammography

Question	Response			
	Prevents the risk of developing	Reduces the risk of developing	**No effect on risk of developing**	Don't know
Does mammography prevent or reduce the risk of developing breast cancer?	26%	31%	37%	6%
	Hardly at all	**By about a quarter**	By half or more	Don't know
How much does mammography reduce mortality for women over 50 who are screened regularly every 2 years for 10 years?	4%	12%	71%	13%

NOTE: Headings in bold and shading indicate the correct or most appropriate answer.

unless it is removed does not need a decision aid to take action. In contrast, a 65-year-old woman diagnosed with low-grade DCIS is likely to welcome a decision aid that allows her (and her physician) to integrate what is known about her personal risk factors with the likely benefits of different treatments. Likewise, a 75-year-old woman may want information that would assess her 10-year likelihood of death from other causes against the likelihood of dying from breast cancer in deciding whether to undergo screening.

Decision aids are tools that assist in choosing between complex alternatives such as determining optimal breast cancer screening strategies or choosing breast cancer treatment options. Sometimes these aids take the form of complex decision analyses, and sometimes they provide baseline probabilistic data in a variety of forms so that patients can better understand tradeoffs between risks and benefits. In the context of screening, formal decision analyses have been used by policymakers to evaluate the societal implications of varying strategies for a variety of tumors. From the perspective of an individual patient, these models can also be useful. However, information about probabilities at varying points in the screening and management process is sometimes more valuable. In the screening situation such information is useful because no screening test is 100 percent sensitive and specific. For example, a positive test for a BRCA1 or BRCA2 mutation does not mean that it is certain a woman will get breast cancer, and conversely, a negative test does not mean she will not. Emerging data on genomic markers and circulating biomarkers suggest that genetic or chemical analyses may help stratify patients into individualized risk categories, but the results are in continual flux and will be difficult to interpret until appropriate longitudinal large-population studies are done. Thus, there is a need to transfer information as clearly as possible to patients as they face decisions about having one or more screening tests for breast cancer.

Effectiveness of Risk Communication and Decision Aids

A large body of research has shown that good communication and strong patient-provider relationships are linked to greater patient satisfaction, and positive health outcomes.[43,55] Moreover, specific provider behaviors such as soliciting patients' opinions, checking patient understanding, and encouraging patients to talk have been linked to reduction of malpractice claims.[47] Poor communication, conversely, was associated with dissatisfaction, conflict, and worse outcomes. Studies suggested that dissatisfied patients tend to opt out of health plans,[21] to change physicians,[44,62] to initiate complaints against physicians,[47] and to be noncompliant with medical recommendations.[31,44]

Women are more likely to get involved in decision making once they are given sufficient information about their medical options.[30] These findings underscore the importance of educating women about the risks and benefits of various options. Studies show that without help, physicians are not consistently doing this well.[8] Although there are some reputable decision aids available on the Internet, as well as risk information provided by the print lay press, there is also an abundance of misinformation to which women are exposed. Messages from direct-to-consumer advertisements about medical tests, procedures, or treatments can also be misleading (see Box 1-3 in Chapter 1). These advertisements tend to overemphasize breast cancer risks to women and the benefits that are likely to accrue if they pursue the medical options the ads publicize.[34] The ads also tend to be fraught with misinformation, such as confusion of clinical benefits with laboratory accuracy.[34,70]

Individualized risk communication tends to improve women's accuracy about their own risk, although different studies have reported that anywhere from 22 to 50 percent of the women studied still overestimate their risk.[12] Edwards and colleagues reviewed 13 studies and concluded that individualized risk communication is also linked to increased participation in mammography screening programs.[26,27] However, many studies have been based on the presumption that the goal of risk communication is to increase participation in screening services, whereas the more important goal is to increase the number of women whose breast cancer is detected early enough to be effectively treated. Indeed, Edwards and his colleagues concluded that, based on the available data, increased use of mammography is not necessarily a consequence of more informed decision making.[26,27,61]

O'Connor and colleagues reviewed 200 decision aids, of which only 30 had been evaluated in methodologically valid clinical studies.[56] Based on those 30 studies, they concluded that the decision aids improved subjects' knowledge about their medical risks—although they did not necessarily influence their medical decisions. For example, the four breast cancer decision aids involved decisions about whether to undergo genetic testing for BRCA mutations. Those decision aids improved the test subjects' understanding of their personal risk, but did not influence whether or not they intended to pursue genetic testing.

Although risk perception is often at odds with actual risk, numerous studies have shown that genetic risk counseling improves people's understanding of their personal risk (reviewed by Hopwood in 2000).[39] A systematic review of studies published from 1980 to 2001 on the effects of genetic counseling and testing for familial breast cancer on women's perception of risk indicated that, overall, genetic counseling and testing appear to produce psychological benefits and to improve accuracy of risk perception, although 22 to 50 percent of the women in the studies reviewed continued to overestimate their risk.[12]

Even straightforward and accurate communication of risk can lead to unintended outcomes. For example, if people are asked to choose between an option that carries a 20 percent risk of dying versus an option that carries an 80 percent chance of survival, the overwhelming majority will opt for the survival option—even though the probable outcomes are identical. The differences in how the options are presented, or framed, are referred to as "loss framing" or "gain framing." Women's responses to information about the value of mammography are similarly affected by how the risks and benefits of mammography are framed.[25] Communication of risk must ensure that women do not mistakenly identify themselves as being at such low risk that they make choices, such as foregoing mammograms entirely, that increase their risks of a preventable death from breast cancer.

SUMMARY

The ultimate purpose of this Institute of Medicine report is to identify better ways to reduce the burden of breast cancer through improving early detection and diagnosis. Because there is so much individual variation in susceptibility to breast cancer, it makes sense to develop more refined screening strategies that provide the greatest possible benefit for individual women. Current screening strategies rely most heavily on age, followed by a history of breast disease. However, the development and progression of breast cancer is driven by biological factors such as genetic inheritance and mutations accumulated during a woman's lifetime. Although much has been learned, research on the genetic risk factors for breast cancer is still in its infancy, but should, in time, increasingly yield the knowledge for individualized risk stratification.

The goal of improved risk assessment is not to increase the use of screening mammography, but rather to identify optimal strategies. For some women, that might mean fewer mammograms. For others, it might mean staying the course and getting annual mammograms after age 50. For still others, it might mean more frequent mammograms or the use of supplemental imaging technologies, such as magnetic resonance imaging or ultrasound, or eventually molecular imaging. The primary goal of national screening programs has been to maximize the number of women who receive regular mammograms, yet it is clear that not all women will benefit equally.

Risk assessment, however, is only the first step. The goal of revising screening strategies necessarily includes revising screening behaviors. Risk must be communicated to individual women (and understood by their physicians) in such a way that they can make informed decisions about screening and their lifestyle. Numerous studies have indicated that a physician's or other provider's referral is the single most important predictor of whether a woman will receive a mammogram. But as discussed earlier, this is correlated with a variety of other factors that influence access to mammography. One example is whether a women who receives a referral is already receiving regular health care and, in most cases, has health insurance, which is itself a major determinant of which women will receive regular mammograms (see section Equal Access in Chapter 3).

To date, the impact of risk communication on informed medical decision making is limited. Even for mammography, which has been the subject of much research on communicating risk, few data show that women are making informed decisions—even within programs to communicate individualized risk.[27] This education is particularly relevant in enabling women to make appropriate decisions about their breast cancer screening because, as discussed earlier, a woman's perception of her breast cancer risk often does not match her actual risk. Risk communication might increase participation in screening mammography for several reasons that are, in fact, contradictory to informed decisions. For example, a woman might be motivated to follow mammography guidelines, because she overestimates her personal risk, or because she overestimates the potential of mammography to reduce her risk.

Many women's health and breast cancer advocates argue that women must be enabled to make informed choices about screening,[4,53,68] but that is not enough. Women and their physicians need better tools for assessing risk. Finally, communicators—physicians, professional societies, national health organizations, breast cancer advocates, and journalists—need a better understanding of how risk should be communicated.

REFERENCES

1. American Cancer Society. 2003. *Breast Cancer Facts and Figures 2003-2004*. Atlanta, GA: American Cancer Society.
2. American Medical Association, CME program publication. 2001. *Identifying and Managing Hereditary Risk for Breast and Ovarian Cancer*.
3. Aro AR, de Koning HJ, Absetz P, Schreck M. 1999. Psychosocial predictors of first attendance for organised mammography screening. *J Med Screen* 6(2):82-88.
4. Baines CJ. 2003. Mammography screening: are women really giving informed consent? *J Natl Cancer Inst* 95(20):1508-1511.
5. Begg CB. 2002. On the use of familial aggregation in population-based case probands for calculating penetrance. *J Natl Cancer Inst* 94(16):1221-1226.
6. Black WC, Nease RF Jr, Tosteson AN. 1995. Perceptions of breast cancer risk and screening effectiveness in women younger than 50 years of age. *J Natl Cancer Inst* 87(10):720-731.
7. Boyd NF, Dite GS, Stone J, Gunasekara A, English DR, McCredie MR, Giles GG, Tritchler D, Chiarelli A, Yaffe MJ, Hopper JL. 2002. Heritability of mammographic density, a risk factor for breast cancer. *N Engl J Med* 347(12):886-894.
8. Braddock CH 3rd, Edwards KA, Hasenberg NM, Laidley TL, Levinson W. 1999. Informed decision making in outpatient practice: time to get back to basics. *JAMA* 282(24):2313-2320.
9. Brekelmans CT, Seynaeve C, Bartels CC, Tilanus-Linthorst MM, Meijers-Heijboer EJ, Crepin CM, van Geel AA, Menke M, Verhoog LC, van den Ouweland A, Obdeijn IM, Klijn JG. 2001. Effectiveness of breast cancer surveillance in BRCA1/2 gene mutation carriers and women with high familial risk. *J Clin Oncol* 19(4):924-930.
10. Burke W, Austin MA. 2002. Genetic risk in context: calculating the penetrance of BRCA1 and BRCA2 mutations. *J Natl Cancer Inst* 94(16):1185-1187.
11. Burke W, Olsen AH, Pinsky LE, Reynolds SE, Press NA. 2001. Misleading presentation of breast cancer in popular magazines. *Eff Clin Pract* 4(2):58-64.
12. Butow PN, Lobb EA, Meiser B, Barratt A, Tucker KM. 2003. Psychological outcomes and risk perception after genetic testing and counselling in breast cancer: a systematic review. *Med J Aust* 178(2):77-81.
13. Carney PA, Miglioretti DL, Yankaskas BC, Kerlikowske K, Rosenberg R, Rutter CM, Geller BM, Abraham LA, Taplin SH, Dignan M, Cutter G, Ballard-Barbash R. 2003. Individual and combined effects of age, breast density, and hormone replacement therapy use on the accuracy of screening mammography. *Ann Intern Med* 138(3):168-175.
14. Cockburn J, Sutherland M, Cappiello M, Hevern M. 1997. Predictors of attendance at a relocatable mammography service for rural women. *Aust N Z J Public Health* 21(7):739-742.
15. Colditz GA, Rosner BA, Chen WY, Holmes MD, Hankinson SE. 2004. Risk factors for breast cancer according to estrogen and progesterone receptor status. *J Natl Cancer Inst* 96(3):218-228.

16. Collaborative Group on Hormonal Factors in Breast Cancer. 2001. Familial breast cancer: collaborative reanalysis of individual data from 52 epidemiological studies including 58,209 women with breast cancer and 101,986 women without the disease. *Lancet* 358(9291):1389-1399.

17. Cotterchio M, Kreiger N, Theis B, Sloan M, Bahl S. 2003. Hormonal factors and the risk of breast cancer according to estrogen- and progesterone-receptor subgroup. *Cancer Epidemiol Biomarkers Prev* 12(10):1053-1060.

18. Culver JB, Hull JL, Levy-Lahad E, Daly MB, Burke W. 2000, March 4. BRCA1 and BRCA2 Hereditary Breast/Ovarian Cancer. Accessed November 20, 2003. Web Page. Available at: http://www.geneclinics.org/servlet/access?db=geneclinics&site= gt&id=8888891&key=pxTA18SOqJ0uZ&gry=&fcn=y&fw=J1fF&filename= /profiles/brca1/index.html.

19. Cummings SR, Duong T, Kenyon E, Cauley JA, Whitehead M, Krueger KA. 2002. Serum estradiol level and risk of breast cancer during treatment with raloxifene. *JAMA* 287(2):216-220.

20. Daly MB, Lerman CL, Ross E, Schwartz MD, Sands CB, Masny A. 1996. Gail model breast cancer risk components are poor predictors of risk perception and screening behavior. *Breast Cancer Res Treat* 41(1):59-70.

21. Davies AR, Ware JE Jr, Brook RH, Peterson JR, Newhouse JP. 1986. Consumer acceptance of prepaid and fee-for-service medical care: results from a randomized controlled trial. *Health Serv Res* 21(3):429-452.

22. de Jong MM, Nolte IM, te Meerman GJ, van der Graaf WT, Oosterwijk JC, Kleibeuker JH, Schaapveld M, de Vries EG. 2002. Genes other than BRCA1 and BRCA2 involved in breast cancer susceptibility. *J Med Genet* 39(4):225-242.

23. Domchek SM, Eisen A, Calzone K, Stopfer J, Blackwood A, Weber BL. 2003. Application of breast cancer risk prediction models in clinical practice. *J Clin Oncol* 21(4):593-601.

24. Domenighetti G, D'Avanzo B, Egger M, Berrino F, Perneger T, Mosconi P, Zwahlen M. 2003. Women's perception of the benefits of mammography screening: population-based survey in four countries. *Int J Epidemiol* 32(5):816-821.

25. Edwards A, Elwyn G, Covey J, Matthews E, Pill R. 2001. Presenting risk information—a review of the effects of "framing" and other manipulations on patient outcomes. *J Health Commun* 6(1):61-82.

26. Edwards A, Unigwe S, Elwyn G, Hood K. 2003. Personalised risk communication for informed decision making about entering screening programs. *Cochrane Database Syst Rev* (1):CD001865.

27. Edwards A, Unigwe S, Elwyn G, Hood K. 2003. Effects of communicating individual risks in screening programmes: Cochrane systematic review. *BMJ* 327(7417):703-709.

28. Ernster VL, Barclay J, Kerlikowske K, Wilkie H, Ballard-Barbash R. 2000. Mortality among women with ductal carcinoma in situ of the breast in the population-based surveillance, epidemiology and end results program. *Arch Intern Med* 160(7):953-958.

29. Ford D, Easton DF, Stratton M, Narod S, Goldgar D, Devilee P, Bishop DT, Weber B, Lenoir G, Chang-Claude J, Sobol H, Teare MD, Struewing J, Arason A, Scherneck S, Peto J, Rebbeck TR, Tonin P, Neuhausen S, Barkardottir R, Eyfjord J, Lynch H, Ponder BA, Gayther SA, Zelada-Hedman M, et al. 1998. Genetic heterogeneity and penetrance analysis of the BRCA1 and BRCA2 genes in breast cancer families. The Breast Cancer Linkage Consortium. *Am J Hum Genet* 62(3):676-689.

30. Ford S, Schofield T, Hope T. 2003. Are patients' decision-making preferences being met? *Health Expect* 6(1):72-80.

31. Francis V, Korsch BM, Morris MJ. 1969. Gaps in doctor-patient communication. Patients' response to medical advice. *N Engl J Med* 280(10):535-540.

32. Frank TS, Deffenbaugh AM, Reid JE, Hulick M, Ward BE, Lingenfelter B, Gumpper KL, Scholl T, Tavtigian SV, Pruss DR, Critchfield GC. 2002. Clinical characteristics of individuals with germline mutations in BRCA1 and BRCA2: analysis of 10,000 individuals. *J Clin Oncol* 20(6):1480-1490.

33. Gail MH, Brinton LA, Byar DP, Corle DK, Green SB, Schairer C, Mulvihill JJ. 1989. Projecting individualized probabilities of developing breast cancer for white females who are being examined annually. *J Natl Cancer Inst* 81(24):1879-1886.

34. Gollust SE, Hull SC, Wilfond BS. 2002. Limitations of direct-to-consumer advertising for clinical genetic testing. *JAMA* 288(14):1762-1767.

35. Goode EL, Ulrich CM, Potter JD. 2002. Polymorphisms in DNA repair genes and associations with cancer risk. *Cancer Epidemiol Biomarkers Prev* 11(12):1513-1530.

36. Grunfeld EA, Ramirez AJ, Hunter MS, Richards MA. 2002. Women's knowledge and beliefs regarding breast cancer. *Br J Cancer* 86(9):1373-1378.

37. Hankinson SE, Willett WC, Manson JE, Colditz GA, Hunter DJ, Spiegelman D, Barbieri RL, Speizer FE. 1998. Plasma sex steroid hormone levels and risk of breast cancer in postmenopausal women. *J Natl Cancer Inst* 90(17):1292-1299.

38. Heine JJ, Malhotra P. 2002. Mammographic tissue, breast cancer risk, serial image analysis, and digital mammography. Part 2. Serial breast tissue change and related temporal influences. *Acad Radiol* 9(3):317-335.

39. Hopwood P. 2000. Breast cancer risk perception: what do we know and understand? *Breast Cancer Res* 2(6):387-391.

40. Huang WY, Newman B, Millikan RC, Schell MJ, Hulka BS, Moorman PG. 2000. Hormone-related factors and risk of breast cancer in relation to estrogen receptor and progesterone receptor status. *Am J Epidemiol* 151(7):703-714.

41. Institute of Medicine. 2001. *Mammography and Beyond: Developing Technologies for the Early Detection of Breast Cancer*. Washington, DC: National Academy Press.

42. Kaklamani VG, Hou N, Bian Y, Reich J, Offit K, Michel LS, Rubinstein WS, Rademaker A, Pasche B. 2003. TGFBR1*6A and cancer risk: a meta-analysis of seven case-control studies. *J Clin Oncol* 21(17):3236-3243.

43. Kaplan SH, Greenfield S, Ware JE Jr. 1989. Assessing the effects of physician-patient interactions on the outcomes of chronic disease. *Med Care* 27(3 Suppl):S110-S127.

44. Kasteler J, Kane RL, Olsen DM, Thetford C. 1976. Issues underlying prevalence of "doctor-shopping" behavior. *J Health Soc Behav* 17(4):329-339.

45. King MC, Marks JH, Mandell JB. 2003. Breast and ovarian cancer risks due to inherited mutations in BRCA1 and BRCA2. *Science* 302(5645):643-646.

46. Kushi LH, Potter JD, Bostick RM, Drinkard CR, Sellers TA, Gapstur SM, Cerhan JR, Folsom AR. 1995. Dietary fat and risk of breast cancer according to hormone receptor status. *Cancer Epidemiol Biomarkers Prev* 4(1):11-19.

47. Levinson W, Roter DL, Mullooly JP, Dull VT, Frankel RM. 1997. Physician-patient communication. The relationship with malpractice claims among primary care physicians and surgeons. *JAMA* 277(7):553-559.

48. McKiernan F, Wiley C. 2002. Measurement of serum estradiol. *JAMA* 287(12):1528.

49. Medstat. 2003. Mammography Use Declines When Breast Cancer Risk is Greatest. Accessed November 2003. Web Page. Available at: http://www.medstat.com/1news/093003.asp.

50. Metcalfe KA, Narod SA. 2002. Breast cancer risk perception among women who have undergone prophylactic bilateral mastectomy. *J Natl Cancer Inst* 94(20):1564-1569.

51. MORI Medicine & Science Research. 2002, October 17. Women See Family History Not Old Age as Greatest Breast Cancer Risk [MORI is an approved survey firm for the British National Health Service]. Accessed May 13, 2003. Web Page. Available at: http://www.mori.com/polls/2002/breakthrough.shtml.

52. Mosca L, Jones WK, King KB, Ouyang P, Redberg RF, Hill MN. 2000. Awareness, perception, and knowledge of heart disease risk and prevention among women in the United States. American Heart Association Women's Heart Disease and Stroke Campaign Task Force. *Arch Fam Med* 9(6):506-515.

53. National Breast Cancer Coalition. 2003, March. Position Statement on Screening Mammography. Accessed November 25, 2003. Web Page. Available at: http://www.natlbcc.org.

54. National Cancer Institute. 2004, March 11. Genetics of Breast and Ovarian Cancer (PDQ(R)). Accessed April 21, 2004. Web Page. Available at: http://www.nci.nih.gov/cancerinfo/pdq/genetics/breast-and-ovarian#Section_1.

55. Nekhlyudov L, Partridge A. 2003. Breast cancer risk communication: challenges and future research directions: workshop report (United States). *Cancer Causes Control* 14(3):235-239.

56. O'Connor AM, Stacey D, Rovner D, Holmes-Rovner M, Tetroe J, Llewellyn-Thomas H, Entwistle V, Rostom A, Fiset V, Barry M, Jones J. 2003. Decision aids for people facing health treatment or screening decisions. *Cochrane Database Syst Rev* (3): CD001431.

57. Rahman N, Stratton MR. 1998. The genetics of breast cancer susceptibility. *Annu Rev Genet* 32:95-121.

58. Rakovitch E, Franssen E, Kim J, Ackerman I, Pignol JP, Paszat L, Pritchard KI, Ho C, Redelmeier DA . 2003. A comparison of risk perception and psychological morbidity in women with ductal carcinoma in situ and early invasive breast cancer. *Breast Cancer Res Treat* 77(3):285-293.

59. Ries LAG, Eisner MP, Kosary CL, Hankey BF, Miller BA, Clegg L, Mariotto A, Fay MP, Feuer EJ, Edwards BK, Editors. 2003. *SEER Cancer Statistics Review, 1975-2000*. Bethesda, MD: National Cancer Institute.

60. Rockhill B, Spiegelman D, Byrne C, Hunter DJ, Colditz GA. 2001. Validation of the Gail et al. model of breast cancer risk prediction and implications for chemoprevention. *J Natl Cancer Inst* 93(5):358-366.

61. Royak-Schaler R, Klabunde CN, Greene WF, Lannin DR, DeVellis B, Wilson KR, Cheuvront B. 2002. Communicating breast cancer risk: patient perceptions of provider discussions. *Medscape Womens Health* 7(2):2.

62. Rubin HR, Gandek B, Rogers WH, Kosinski M, McHorney CA, Ware JE Jr. 1993. Patients' ratings of outpatient visits in different practice settings. Results from the Medical Outcomes Study. *JAMA* 270(7):835-840.

63. Rubin R. 2003, November 10. New agony over breast cancer. *USA TODAY*. P. 5.

64. Singletary SE. 2003. Rating the risk factors for breast cancer. *Ann Surg* 237(4):474-482.

65. Stahlberg C, Pedersen AT, Lynge E, Andersen ZJ, Keiding N, Hundrup YA, Obel EB, Ottesen B. 2004. Increased risk of breast cancer following different regimens of hormone replacement therapy frequently used in Europe. *Int J Cancer* 109(5):721-727.

66. Taylor MRG. 2001. Genetic testing for inherited breast and ovarian cancer syndromes: important concepts for the primary care physician. *Postgrad Med J* 77(903):11-15.

67. Theisen C. 2003. For patients, prediction of cancer risk can be worrisome. *J Natl Cancer Inst* 95(18):1360-1361.

68. Thornton H, Edwards A, Baum M. 2003. Women need better information about routine mammography. *BMJ* 327(7406):101-103.

69. Ursin G, Ma H, Wu AH, Bernstein L, Salane M, Parisky YR, Astrahan M, Siozon CC, Pike MC. 2003. Mammographic density and breast cancer in three ethnic groups. *Cancer Epidemiol Biomarkers Prev* 12(4):332-338.

70. Woloshin S, Schwartz LM, Tremmel J, Welch HG. 2001. Direct-to-consumer advertisements for prescription drugs: what are Americans being sold? *Lancet* 358(9288): 1141-1146.

71. Wooster R, Weber BL. 2003. Breast and ovarian cancer. *N Engl J Med* 348(23):2339-2347.

72. Yaffe MJ, Boyd NF, Byng JW, Jong RA, Fishell E, Lockwood GA, Little LE, Tritchler DL. 1998. Breast cancer risk and measured mammographic density. *Eur J Cancer Prev* 7(Suppl 1):S47-S55.

73. Ziv E, Shepherd J, Smith-Bindman R, Kerlikowske K. 2003. Mammographic breast density and family history of breast cancer. *J Natl Cancer Inst* 95(7):556-558.

5

Biologically Based Technologies

Advances in molecular biology are gradually revealing the biological processes underlying the individual predisposition to breast cancer, its early development, and its progression from benign to invasive to lethal. As our understanding of cancer biology grows, so does the potential to turn that knowledge into technologies that are not limited to screening, prognosis, monitoring, or even treatment, but which inform every aspect of patient care. The three areas of biologically based technologies discussed in this chapter—cancer biomarkers, molecular profiles, and molecular imaging—hold the promise of revolutionizing breast cancer detection and management.

Instead of competing with mammography, biologically based technologies for breast cancer detection are currently poised to serve as its adjuncts. Molecular biomarkers or profiles of breast cancer will need to be linked with imaging information to define tumor size and location. Among the most important recent insights into breast cancer biology is the recognition that cancer can arise through various sequences of events, and through the actions of many genes with small but additive effects.[35] While some researchers are seeking these genes (or their products) one by one, investigating the most promising candidates as potential biomarkers for breast cancer, others are examining overall patterns of gene expression associated with breast cancer risk or prognosis. Whatever the method of discovery, however, the final result is likely to reflect a highly individual molecular profile, characterized by both tumor and patient heterogeneity.

A major goal of these efforts is the development of blood tests to detect specific types of cancer. It is important to recognize, however, that the value of such a test depends on existing options. For example, the development of a test for ovarian cancer, even one that is not highly accurate, could save many lives because there is no existing technique to detect early stage ovarian cancer. In contrast, a comparable test for breast cancer would be unlikely to save lives unless it is more sensitive or specific than mammography and gave localization information or was paired with mammography.

Recent headlines to the contrary, it will be many years—if ever—before blood tests replace mammograms. The most obvious reason is that a blood test would measure biomarkers (usually proteins) that have been released from cancerous tissue into the general blood circulation, which means they are highly diluted in the midst of a multitude of other proteins, and are a long way from their source. A blood test would have to be able to measure trace quantities of any biomarkers and, at best, a blood test would indicate that cancer was present somewhere in the body, but not where—unless the biomarkers were found only in breast tissue, which puts yet another restriction on possible tests. For example, a problem could arise if it was so sensitive that only a few cancer cells would result in a positive test. The cancer could not be physically located with current imaging technology within the breast and thus true positives could not be distinguished from false positives.

No existing blood test—for breast or any other cancer—rivals mammography as a screening method. Mammography has an acceptable sensitivity, and despite its modest specificity, it locates the tumor for definitive biopsy. Furthermore, mammograms provide richer data than would be possible from a low-dimensional biochemical assay that measures only one or a few substances; improvements described in Chapter 3 have the potential to increase the information available from mammography.

Many different biologically based approaches to detecting breast cancer are in development, but they face many of the same challenges if they are to become truly useful for improving outcomes for breast cancer patients. Certain themes recur throughout this chapter in the discussions of the different types of biologically based cancer detection technologies:

- Biological methods may prove to be advantageous for screening high-risk populations, but are not likely to replace mammography.
- Nonimaging biological techniques must be linked to imaging methods that can localize the cancer.
- Statistical methods necessary for definitive analysis of large genomic and proteomic data sets are not yet defined or standardized.
- Assays to detect cancer must account for the variability that exists among tumor types and among patients in order to be effective for widespread use.

- New technologies should be developed in conjunction with experts in the current best practices for breast cancer detection and diagnosis.
- Novel diagnostic approaches need to be validated in large-scale clinical studies.

CLUES TO BREAST CANCER: INDIVIDUAL BIOMARKERS

Broadly defined, a biomarker is an objectively measurable characteristic that can be evaluated as an indicator of normal biological processes, disease, or response to therapeutic intervention.[15,65] The search for biomarkers of breast cancer should not be confused with the search for inherited, or germ-line, mutations that affect the likelihood of developing breast cancer. Although the discovery of such mutations is important to assess breast cancer *risk* and may, ultimately, lead to the identification of the causes of breast cancer, the presence of such mutations does not indicate or predict the *presence* of breast cancer in an individual.

Biomarkers are being sought—and some have been identified—across a wide spectrum of events in the development of breast cancer, as shown in Table 5-1. The clinical use of breast cancer biomarkers is currently limited largely to prognosis, predicting response to therapy, and monitoring patients with diagnosed malignancy, but biomarkers hold considerable potential for risk assessment, screening, diagnosis, and the identification of therapeutic targets.[11,18,38,44,55,58,65] Fulfilling that potential will not be easy. There are considerable biological and technical challenges to both the discovery and development of assays to detect early events in cancer development.[18,44,55]

The search for cancer biomarkers is proceeding along parallel paths: the "hypothesis-driven" assessment of candidate genes or proteins and the "discovery-based" comparison of gene expression and proteomic profiles.[55,58] The potential uses and limitations of bioassays based on individual biomarkers for breast cancer are reviewed in this chapter. Molecular profiles of breast cancer, as revealed by DNA microarrays and proteomic analysis, are also discussed later in this chapter.

Biomarker Assays May Complement Mammography

Research on cancer detection has long been inspired by the search for a single, specific biomarker: a molecule or compound produced at such high levels by newly malignant or premalignant cells that it could be detected in an easily obtained fluid or tissue sample. This ideal marker would appear in all patients with a specific type of cancer and be absent or below a definable threshold in individuals without the disease. Its concentration in the sampled

TABLE 5-1 Biomarkers of Events in the Development of Breast Cancer: Their Potential Uses and Limitations

Event	Potential Use for Biomarkers	Progress to Date	Key Limitations
Germ-line mutations[27]	Risk indicator	Several mutations identified; genetic testing available for BRCA1 and BRCA2	Account for only 10 percent of breast cancers
Genetic polymorphisms[27,44]	Risk indicator	Some candidate polymorphisms identified; thousands of single nucleotide polymorphisms (SNPs) have been mapped	Validation difficult due to genetic diversity among different ethnic populations and the need to measure cumulative effects of multiple SNPs
Somatic genetic alterations[27]	Risk indicator; screening; diagnosis; prognosis	Loss of heterozygosity (LOH) at several loci associated with premalignant disease, as well as early and late-stage breast cancer	Unknown which, if any, LOH events are specific to invasive or metastatic cancer
Epigenetic changes (e.g., methylation) in breast cells[14,57,67]	Risk indicator; screening; diagnosis; prognosis; therapeutic target	Research correlating methylation patterns at key loci with breast cancer presence and stage	Validation will require large-scale longitudinal studies and comprehensive cancer registry data
Altered gene expression in breast cells[18,25,36,67]	Screening; diagnosis; prognosis; choosing therapy; monitoring outcome	Studies under way on several overexpressed and underexpressed genes in breast tumor tissue; estrogen receptor status predicts response to antiestrogen therapy	Validation will require large-scale longitudinal studies and comprehensive cancer registry data

Changes in protein signaling pathways in breast cells[36]	Screening; diagnosis; prognosis; choosing therapy; monitoring outcome	Clinical trials underway in breast cancer patients before, during, and after therapy	Population heterogeneity reduces sensitivity and complicates standardization; sampling involves microdissection
Changes in individual serum markers[18]	Screening; diagnosis; prognosis; monitoring outcome	Preliminary findings indicate prognostic benefits of monitoring a mucin, CA 15-3, which has received FDA approval for the detection of recurrent breast cancer	Typically lack sensitivity for early malignancy and organ specificity; not elevated in all patients
Changes in serum protein/peptide profile[36]	Secondary screening; diagnosis; prognosis; choosing therapy; monitoring outcome	Research under way to improve ovarian cancer diagnosis	Low sensitivity and specificity; population heterogeneity
Angiogenesis[5,22]	Risk indicator, prognosis, choosing therapy	Research on several angiogenesis-related receptors being conducted to develop a possible treatment	Validation will require large-scale longitudinal studies. Main focus is currently on developing therapeutics
Invasion and metastasis[18,25,36,67]	Prognosis	Candidate proteases and inhibitors have been identified; prognostic benefit of urokinase plasminogen activator for node-negative breast cancer confirmed in large prospective randomized trial	Lack of effective therapy for metastatic breast cancer

---

BOX 5-1
CA 15-3

The CA 15-3 protein is a member of the family of proteins known as mucins, whose normal function is cell protection and lubrication. It plays a role in reducing cell adhesion and is found throughout the body. Elevated levels in breast cancer tissue may be involved in metastasis. CA 15-3 levels can also be elevated in patients with other cancers (lung, colorectal, ovarian, pancreatic) or because of hepatitis or cirrhosis of the liver.

---

fluid would increase or decrease as the cancer progresses or regresses and could be determined by a simple, reliable, inexpensive assay.

Individual biomarkers currently in clinical and experimental use fall far short of this ideal, however. (See Table 5-1 for a summary of potential issues and limitations of biomarkers for specific events in the development of breast cancer.) Most are synthesized by normal as well as malignant tissues and are only rarely elevated in premalignant or early stage disease. For example, in cancerous breast tissue high levels of the protein CA 15-3 are produced, but usually not until the cancer has reached an advanced stage (Box 5-1).[18] Few of the biomarkers in use today are found among all patients with a particular type of cancer, and with the exception of prostate specific antigen, none are organ-specific.[18]

Absent an ideal biomarker, it is likely that any biomarker-based assay used as a primary screen for breast cancer in normal-risk populations will produce significant numbers of false positives. However, biomarker-based screening may prove to be a practical means of screening women at high risk for breast cancer for premalignant disease and/or occult cancer. Such an assay could detect clusters of proliferating cells at a preclinical stage, as well as cell clusters that may never require treatment. With the discovery of additional or better markers, bioassays may eventually be developed that not only detect the presence of breast cancer or precancer, but also predict clinical course.

As with mammographic screens, the performance of a biomarker assay should increase as additional time points are taken, particularly if the marker(s) reflect disease burden. This is true of existing biomarker assays for prostate, ovarian, and colon cancer. Therefore, although it may be unreasonable to expect that a single assay measurement can replace mammographic screening, multiple measurements taken over time that show a consistent rise in value could be indicative of an enlarging mass. This type of algorithm is likely to be the first implementation for biomarkers in breast cancer screening.

Biomarker assays could also be used to aid the decision-making process for biopsy following a suspicious mammogram, if the bioassay reduced the number of false positives (increased specificity) without sacrificing sensitivity. Reliance on such an assay in cases of questionable mammographic results (for example, BI-RADS® 3-4) would be prudent only if the positive predictive value of the assay is extremely high, particularly when the result is to forgo biopsy. This is especially critical in the United States, where biopsy is the current standard of care for virtually every suspicious lesion. Bioassays may also be performed on the sample of suspicious cells obtained at biopsy in order to inform treatment decisions, but such tests will not supplant pathological examination of the biopsied tissue sample for the primary diagnosis.

As long as biomarkers continue to have low sensitivity and specificity, their use in primary diagnosis will be limited, and histological examination of biopsied tissue will remain the gold standard. But even then, biomarkers are likely to be useful as adjunct to other procedures, including:

- Differential diagnosis or prognosis, such as distinguishing among types of ductal carcinoma in situ;
- Assistance in the choice of therapy and evaluation of its outcome; or
- Monitoring patients with ongoing disease before or after therapy.

Results of preliminary studies suggest that pre-operative serum levels of CA 15-3 are as good, if not better, predictors of patient outcome than traditional measures such as tumor size and nodal status.[18] Tissue levels of estrogen and progesterone receptors and the erbB2 receptor, as determined by immunohistochemical analysis, are considered in the selection of therapy.[18,42] CA 15-3, approved in 1997 by the Food and Drug Administration (FDA) for the detection of recurrent breast cancer, may also prove useful in monitoring response to therapy for metastatic breast cancer.[18]

Roadblocks to Biomarker Discovery and Development

The path to biomarker-based assays for breast cancer, and particularly for the early detection of the disease, is far from smooth. The considerable challenge of identifying highly sensitive and specific screens that rival the effectiveness of mammography is made more difficult by biological heterogeneity among humans, as well as among cancers, and even among different cell populations within a single tumor.[55] A successful bioassay for breast cancer will need to overcome variability associated with cancers of different histologic types, expression patterns within histologic types, additional (noncancerous) patient conditions, and intrinsic human biochemistry. For now, as noted by Kenneth Pritzker, "our conceptual framework of cancer biology remains inadequate to recognize the ideal or optimal biomarker for most cancers."[55]

Guiding principles for the validation of promising biomarkers have been developed by the National Cancer Institute's (NCI's) Early Detection Research Network (Box 5-2). Shown in Table 5-2, these principles define a process for selecting biomarkers with sufficient positive predictive value that they can be used for population screening.[44] Navigating this process will require extensive and unprecedented collaboration among industry,

---

BOX 5-2
Early Detection Research Network

The NCI's Early Detection Research Network (EDRN) was founded in 2000 to facilitate biomarker discovery and validation through the collaboration among government, academia, and industry. The EDRN was established to set standards for the development and evaluation of biomarkers and guide the process of biomarker discovery in an effort to produce a useful population-screening tool.

The goals of the EDRN include:
- Development and testing of promising biomarkers or technologies
- Evaluation of promising, analytically proven biomarkers or technologies
- Collaboration among academic and industrial leaders in molecular biology, molecular genetics, clinical oncology, computer science, public health, and clinical application for early cancer detection
- Collaboration and rapid dissemination of information among awardees

The research network consists of three components:
- **Biomarker Discovery Laboratories** are responsible for the development and characterization of new biomarkers or the refinement of existing biomarkers. There are currently 18 facilities involved in this research.
- **Biomarker Validation Laboratories** serve as a network resource for clinical and laboratory validation of biomarkers, which includes technological development, quality control, refinement, and high throughput. The EDRN includes three validation facilities.
- **Clinical Epidemiological Centers** conduct clinical and epidemiological research regarding the clinical application of biomarkers. There are nine facilities responsible for this research.

A fourth component, the **Data Management and Coordinating Center** located at the Fred Hutchinson Cancer Research Center, is responsible for coordinating the EDRN research activities in order to develop a common database for network research.

For more information see: http://www3.cancer.gov/prevention/cbrg/edrn/.

TABLE 5-2 Guiding Principles Used in Biomarker Validation[44]

Phase	Results
Phase 1: Preclinical exploratory	Promising directions identified
Phase 2: Clinical assay and validation	Clinical assay detects established disease
Phase 3: Retrospective longitudinal	Biomarker detects preclinical disease and a "screen positive" rule defined
Phase 4: Prospective screening	Extent and characteristics of disease detected by the test and the false referral rate are identified
Phase 5: Cancer control	Impact of screening on reducing burden of disease on population is quantified

NOTE: The phases of research are ordered according to the strength of evidence that each phase provides in favor of the biomarker, from the weakest to the strongest. In general the results of earlier phases are necessary to design later phases. In some cases, where discovery of the biomarker establishes the method of detection, such as surface-enhanced laser desorption, then Phase I is skipped.

academia, and government, each of which controls resources essential to the development of clinically significant biomarkers.[44,66] New legislation may be needed to provide incentives for cooperation between the pharmaceutical industry, which has identified hundreds to thousands of potential biomarkers for early cancer detection, and medical schools and research institutes possessing tissue banks, cell lines, and other reagents necessary to test these candidates.[44] Increased effort is being made to sample tissues with precancerous and early stage disease due to their crucial role in testing biomarkers for cancer screening; such specimens are currently underrepresented in tissue banks.[42]

Once a promising biomarker is identified, researchers must address the technical challenges of developing a viable assay. The procurement, handling, and storage of fluid or tissue sample warrants careful consideration, because minor differences in these procedures may introduce systematic but unknown biases. However, it will be difficult to specify precise parameters for handling samples until the effects of inconsistencies on a given bioassay can be determined.

Further progress toward biomarker-based screening will require large-scale, longitudinal studies to evaluate the ability of a given screen to reduce cancer deaths and/or increase survival. Existing cancer registry data are woefully inadequate for this purpose, but more extensive information gathering may be hampered by the Health Insurance Portability and Accountability Act (HIPAA) and other legislation to protect patient confidentiality. (For more about HIPAA, see Chapter 6.) There is also a need to define statistical and inferential criteria for the evaluation of biomarker candidates for cancer screening, so that their efficacy can be measured against competing technologies.[65] This comparison will ultimately hinge on the ability of the candidate technologies to reduce cancer mortality through the early detection of treatable disease.

If serum markers are shown to have promise in breast cancer studies such as these, the concept that a blood test can actually reduce cancer mortality should ultimately be evaluated in a randomized trial with cancer mortality as the endpoint, as was required in the pioneering studies of radiologic screening using mammography. Such a study would require resources similar to the mammography trials, namely tens of thousands of participants and lengthy follow-up. Methodologic issues in evaluating breast cancer screening tests are further discussed in Chapter 6.

PROFILES OF BREAST CANCER:
GENOMICS AND PROTEOMICS

Until the early 1990s, the search for cancer biomarkers proceeded through the one-by-one investigation of candidate genes and proteins. The advent of high-throughput techniques capable of screening thousands of genes and, more recently, proteins, has made possible broad comparisons of cancerous and normal cells, revealing new biomarker candidates and introducing the possibility that patterns of gene expression or protein profiles could themselves serve as cancer biomarkers.[51,58,69] DNA microarrays, consisting of thousands of DNA oligonucleotides (short sequences of DNA) or cDNAs (complete gene sequences of DNA reverse-transcribed from RNA templates) spotted in fixed locations are used to screen samples via hybridization (joining of two complementary strands of nucleic acid). Various applications of this technique can identify cancer-related changes in gene activity and reveal qualitative and quantitative variations in genomic DNA that occur during tumor formation.

Additional high-throughput methods focus on cancer-induced changes in protein pathways and populations, both within the tumor cell and at the tumor-host interface.[37,51] These techniques scan the proteome—the protein equivalent of the genome—of affected cells and tissues for cancer biomarkers. Protein microarrays, which are an analogous technology to DNA microarrays, enable researchers to screen many proteins simultaneously for function and amplification.[69] Serum proteomic profiling, the analysis of disease-related changes in proteins circulating in the blood, reveals patterns that may ultimately be used to detect cancer, identify therapeutic targets, and monitor response to therapy.[51]

Expression Profiles of Breast Cancer

The disruption of cell growth and survival pathways that lead to cancer occurs through multiple, cumulative genetic and epigenetic changes that in turn alter gene expression.[2] While all breast tumors reflect changes common to malignant tissue, such as disordered cell cycle control, apoptosis (programmed cell death), adhesion and motility, and angiogenesis (new blood vessel formation), each tumor presents a unique pattern of gene expression (reviewed by Chung and colleagues in 2002).[13] By classifying tumors according to their expression profiles, as revealed by microarrays, researchers hope to create a taxonomy that will improve prognosis and better predict each patient's response to available therapies.[13,28]

Expression microarrays can analyze gene expression levels in a single sample or compare the expression of thousands of genes between two different cell types or tissue samples, such as malignant and normal breast tissues. Although the technology is still in its infancy, expression-based classifications for many types of tumors, including breast cancers, have already been developed through microarray analysis.[1,13,81] For example, researchers identified five distinct subtypes of breast tumors derived largely from patients with infiltrating ductal carcinoma.[49,63] This approach to detecting tumor classes based on *a priori* similarities in expression signature is known as "unsupervised" analysis.

A contrasting approach, "supervised analysis," directly examines the relationship between gene expression profiles and a clinically determined variable, such as breast cancer prognosis. Van't Veer and colleagues determined expression patterns of 98 primary breast tumors from lymph node-negative patients less than 55 years of age using oligonucleotide microarrays of 25,000 genes.[74] Based on the clinical outcome of these patients, the researchers identified a set of 70 genes with expression patterns that closely predicted patient prognosis. A poor prognosis was associated with increased expression of genes associated with cell cycle control, invasion, angiogenesis, and signal transduction. A subsequent study tested the 70-gene prognosis profile in microarrays from 295 patients under age 53 with primary breast cancers with and without lymph node involvement. In this group of patients, the prognosis profile outperformed other standard criteria—including age, tumor size and histology, and the involvement of axillary lymph nodes—in predicting outcome.[73] The next step should be to conduct studies in larger and more representative groups of breast cancer patients to determine whether these encouraging initial results prove to be reliable in clinical practice.[30] However, despite the lack of evidence from true prospective clinical trials, versions of this test (Oncotype DX) are already on the market in the United States and The Netherlands. The test became available in the United States in early 2004 without having been approved by the

FDA because the device was marketed as a laboratory service rather than a diagnostic kit.[24]

Although expression microarray analysis is likely to identify clinically significant diagnostic and prognostic markers for breast cancer, the technology may not be well suited to the clinic.[13] Microarray analysis as currently performed is too expensive for routine clinical use, and RNA is difficult to recover from biopsy specimens, which are normally fixed in formalin and embedded in paraffin for histological analysis and preservation.[33,82] However, once subsets of clinically significant genes are identified via expression microarray analysis, other faster and less expensive techniques could be used in diagnostic tests. For example, researchers at Johns Hopkins University used expression microarray analysis to identify a large number of genes that were overexpressed in breast cancers.[67] This group was further narrowed to a group of 35 potential tumor suppressor genes, selected on the basis of hypermethylation, and then to a panel of 3 genes that were highly and specifically correlated with early stage breast cancer. The markers are measured, via methlyation-specific polymerase chain reaction (PCR), in breast cells obtained by ductal lavage (described in Appendix A). Large clinical trials are currently under way to test the ability of this panel of markers to detect early stage breast cancer in asymptomatic women, as well as in women who are at high risk for primary and recurrent breast cancer.[17,21]

Cancer Clues Throughout the Genome

Mutations in DNA repair genes that normally protect the body against cancer-related mutations often result in chromosome loss, breakage, and gene amplification.[2] The number and location of these "hits" to the genome strongly influence a person's risk for developing cancer and, if malignancy occurs, its relative aggressiveness. A technique called microarray comparative genomic hybridization (CGH), which detects and maps cancer-related changes in DNA copy number, is therefore being pursued for clinical use in cancer prognosis. Microarray CGH is performed by hybridizing large pieces of sample genomic DNA to arrays spotted with DNA from a spectrum of known chromosomal locations. Differences in hybridization between, for example, normal ductal epithelial cells and biopsied breast tumor cells indicate key regions of chromosomal damage associated with the development of individual tumors. Unlike RNA-based expression analysis, DNA-based microarray CGH can be performed on formalin-fixed tissue such as archival biopsy material and therefore is more adaptable to routine pathology practice.[33]

In breast tumors, microarray CGH frequently reveals the loss of whole or partial chromosome arms, gene amplification, and erosion of the ends of chromosomes, characteristics that may provide prognostic and/or diagnostic markers for breast cancer.[2] For example, amplification of the erbB2 gene, as detected by microarray CGH, strongly correlates with increased gene expression. ErbB2 protein levels, which have been shown to predict breast cancer response to Herceptin therapy, are currently measured by immunohistochemical analysis of biopsied tumor tissue, but erbB2 copy number may prove a simpler and more sensitive indicator of Herceptin susceptibility.[2,4,48] The further identification of dysfunctional genes in breast tumors by microarray CGH may enable the design of therapies targeting those genes, as well as tests to reveal genetic changes that make tumors resistant to certain therapies, such as defects in DNA repair genes associated with cisplatin resistance. (Herceptin and cisplatin are intravenously administered anticancer drugs.[2])

Researchers have also used microarrays to search the genome for disease-associated patterns of single nucleotide polymorphisms[a] (SNPs) and for loss of heterozygosity (LOH)[b] (reviewed by Singletary, 2003).[62] Both characteristics reflect somatic changes that are thought to occur early in cancer development, and thus hold potential for risk assessment or early detection. As with aberrations in DNA copy number, the analysis of SNP and LOH patterns in breast tumors may provide the basis for the prognostic and therapeutic classification schemes, as well as leads for the development of targeted therapies.

Signaling Circuits Gone Haywire

Cancer alters the signaling circuitry that governs cell growth and death by changing the expression level, post-translational processing, and functional modification (such as phosphorylation) of key proteins (Box 5-3).[51,69] None of these parameters can be measured reliably, if at all, by expression profiling. Thus researchers have developed versions of protein microarrays that can simultaneously measure the concentration and phosphorylation state of thousands of individual proteins. The reverse-phase protein array consists of a nitrocellulose slide onto which tumor cell proteins—potentially from hundreds of patients—are applied in a range of dilutions, then probed with antibodies to phosphorylated forms of known signaling proteins.[51] The specifically bound antibodies can be located and quantified by chemiluminescent, fluorescent, or colorimetric methods.

---

[a]An SNP is defined as a variation of a specific nucleotide that is present in over 1 percent of the population.

[b]LOH results from a mutation resulting in the absence or loss of one of the normal two forms of a gene from one of a chromosome pair for tumor DNA as compared to nontumor DNA in the same subject.

BOX 5-3
How Genetic Mutations Can Disrupt
Control of Cellular Functions

There are many other ways that cell functions are altered, but these are especially pervasive and underlie the regulations of processes such as cell division, cell movements, and cell death—each of which are critical elements in cancer development and progression.

Alterations in gene copy number, or changes in the number of copies of individual genes, are key genetic events in the development and progression of human cancers. At least 12 percent of all the variation in gene expression among the breast tumors is directly attributable to underlying variation in gene copy number.[54] Widespread DNA copy number alteration can lead directly to global deregulation of gene expression, which may contribute to the development or progression of cancer.

Post-translational processing refers to the chemical modification of a protein after it has been synthesized, or translated. These modifications impart specialized functions upon the resultant proteins. Examples include the addition of glycosyl groups (glycosylation) or acetyl groups (acetylation) to a protein.

Phosphorylation is a post-translation modification that refers to the attachment of a phosphoryl group (PO_4) onto a protein. Many proteins remain inactive until they are phosphorylated, thus phosphorylation is a critical element in the control of cellular functions.

A comparison of the phosphorylation states of signaling proteins involved in growth factor and apoptosis pathways in breast epithelial cells from a total of 150 patients with either normal, premalignant, or cancerous results indicated that patient survival was correlated with the phosphorylation of two key signaling proteins.[36] However, the overall signaling protein profile determined for each patient was sufficiently unique to resist comparison, except possibly with subsequent profiles of the same patient, over time or following therapy.

The promise of protein microarrays lies in their potential to identify the specific, highly individual cancer-related changes in each patient's signaling circuitry—perhaps at an earlier stage than is currently feasible—and on the basis of that information, select the best possible treatment. It may also be possible to identify and target each of several different altered signaling proteins in a single tumor. The additive effect of this "combinatorial" treatment might require smaller amounts of each drug used, thereby reducing the toxic effects of therapy.[51] A drug aimed at a single molecular target to inhibit cell proliferation rather than, as is often the case currently, unselectively destruction of cells will likely also prove less toxic to the normal cells of the body. However, because the vast majority of signaling proteins remain to be identified, and their role in cell growth and death characterized, the future utility of protein microarrays in cancer detection and treatment depends on an expanding knowledge of the molecular basis of cancer. Current protein microarrays can display less than 10 percent of the total cell proteome;[33] however, as key diagnostic and prognostic protein markers are identified and validated, they could be incorporated into smaller, more selective arrays. In addition, the inherent instability of proteins and the difficulty of producing consistent, reproducible results in protein-binding assays present significant technical roadblocks to the development of protein microarrays for clinical use.[51]

Serum Signatures of Cancer

Proteins, protein fragments, and metabolites from every tissue that blood flows though, accumulate in the serum. Some of these molecules, if derived from a tumor or its host organ, could serve as markers for malignant transformation or tumor-host interactions.[51] Serum proteomic profiling, a high-throughput technique, reveals patterns comprising many individual proteins, the identities of which remain unknown (described in Appendix A). As with gene expression profiles, proteomic patterns can be analyzed using unsupervised methods to reveal groups of related proteins that can form the basis of taxonomic categories, or using supervised methods that relate protein patterns to a clinically determined variable, such as survival. Often these analyses are performed by artificial intelligence systems capable of handling vast amounts of data: A typical proteomic profile can include more than 15,000 data points.

Serum proteomic profiling could be used to identify novel biomarker candidates for characterization by conventional methods, but the great promise of the technology lies in the possibility of using a discriminating pattern within a patient's profile to diagnose cancer and monitor the results of treatment.[36,50] If this were possible, a profile might be obtained following a suspicious mammogram to inform a decision to biopsy, or in the event of a positive biopsy, a proteomic profile might be used to inform therapeutic choices. With even more exacting validation, serum proteomic profiling could be used to screen high-risk patients for early signs of cancer. Serum profiles of 50 ovarian cancer patients and 50 unaffected women have already been used to develop a discriminating pattern, formed by a subset of small proteins and peptides in the serum, that could discriminate ovarian cancer from noncancer.[50] Follow-up results of this study incorporating 250 patients determined the sensitivity (rate of true negatives) and specificity (rate of true positives) were both 99 percent for stage I ovarian cancer.[36]

Although these results are encouraging for the early detection of ovarian cancer, for which no screen exists, they are far from competitive with mammography, particularly given the much higher population prevalence of breast cancer as compared with ovarian cancer. However, to explore the possibility of serum proteomic profiling as a supplement to biopsy, an initial study was performed on serum samples from 317 patients who received breast biopsies. A training set, consisting of sera from 43 patients with benign lesions and 58 with breast cancer, was used to identify a discriminating pattern, which, when blind-tested on the remaining 216 samples, detected breast cancer with 90 percent sensitivity and benign lesions with 71 percent specificity.[36] These results suggest the feasibility of using this methodology as a supplement to biopsy, as well as the need for significant improvement in the accuracy of proteomic diagnosis before it could be substituted for the actual results of biopsy. However, a serum proteomic test will only reveal certain biological characteristics of a tumor; other characteristics such as the size, shape, and location of the tumor remain unknown when using only a serum test. Therefore, in using this technique, lesions will most likely still have to be imaged by modalities such as mammogram, ultrasound, and magnetic resonance imaging (MRI), for effective treatment.

Barriers to Clinical Use of Molecular Profiles

In addition to previously described technical challenges to the clinical adaptation of DNA and protein microarrays and of serum proteomic profiling, these high-throughput, biologically based technologies face several barriers to development for the detection, diagnosis, or monitoring of cancer. Two largely unmet requirements stand out: to validate a strong and reliable link between profile characteristics and clinical outcomes and to create reliable, cost-effective profiling methods that can be performed in the clinical setting.[52]

The accurate analysis and correct interpretation of data from high-throughput experiments, key factors in establishing the clinical significance of molecular profiles, are far from ensured. Many sources of noise can obscure the results of these experiments. Results generated by DNA microarrays, for example, may be influenced by methods of sample storage, preparation, and labeling; by spot location on the array; or by imperfections in the array itself. These problems were clearly illustrated in a recent study in which samples from the same tissue, analyzed with different DNA microarray technologies (cDNA versus oligonucleotide), produced different gene expression profiles.[32] In the case of serum proteomic profiling, where the identity of the specific proteins is unknown, minor differences in specimen procurement and subsequent handling may introduce systematic but undetectable biases into profiles.

Thus it is perhaps not surprising that statisticians have warned of significant potential for error in the analysis of voluminous genomic and proteomic data.[52] Even experts in the field disagree on the merits of the various statistical methods employed to bring molecular profiles into focus.[26,70,76] Some argue that there is no "right" way to analyze molecular profiles, only the best choice based on the characteristics of the data and the scientific questions being asked.[70,76] Thus, the more detailed our understanding of cancer biology is, the better informed such choices will be.

In the meantime, work is under way to resolve and refine statistical methods applied to microarray data, including gatherings of experts and standard-setting efforts by data repositories and professional journals. The annual meeting of the Critical Assessment of Microarray Data Analysis, first held in 2000, features direct competition among analytical methods. To support public use and dissemination of gene expression data, the National Center for Biotechnology Information, an arm of the National Library of Medicine, is building an expression data repository and online resource for data storage and retrieval. To facilitate comparisons of gene expression data from different sources, submissions to the repository must meet standards for data representation, experimental controls, and analysis. Although initial publications of DNA microarray results featured little if any statistical analysis, major journals, most notably *Nature*, recently have begun to impose publication standards for such data.[3]

The resolution of technical, interpretive, and statistical issues will help move molecular profiles to the clinic, but not before these technologies have been shown to reduce cancer deaths or increase survival in large-scale clinical trials. This process is likely to be hindered by the same constraints (lack of cancer registry data, restricted information gathering under HIPAA) as the validation of individual biomarkers, but perhaps even more to the need to demonstrate the utility of complex patterns without knowledge of their underlying biology, and to reliably reproduce profiles on a large scale.[52] There are several methods of proteomic profiling and, for now, there are controversies about which methods are best. Indeed, many findings of very high accuracy are not confirmed by subsequent studies using other methods.

"This may be one of the greatest challenges this field currently faces," according to researcher Emmanuel Petricoin.[52] "Scientific consensus and standards are needed to develop, to evaluate, and to accept new statistical models for establishing the significance of linking gene and protein pattern analyses to more conventional diagnostic endpoints or outcomes." It may be necessary, he concludes, to agree on different degrees of validation, depending on an individual product's intended purpose, its stage of development, and the role of profile data in the evaluation of the product's performance.

Finally, all molecular profiles have an important limitation: Although they may detect signals indicating the presence of cancer or its precursors somewhere in the body, they cannot locate the source of those signals. Thus a molecular profile, like any individual cancer biomarker, must be paired with an imaging technique such as mammography, histochemistry, or—in the future—molecular imaging, a biologically based technology described in the next section of this chapter.

PICTURES OF BREAST CANCER:
MOLECULAR IMAGING

Along with the promise of bioassays and therapies directed at the molecular roots of breast cancer comes a need to locate incipient disease, determine its extent, and monitor response to therapy, all at the molecular level.[68] Molecular imaging, the in vivo measurement, characterization, and quantification of biological processes at the cellular and subcellular level, completes the picture of molecular medicine sketched in this chapter.[41,68,77] The ability to "see" the molecular signatures of breast cancer is critical to fulfilling biologically based technologies' promise of earlier detection and better disease management.

Today, the vast majority of breast cancers are detected with mammography and other imaging methods that measure nonspecific physical, physiological, anatomic, or metabolic phenomena such as electron density, acoustic interfaces, or temperature.[41,53] While conventional images can sometimes differentiate pathological from normal tissue, molecular images can identify specific events—such as altered gene expression or changes in the proteome—that cause disease. In the future, molecular images will also play a key role in monitoring therapeutic response to biologically or molecularly based cancer treatment. Targeted molecular therapies are likely to inhibit cell proliferation rather than kill tumor cells, so their impact cannot be judged by radiological measures of tumor size.[9] Gene therapy will necessitate tracking the transgene's location, level of expression, and duration of effect.[41] To gauge the success of anti-angiogenesis drugs, clinicians will need to measure changes in the number or viability of the blood vessels that feed tumors.[68]

Molecular imaging could one day be used throughout the cancer care pathway, to detect early stage alterations in gene expression, to guide therapeutic choices, and to evaluate and adjust treatment protocols.[53] Ultimately, researchers envision molecular image-guided therapy systems to treat cancer as soon as it is found.[68] However, the development of molecular imaging for breast cancer faces many of the same hurdles described for biomarkers and molecular profiles, particularly the need for deeper knowledge of cancer biology and the ability to evaluate new technologies in large-scale epidemiological trials. Most of the technologies described in this chapter are currently being tested in animal models. Despite their distance from clinical use, their promise is immense: to revolutionize cancer medicine at every stage of patient care.

Functional Images Reveal Biological Processes

Molecular imaging is a high-resolution form of functional imaging, which reveals physiological, cellular, or molecular processes in living tissue.[41,77] Existing functional imaging technologies depict cancer-associated physiological processes—such as glucose metabolism, oxygen consumption, and blood flow—in vivo and in real time. A few such technologies have been clinically approved for cancer imaging, including the detection of radiolabeled fluorodeoxyglucose by positron emission tomography, which provides a somewhat nonspecific, but interpretable, indicator of tumor metabolism. Similarly, optical imaging of near-infrared absorption by hemoglobin appears to correlate with malignancy.[45] This technique, called diffuse optical tomography, is currently being tested in clinical trials.

In scintimammography, tracers such as 99mTc-Sestamibi are injected intravenously and then visualized using gamma camera/single-emission photon emisison computed tomography (SPECT) imaging of the breasts. Although it has not been evaluated as a viable screen for breast cancer, this technology has been found to detect the expression of a key multidrug resistance gene in tumors. Therefore scintimammography could potentially be used for prognosis (because multidrug resistance is an indicator of poor prognosis) and to guide therapeutic choices.[53]

Ultrasound can be used to assess blood flow in tumors, but in its present form, cannot reliably distinguish benign from malignant lesions.[20] However, targeted ultrasonic agents are being developed to provide high-contrast images for specific cell surface receptors.[34,41] In this guise, ultrasound would become a true molecular imaging technology—a technology cultivated much as other molecular imaging methods to be described, through parallel advances in probe and imaging design.

Molecular Probes Amplify Biological Signals

The biological processes targeted by molecular imaging are also key to cancer therapy: signal transduction, cell cycle regulation, multidrug resistance, angiogenesis, apoptosis, and telomerase expression (Table 5-3).

To visualize these processes in action, molecular probes may need to penetrate vascular, tissue, and cell membrane barriers, and they must be biocompatible.[9] The smallest possible probes, at low concentration, stand the greatest chance of success against these odds. However, with target molecules at extremely low (picomolar) concentrations or even lower, molecular imaging probes must also bind specifically; thus for some applica-

174 SAVING WOMEN'S LIVES

TABLE 5-3 Molecular Imaging in Breast Cancer Targets and Agents[53]

Target	Imaging Agent	Imaging Modality	Current Status
Glucose transporter-1 (Glut 1)	Fluorodeoxyglucose (FDG)	PET	Clinically approved
Hexokinase 1	FDG	PET	Clinically approved
Multidrug resistance 1 P-glycoprotein (MDR1 Pgp)	^{99m}Technetium	SPECT	Clinically verified
Estrogen receptors (ERs)	Fluoroestradiol	PET	Clinically verified
Vasoactive intestinal peptide receptors	Labeled peptides	SPECT/PET	Preclinical/ early clinical
Met tyrosine kinase	HGF/SF[60]	Blood oxygenation level dependent MRI	Preclinical/ early clinical
Sigma-2 receptors	Iodobenzamide	SPECT/PET	Preclinical/ early clinical
Na$^+$/I$^-$ symporter (NIS)	$^{131/125}$Iodine	SPECT	Preclinical/ early clinical
Mucin-1 glycoprotein (MUC1)	Pre-targeting antibody fragments	PET	Preclinical/ early clinical
Cell proliferation activities	Fluorothymidine (FLT)	PET	Preclinical/ early clinical
Cathepsin D	Cy-CDF-PGC[72c]	NIR Optical	Preclinical/ early clinical
MMP2	C-PGC[79d]	NIR Optical	Preclinical/ early clinical

[c]Cy5.5 Cathepsin D Sensitive Peptide Protected Graft Copolymer.
[d]Cy5.5 Poly L-Lysine Methoxypolyethylene Glycol.

tions, larger molecules with high affinities for their targets, such as antibodies or recombinant proteins, make superior probes.[9,41,53]

Low target concentrations also mean that molecular affinity probes must produce a strong signal, a challenge that has been met by attaching the target-binding affinity component to a signaling component.[41] The signal may be produced by a radioisotope, as detected by PET or another tomographic method; by a paramagnetic atom, as revealed by molecular resonance imaging; or by a fluorochrome, as visualized by imaging. (See Appendix A for description of these technologies.) Some nonradiolabeled probes send a signal only after being biochemically "turned on" by enzymatic activity that occurs upon target binding.[41,78] Such activatable imaging probes reduce background noise caused by nonspecific probe binding.

Molecular probes have already revealed a variety of cancer-related processes—so far, mostly in experimental animals—in unprecedented detail. These include events and features occurring in the extracellular milieu, such as the activity of cathepsins B and H in breast and other cancers; at the cell surface, such as tumor receptors, multidrug resistance transporters, and membrane phospholipids associated with apoptosis; within the cell, such as DNA replication; and even oncogene activity within the nucleus.[7,8,10,16,39,41,61,75,83]

Imaging Technologies Bring Probes into Focus

In addition to probes that bind specifically to their targets and produce clear signals, noninvasive molecular imaging techniques are being developed that can distinguish between probe signals and non-specific "noise" from other biological activity within the body. Molecular imaging technologies include radiological methods, such as positron emission tomography (PET) and single-emission photon emission computed tomography (SPECT); optical imaging approaches for fluorescent or bioluminescent probes; and MRI and magnetic resonance spectroscopy (MRS) (see Table 5-4).

Radiological Imaging

PET-based molecular imaging could eventually be used to diagnose a variety of molecular or genetic diseases, to predict a patient's response to a particular molecular therapy, and, if a molecular therapy is chosen, to determine whether it reaches its target and is effective.[12] Researchers have used PET with molecular probes to track gene expression in living animals; in addition to taking the technology one step closer to monitoring gene therapy in humans, mouse models such as these could be used to assess new drugs.[12,41] Like PET, SPECT, a similar technology that visualizes a different

TABLE 5-4 Characteristics of Various Molecular Imaging Modalities in Animal Studies

Imaging Technique	Portion of EM Spectrum Used	Spatial Resolution*	Tissue Penetration Depth	Type of Probe	Amount of Probe Used	Cost Ranking[e]
Positron emission tomography (PET)	High-energy gamma rays	1-2 mm	No limit	Radiolabeled	Nanograms	$$$$
Single photon emission computed tomography (SPECT)	Low-energy gamma rays	1-2 mm	No limit	Radiolabeled	Nanograms	$$$
Optical bioluminescence imaging	Visible light	3-5 mm[f]	1-2 cm	Activatable	Micrograms to milligrams	$$
Optical fluorescence	Visible light or near-infrared	2-3 mm[g]	<1 cm[h]	Activatable	Micrograms to milligrams	$-$$
Magnetic resonance imaging (MRI)	Radiowaves	25-100 μm	No limit	Activatable	Micrograms to milligrams	$$$$
Computed tomography (CT)	X-rays	50-200 μm	No limit	Under study	Not applicable	$$
Sonography	High-frequency sound waves	50-500 μm	Millimeters to centimeters	Limited activatable	Micrograms to milligrams	$$

*These values are for microPET and microSPECT which are used in animal studies. Most PET results in humans have spatial resolution of about 6-8 mm, with newer models being 5-6 mm. SPECT resolution for humans is about 10 mm.
eIncludes cost of equipment and cost per study.
fResolution is tissue depth dependent.
gFluorescence tomography may have better resolution.
hFluorescence tomography can likely image at greater depths (2-6 cm).
SOURCE: Adapted from Massoud and Gambhir, 2003.

range of isotopes, is currently used in functional imaging.[42] PET is more adaptable to molecular imaging, however, because the positron-emitting isotopes it employs are more easily incorporated into probes than the gamma-emitting isotopes visualized by SPECT.[41]

"It is clear that the first gene imaging to obtain FDA approval will be with PET, because the imaging probes are used in such low amounts that they will not produce pharmacologic or physiologic effects," according to Michael Phelps, chair of molecular and medical pharmacology at the University of California at Lost Angeles.[9] PET imaging probes are also relatively easy to construct, because drugs or existing molecules known to interact with a specific target can be modified with a radiolabel with minimal perturbation.[41] But even if a PET-based molecular imaging technology gains clinical approval in the near future, it is not likely to be widely adopted without the introduction of less-expensive PET scanners with better resolution and sensitivity.[12]

Another development likely to boost the clinical value of molecular imaging with PET is the advent of "multimodality" imaging systems combining PET scans—which do not clearly reveal the anatomy of regions of probe uptake—with high-resolution x-ray computed tomography (CT) imaging.[12] PET/CT scanners are already in clinical use for functional imaging.[12,41,71] Work is also under way to develop combined PET and MRI; however, although MRI provides better soft-tissue contrast than CT, it will be more technically challenging to integrate with PET. Researchers are exploring additional combinations of optical, radiological, MRI, and CT techniques capable of producing truly multimodal images.[6,29,41]

MRI

Functional MRI was introduced as an imaging technique in the 1970s, but was not widely used to detect breast cancer until the late 1990s.[19] Although orders of magnitude less sensitive than PET or optical techniques, molecular resonance has attracted the attention of molecular imaging researchers because of its higher spatial resolution and simultaneous depiction of molecular and anatomical information.[9,41] Antibody- and protein-based MRI probes have been used to visualize cell-surface molecules including cancer antigens and a protein associated with apoptosis.[23,31,41,59,83] Novel cancer therapies containing gadolinium, a paramagnetic species commonly used in magnetic resonance applications, could be tracked with MRI to image tumors and monitor their uptake of the labeled drugs over the course of treatment.[19] Activatable MRI agents for visualizing intracellular processes are possible, but only if the large target-binding molecules used in current probes can be replaced by smaller ones or made penetrable to cell membranes.[9] This constraint, for example, challenges work in progress on an MRI-based reporter system employing the intracellular enzyme beta-galactosidase.[53]

Optical Imaging

Optical imaging will be widely adopted because its capabilities exceed those of other imaging technologies, according to Ralph Weissleder, director of the Center for Molecular Imaging Research at Massachusetts General Hospital.[9] By identifying cancer-related alterations in gene expression, optical imaging will permit early diagnosis, "perhaps before morphological or clinical signs of disease can be seen," he says. Yet, as abnormalities are detected earlier, confirming the presence of cancer for a definitive diagnosis will become more difficult. Optical technology presents the possibility of using multiple probes, each with a distinct spectrum, to monitor several events or molecular species simultaneously.[41,77] Promising optical techniques for molecular imaging feature targeted bioluminescent probes, near-infrared (IR) fluorochromes (including activatable probes), and red-shifted fluorescent proteins.[41,80]

Bioluminescent probes emit light that is essentially free of background, and are therefore attractive because they can be detected at very low concentrations.[41] However, viable technology has yet to be developed for bioluminescent imaging in the human body, and this strategy would still require injecting mass levels of substrates, such as D-Luciferin, into the body.[41] Fluorescent probes have higher background, but offer two advantages: they can be used as reporters in both live and fixed tissues, and they can often be visualized without the addition of a substrate.[64]

Fluorescent probes that emit in the near IR have maximal tissue penetration and minimal background fluorescence.[41] An activatable near-IR probe has been used in vivo to monitor activity of cathepsin D, an extracellular protease that is overexpressed in many tumors.[41,53,68] Fluorescence-mediated tomography, an approach that is still in its infancy, is being developed to penetrate further than is possible with existing near-IR methods.[41,46,47] Multimodality probes that are capable of fluorescence and bioluminescence are also under active investigation.

Multidisciplinary Research Is Key to
Bringing Molecular Imaging to the Clinic

A review article by Massoud and Gambhir (2003) identifies the following goals for molecular imaging, leading from the research laboratory to the clinic:

- To develop noninvasive in vivo imaging methods that reflect specific cellular and molecular processes, such as gene expression and protein-protein interactions
- To monitor multiple molecular events in concert
- To follow trafficking and targeting of cells
- To optimize drug and gene therapy
- To image drug effects at the molecular and cellular level
- To assess the molecular pathology of disease progression

Meeting these goals and translating that achievement into rapid, reproducible and quantitative clinical technologies will be a critical step toward the molecular management of cancer.

Many basic questions remain to be answered in the course of developing and refining molecular imaging technologies. Overcoming the theoretical and practical challenges of biocompatibility, barriers to probe delivery, and signal amplification will require continued research.[40,41] Investigators are concentrating their efforts on selecting appropriate cellular and subcellular imaging targets, probing the development and delivery, amplification strategies for targets at nanomolar to picomolar concentrations, and the development of high-resolution, real-time imaging systems that can ultimately be used in humans.[41,77,80]

If the potential of molecular imaging is fulfilled, imaging will influence all aspects of cancer care, from diagnosis to treatment evaluation, and will play an increased role in the development of new molecular therapies. Researchers are already looking beyond the previously described imaging technologies to the design of molecular biosensors that can be injected into the bloodstream to find and destroy cancer cells. Advances such as these can only be achieved through collaborative, multidisciplinary research that brings together molecular and cellular biologists, imaging scientists, nanotechnologists, and cancer clinicians. Consequently, a key online resource, Molecular Imaging Central, has been created to provide links among the various areas of research in molecular imaging, background information on different types molecular imaging, as well as highlighting the latest research findings. Supporting agencies for such research include the NCI, which funds a variety of molecular imaging initiatives (see Box 5-4). Bridging these disparate fields is perhaps the greatest challenge to the development of molecular imaging, but one which, if met, could establish a new research paradigm for the advancement of molecular medicine.

**BOX 5-4
National Cancer Institute Support for
Molecular Imaging Research[43]**

The following NCI initiatives foster advances in functional and molecular imaging:

In Vivo Cellular and Molecular Imaging Centers: Bring together experts from diverse scientific and technological backgrounds to conduct multidisciplinary research on cellular and molecular imaging in cancer. Five Centers established as of 2002; support provided for 14 potential sites, including a site for researching functional imaging of low-activity genes.

Novel Imaging Technologies Program: Supports collaboration of academic scientists with industry and foreign institutes to create unique imaging technology, including the next generation of PET/CT scanner for improved localization and evaluation of difficult-to-locate cancers and therapeutic monitoring.

Clinical Imaging Drugs and Enhancers Program: Fosters the development of new imaging contrast agents and molecular probes to improve cancer diagnosis and treatment. Several agents or probes currently in development for measuring blood vessel formation and cell death, evaluating cell growth, and enhancing visualization of various cancers.

Molecular Imaging Database (MOLI): A publicly available imaging database intended to help researchers develop new imaging agents and to help clinicians find existing agents for imaging specific cancers. The database is expected to be released in mid-2004.

Clinical Trial Cooperative Groups: Networks of healthcare professionals affiliated with medical schools, teaching hospitals, and community-based cancer treatment centers who encourage movement of promising imaging advances from discovery and development to clinical use (e.g., American College of Radiology Imaging Network).

Cancer Therapy Evaluation Program: Exploring the use of imaging as a biomarker or surrogate marker for cancer, instead of biopsy, to monitor treatment effectiveness.

Mouse Models of Human Cancer Consortium: Includes researchers who are developing novel imaging modalities for use in preclinical studies.

Small Animal Imaging Resource Program: Resource to allow scientists from different disciplines to use small animal imaging technology, including molecular imaging.

NOVEL IN VITRO DIAGNOSTIC TESTS POSE
UNIQUE REGULATORY CHALLENGES

Innovative in vitro diagnostics, such as tests for genetic susceptibility to various diseases, pose a new spectrum of regulatory challenges. These include overcoming both the inexperience of the FDA with such cutting-edge technology and the inexperience of the budding companies that are developing it, as well as narrowing down the complex genetic data being generated, and providing uniformity in analysis and testing.

The FDA is currently in a learning mode about genomics and proteomics. These methods use patterns in the activation of specific genes or production of specific proteins to help determine the diagnosis, prognosis, or risk of developing various diseases. New products from these endeavors have emerged in significant numbers only in the past decade.

In the past 3 years, the agency has had about 50 presentations about this technology from industry, academia, or the government. The FDA's in vitro diagnostics office has an internal "Omics" working group that has met periodically over the last 3 years to discuss new developments in the field and to interact with their counterparts in the FDA's Center for Drug Evaluation and Research, and the agency released a guidance document for pharmacogenetics and pharmacogenomics in November 2003.

Hundreds or thousands of results are generated by genomic and proteomic tests for each specimen as opposed to one result per sample in the conventional diagnostic tests that the FDA is used to seeing. Regulation of these array tests will be much easier if manufacturers of genomic or proteomic tests can reduce the amount of data required for a given diagnostic determination. Regulatory submissions for such diagnostics include imprecise measurements of every analyte and a lack of standardization in the analysis approach. These technologies are so new that clear standards have not yet emerged, which means that the FDA must not only conduct its usual evaluation for adherence to established methodological and analytic standards, but it must evaluate the validity of new methods as they are evolving.

SUMMARY

The biological revolution in breast cancer detection and management is under way, but it is likely to proceed slowly and by degrees. Significant progress has been made toward the identification of key breast cancer biomarkers, as well as aggregate profiles of breast cancer in the genome, transcriptome, and proteome; the theoretical promise of molecular imaging is beginning to be realized in animal models. When molecular medicine for breast cancer first enters the clinic, it will most likely come in the form of techniques to monitor therapeutic response and recurrence. The use of molecular screening technologies, such as blood tests for routine screening of normal-risk, symptom-free women, likely lies in the more distant future. Measures of recurrence or response to therapy are intrinsically easier to develop than screening tests, because each woman can serve as her own reference point for changes that can be measured over days or months. In contrast, a screening test needs to provide interpretable results based on a single time point.

Even further in the future, researchers envision individualized management of each case of breast cancer, based on its specific molecular characteristics. "We'll have a roadmap, a wiring diagram of the deranged cellular circuitry of each patient's cancer, not just a named diagnosis, but a molecular profile," according to Lance Liotta of the NCI. "Instead of choosing therapy by a category of disease, we'll use combination therapy tailored to the individual molecular profile of the tissue, the tumor microenvironment, and the cancer. Instead of single targets and single therapeutic agents, we'll have multiple targets all along the length of key signal transduction pathways, both intracellular and extracellular, at the tumor-host interface. And finally, instead of determining efficacy by waiting for a change in tumor size or recurrence, we'll have direct monitoring of cellular targets before, during, and after therapy by biopsy—or ideally by molecular imaging or serum proteomics—to monitor changes that are going on in the tissue microenvironment following treatment." However, the nonimaging biological techniques must be linked to additional procedures that can localize the cancer and examine its pathology. In addition, the problem of a test being too sensitive—detecting cancer before it could be physically located with current imaging technology—could be traumatic for patients. True positives would thus be indistinguishable from false positives and create a high level of anxiety among women with a positive test.

Fulfilling the potential of molecular medicine for breast and other cancers will require collaboration between molecular biologists and scientists from a broad spectrum of disciplines. It will fall to epidemiologists and biostatisticians to guide the rational design of biologically based cancer diagnostics, to establish their significance and reproducibility, and, in the case of clinical epidemiologists, to adapt them for routine clinical use.[56] Ultimately, they will have to develop standardized statistical methods for analysis of large genomic and proteomic data sets. Once these new biologically based detection and diagnostic tools have been developed, they will need to be tested for safety and effectiveness beyond the research setting in multicenter clinical trials. Yet, a lack of regulatory standards for the validation of novel diagnostic tests may hinder clinical trials by making them more difficult to design and the results more challenging to interpret. Finally, these tools will not be used in isolation but will become part of an arsenal of tools—each with distinctive capacities and caveats. Developing evidence-based systems for integrating this new technology will require attention at all levels of the health care system—physicians, payers, purchasers, and patients.

REFERENCES

1. Ahr A, Holtrich U, Solbach C, Scharl A, Strebhardt K, Karn T, Kaufmann M. 2001. Molecular classification of breast cancer patients by gene expression profiling. *J Pathol* 195(3):312-320.
2. Albertson DG. 2003. Profiling breast cancer by array CGH. *Breast Cancer Res Treat* 78(3):289-298.
3. Anonymous. 2002. Microarray standards at last. *Nature* 419(6905):323.
4. Baselga J. 2001. Herceptin alone or in combination with chemotherapy in the treatment of HER2-positive metastatic breast cancer: pivotal trials. *Oncology* 61(Suppl 2):14-21.
5. Beenken SW, Bland KI. 2002. Biomarkers for breast cancer. *Minerva Chir* 57(4):437-448.
6. Bogdanov A Jr, Weissleder R. 1998. The development of in vivo imaging systems to study gene expression. *Trends Biotechnol* 16(1):5-10.
7. Bremer C, Tung CH, Bogdanov A Jr, Weissleder R. 2002. Imaging of differential protease expression in breast cancers for detection of aggressive tumor phenotypes. *Radiology* 222(3):814-818.
8. Bremer C, Tung CH, Weissleder R. 2001. In vivo molecular target assessment of matrix metalloproteinase inhibition. *Nat Med* 7(6):743-748.
9. Brice J. 2001. Molecular imaging transports diagnosis to the next level. *Diagnostic Imaging* Special Edition(July):8-15.
10. Chen WS, Luker KE, Dahlheimer JL, Pica CM, Luker GD, Piwnica-Worms D. 2000. Effects of MDR1 and MDR3 P-glycoproteins, MRP1, and BCRP/MXR/ABCP on the transport of (99m)Tc-tetrofosmin. *Biochem Pharmacol* 60(3):413-426.
11. Chen Y, Yakhini Z, Ben-Dor A, Dougherty E, Trent JM, Bittner M. 2001. Analysis of expression patterns: the scope of the problem, the problem of scope. *Dis Markers* 17(2):59-65.
12. Cherry SR, Physics World. Watching Biology in Action. June 2002. Accessed January 6, 2003. Web Page. Available at: http://physicsweb.org/article/world/15/6/7.
13. Chung EJ, Sung YK, Farooq M, Kim Y, Im S, Tak WY, Hwang YJ, Kim YI, Han HS, Kim JC, Kim MK. 2002. Gene expression profile analysis in human hepatocellular carcinoma by cDNA microarray. *Mol Cells* 14(3):382-387.
14. Cui H, Cruz-Correa M, Giardiello FM, Hutcheon DF, Kafonek DR, Brandenburg S, Wu Y, He X, Powe NR, Feinberg AP. 2003. Loss of IGF2 imprinting: a potential marker of colorectal cancer risk. *Science* 299(5613):1753-1755.
15. De Gruttola VG, Clax P, DeMets DL, Downing GJ, Ellenberg SS, Friedman L, Gail MH, Prentice R, Wittes J, Zeger SL. 2001. Considerations in the evaluation of surrogate endpoints in clinical trials: summary of a National Institutes of Health workshop. *Control Clin Trials* 22(5):485-502.
16. Dewanjee MK, Ghafouripour AK, Kapadvanjwala M, Dewanjee S, Serafini AN, Lopez DM, Sfakianakis GN. 1994. Noninvasive imaging of c-myc oncogene messenger RNA with indium-111-antisense probes in a mammary tumor-bearing mouse model. *J Nucl Med* 35(6):1054-1063.

17. Dooley WC, Ljung BM, Veronesi U, Cazzaniga M, Elledge RM, O'Shaughnessy JA, Kuerer HM, Hung DT, Khan SA, Phillips RF, Ganz PA, Euhus DM, Esserman LJ, Haffty BG, King BL, Kelley MC, Anderson MM, Schmit PJ, Clark RR, Kass FC, Anderson BO, Troyan SL, Arias RD, Quiring JN, Love SM, Page DL, King EB. 2001. Ductal lavage for detection of cellular atypia in women at high risk for breast cancer. *J Natl Cancer Inst* 93(21):1624-1632.

18. Duffy MJ. 2001. Clinical uses of tumor markers: a critical review. *Crit Rev Clin Lab Sci* 38(3):225-262.

19. Esserman L, Wolverton D, Hylton N. 2002. Magnetic resonance imaging for primary breast cancer management: current role and new applications. *Endocr Relat Cancer* 9(2):141-153.

20. Esserman LJ. 2002. New approaches to the imaging, diagnosis, and biopsy of breast lesions. *Cancer J* 8(Suppl 1):S1-S14.

21. Evron E, Dooley WC, Umbricht CB, Rosenthal D, Sacchi N, Gabrielson E, Soito AB, Hung DT, Ljung B, Davidson NE, Sukumar S. 2001. Detection of breast cancer cells in ductal lavage fluid by methylation-specific PCR. *Lancet* 357(9265):1335-1336.

22. Fabian CJ, Kamel S, Zalles C, Kimler BF. 1996. Identification of a chemoprevention cohort from a population of women at high risk for breast cancer. *J Cell Biochem Suppl* 25:112-122.

23. Flacke S, Fischer S, Scott MJ, Fuhrhop RJ, Allen JS, McLean M, Winter P, Sicard GA, Gaffney PJ, Wickline SA, Lanza GM. 2001. Novel MRI contrast agent for molecular imaging of fibrin: implications for detecting vulnerable plaques. *Circulation* 104(11):1280-1285.

24. Garber K. 2004. Genomic medicine. Gene expression tests foretell breast cancer's future. *Science* 303(5665):1754-1755.

25. Gruvberger S , Ringner M, Chen Y, Panavally S, Saal LH, Borg A, Ferno M, Peterson C, Meltzer PS. 2001. Estrogen receptor status in breast cancer is associated with remarkably distinct gene expression patterns. *Cancer Res* 61(16):5979-5984.

26. Hollon T. 2002. Classifying breast cancer models. *The Scientist* 16(17):20-24.

27. Institute of Medicine. 2001. *Mammography and Beyond: Developing Technologies for the Early Detection of Breast Cancer*. Washington, DC: National Academy Press.

28. Jeffrey SS, Pollack JR. 2003. The diagnosis and management of pre-invasive breast disease: promise of new technologies in understanding pre-invasive breast lesions. *Breast Cancer Res* 5(6):320-328.

29. Josephson L, Kircher MF, Mahmood U, Tang Y, Weissleder R. 2002. Near-infrared fluorescent nanoparticles as combined MR/optical imaging probes. *Bioconjug Chem* 13(3):554-560.

30. Kallioniemi A. 2002. Molecular signatures of breast cancer—predicting the future. *N Engl J Med* 347(25):2067-2068.

31. Kang HW, Josephson L, Petrovsky A, Weissleder R, Bogdanov A Jr. 2002. Magnetic resonance imaging of inducible E-selectin expression in human endothelial cell culture. *Bioconjug Chem* 13(1):122-127.

32. Kuo WP, Jenssen TK, Butte AJ, Ohno-Machado L, Kohane IS. 2002. Analysis of matched mRNA measurements from two different microarray technologies. *Bioinformatics* 18(3):405-412.

33. Lakhani SR, Ashworth A. 2001. Microarray and histopathological analysis of tumours: the future and the past? *Nat Rev Cancer* 1(2):151-157.

34. Lanza GM, Wickline SA. 2001. Targeted ultrasonic contrast agents for molecular imaging and therapy. *Prog Cardiovasc Dis* 44(1):13-31.

35. Lewis R. 2002. Breast cancer: the big picture emerges. *The Scientist* 17(3):24-25.

36. Liotta L. 2003. Deciphering the molecular signatures of breast cancer. *Institute of Medicine Workshop on New Technologies for the Early Detection and Diagnosis of Breast Cancer.* Washington, DC: The Institute of Medicine of the National Academies.

37. Liotta LA, Kohn EC. 2001. The microenvironment of the tumour-host interface. *Nature* 411(6835):375-379.

38. Liotta LA, Kohn EC, Petricoin EF. 2001. Clinical proteomics: personalized molecular medicine. *JAMA* 286(18):2211-2214.

39. Mahmood U, Tung CH, Bogdanov A Jr, Weissleder R. 1999. Near-infrared optical imaging of protease activity for tumor detection. *Radiology* 213(3):866-870.

40. Mahmood U, Weissleder R. 2002. Some tools for molecular imaging. *Acad Radiol* 9(6):629-631.

41. Massoud TF, Gambhir SS. 2003. Molecular imaging in living subjects: seeing fundamental biological processes in a new light. *Genes Dev* 17(5):545-580.

42. Nass SJ, Henderson IC, Lashof JC. 2001. *Mammography and Beyond: Developing Technologies for the Early Detection of Breast Cancer.* Washington, DC: National Academy Press.

43. National Cancer Institute. Cancer Imaging and Molecular Sensing. 2004. *The Nation's Investment in Cancer Research: A Plan and Budget Proposal for Fiscal Year 2004.* Bethesda, MD: National Cancer Institute. Bypass Budget.

44. Negm RS, Verma M, Srivastava S. 2002. The promise of biomarkers in cancer screening and detection. *Trends Mol Med* 8(6):288-293.

45. Ntziachristos V, Chance B. 2001. Probing physiology and molecular function using optical imaging: applications to breast cancer. *Breast Cancer Res* 3(1):41-46.

46. Ntziachristos V, Tung CH, Bremer C, Weissleder R. 2002. Fluorescence molecular tomography resolves protease activity in vivo. *Nat Med* 8(7):757-760.

47. Ntziachristos V, Weissleder R. 2002. Charge-coupled-device based scanner for tomography of fluorescent near-infrared probes in turbid media. *Med Phys* 29(5):803-809.

48. Pauletti G, Godolphin W, Press MF, Slamon DJ. 1996. Detection and quantitation of HER-2/neu gene amplification in human breast cancer archival material using fluorescence in situ hybridization. *Oncogene* 13(1):63-72.

49. Perou CM, Sorlie T, Eisen MB, van de Rijn M, Jeffrey SS, Rees CA, Pollack JR, Ross DT, Johnsen H, Akslen LA, Fluge O, Pergamenschikov A, Williams C, Zhu SX, Lonning PE, Borresen-Dale AL, Brown PO, Botstein D. 2000. Molecular portraits of human breast tumours. *Nature* 406(6797):747-752.

50. Petricoin EF, Ardekani AM, Hitt BA, Levine PJ, Fusaro VA, Steinberg SM, Mills GB, Simone C, Fishman DA, Kohn EC, Liotta LA. 2002. Use of proteomic patterns in serum to identify ovarian cancer. *Lancet* 359(9306):572-577.

51. Petricoin EF, Zoon KC, Kohn EC, Barrett JC, Liotta LA. 2002. Clinical proteomics: translating benchside promise into bedside reality. *Nat Rev Drug Discov* 1(9):683-695.

52. Petricoin EF 3rd, Hackett JL, Lesko LJ, Puri RK, Gutman SI, Chumakov K, Woodcock J, Feigal DW Jr, Zoon KC, Sistare FD. 2002. Medical applications of microarray technologies: a regulatory science perspective. *Nat Genet* 32(Suppl):474-479.

53. Piwnica-Worms D. 2003. Molecular Imaging. *Institute of Medicine Workshop on New Technologies for the Early Detection and Diagnosis of Breast Cancer.* Washington, DC: The Institute of Medicine of the National Academies.

54. Pollack JR, Sorlie T, Perou CM, Rees CA, Jeffrey SS, Lonning PE, Tibshirani R, Botstein D, Borresen-Dale AL, Brown PO. 2002. Microarray analysis reveals a major direct role of DNA copy number alteration in the transcriptional program of human breast tumors. *Proc Natl Acad Sci USA* 99(20):12963-12968.

55. Pritzker KP. 2002. Cancer biomarkers: easier said than done. *Clin Chem* 48(8):1147-1150.

56. Ransohoff DF. 2002. Challenges and opportunities in evaluating diagnostic tests. *J Clin Epidemiol* 55(12):1178-1182.

57. Ransohoff DF. 2003. Cancer. Developing molecular biomarkers for cancer. *Science* 299(5613):1679-1680.

58. Ransohoff DF. 2003. Gene-expression signatures in breast cancer. *N Engl J Med* 348(17):1715-1717.

59. Remsen LG, McCormick CI, Roman-Goldstein S, Nilaver G, Weissleder R, Bogdanov A, Hellstrom I, Kroll RA, Neuwelt EA. 1996. MR of carcinoma-specific monoclonal antibody conjugated to monocrystalline iron oxide nanoparticles: the potential for noninvasive diagnosis. *Am J Neuroradiol* 17(3):411-418.

60. Shaharabany M, Abramovitch R, Kushnir T, Tsarfaty G, Ravid-Megido M, Horev J, Ron R, Itzhak Y, Tsarfaty I. 2001. In vivo molecular imaging of met tyrosine kinase growth factor receptor activity in normal organs and breast tumors. *Cancer Res* 61(12):4873-4878.

61. Shields AF, Grierson JR, Dohmen BM, Machulla HJ, Stayanoff JC, Lawhorn-Crews JM, Obradovich JE, Muzik O, Mangner TJ. 1998. Imaging proliferation in vivo with. *Nat Med* 4(11):1334-1336.

62. Singletary SE. 2003. Rating the risk factors for breast cancer. *Ann Surg* 237(4):474-482.

63. Sorlie T, Perou CM, Tibshirani R, Aas T, Geisler S, Johnsen H, Hastie T, Eisen MB, van de Rijn M, Jeffrey SS, Thorsen T, Quist H, Matese JC, Brown PO, Botstein D, Eystein Lonning P, Borresen-Dale AL. 2001. Gene expression patterns of breast carcinomas distinguish tumor subclasses with clinical implications. *Proc Natl Acad Sci USA* 98(19):10869-10874.

64. Spergel DJ, Kruth U, Shimshek DR, Sprengel R, Seeburg PH. 2001. Using reporter genes to label selected neuronal populations in transgenic mice for gene promoter, anatomical, and physiological studies. *Prog Neurobiol* 63(6):673-686.

65. Srivastava S, Gopal-Srivastava R. 2002. Biomarkers in cancer screening: a public health perspective. *J Nutr* 132(8 Suppl):2471S-2475S.

66. Srivastava S, Kramer BS. 2000. Early detection cancer research network. *Lab Invest* 80(8):1147-1148.

67. Sukumar S. 2003. The Search for Breast Cancer Biomarkers. *Institute of Medicine Workshop on New Technologies for the Early Detection and Diagnosis of Breast Cancer.* Washington, DC: The Institute of Medicine of the National Academies.

68. Tempany CM, McNeil BJ. 2001. Advances in biomedical imaging. *JAMA* 285(5):562-567.

69. Templin MF, Stoll D, Schrenk M, Traub PC, Vohringer CF, Joos TO. 2002. Protein microarray technology. *Drug Discov Today* 7(15):815-822.

70. Tilstone C. 2003. DNA microarrays: vital statistics. *Nature* 424(6949):610-612.

71. Townsend DW, Cherry SR. 2001. Combining anatomy and function: the path to true image fusion. *Eur Radiol* 11(10):1968-1974.

72. Tung CH, Bredow S, Mahmood U, Weissleder R. 1999. Preparation of a cathepsin D sensitive near-infrared fluorescence probe for imaging. *Bioconjug Chem* 10(5):892-896.

73. van de Vijver MJ, He YD, van't Veer LJ, Dai H, Hart AA, Voskuil DW, Schreiber GJ, Peterse JL, Roberts C, Marton MJ, Parrish M, Atsma D, Witteveen A, Glas A, Delahaye L, van der Velde T, Bartelink H, Rodenhuis S, Rutgers ET, Friend SH, Bernards R. 2002. A gene-expression signature as a predictor of survival in breast cancer. *N Engl J Med* 347(25):1999-2009.

74. van't Veer LJ, Dai H, van de Vijver MJ, He YD, Hart AA, Bernards R, Friend SH. 2002. Expression profiling predicts outcome in breast cancer. *Breast Cancer Res* 5(1):57-58.

75. Virgolini I. 2000. Peptide Imaging. *Diagnostic Nuclear Medicine*. Berlin: Springer-Verlag. Pp. 135-158.

76. Weinstein JN, Scherf ULJ, Nishizuka SGF, Bussey AK, Kim SSL, Tanabe L, Richman S, Alexander J, Kouros-Mehr H, Maunakea A, Reinhold WC. 2002. The bioinformatics of microarray gene expression profiling. *Cytometry* 47:46-49.

77. Weissleder RM. 1999. Molecular imaging: exploring the next frontier. *Radiology* 212(3):609-614.

78. Weissleder RM. 2002. Scaling down imaging: molecular mapping of cancer in mice. *Nature Rev Cancer* 2:1-8.

79. Weissleder RM, Tung CH, Mahmood U, Bogdanov A Jr. 1999. In vivo imaging of tumors with protease-activated near-infrared fluorescent probes. *Nat Biotechnol* 17(4):375-378.

80. Weissleder RM. 2001. Molecular imaging. *Radiology* 219:316-333.

81. West M, Blanchette C, Dressman H, Huang E, Ishida S, Spang R, Zuzan H, Olson JA Jr, Marks JR, Nevins JR. 2001. Predicting the clinical status of human breast cancer by using gene expression profiles. *Proc Natl Acad Sci USA* 98(20):11462-11467.

82. Yaffe MJ, Boyd NF, Byng JW, Jong RA, Fishell E, Lockwood GA, Little LE, Tritchler DL. 1998. Breast cancer risk and measured mammographic density. *Eur J Cancer Prev* 7(Suppl 1):S47-S55.

83. Zhao M, Beauregard DA, Loizou L, Davletov B, Brindle KM. 2001. Non-invasive detection of apoptosis using magnetic resonance imaging and a targeted contrast agent. *Nat Med* 7(11):1241-1244.

6

The Necessary Environment for Research and Development

While the public impatiently awaits new technologies and headlines, medical researchers bemoan the "national crisis." The crisis is not in discovery and invention, but rather in getting those discoveries to the public.

RN Rosenberg, *JAMA* 2003

asic research lays the foundation for the discovery and invention of new medical technologies, but the path from discovery to adoption is long and often full of unexpected turns. The value of any new technology must be demonstrated through a series of increasingly stringent steps, each of which can take years.[a] Figure 6-1 illustrates the pathway of medical technology development from discovery to adoption in clinical practice.

Once a technology reaches the prototype, or investigational, stage, it is typically tested in small clinical studies, usually involving fewer than 50 subjects. In most cases, a technology must pass Food and Drug Administration (FDA) review for safety and effectiveness before it can be marketed. Because most technologies are affordable only if they are covered by health care insurance, most will not be adopted in clinical practice unless their use is deemed "reasonable and necessary," by either the Centers for Medicare & Medicaid Services (CMS) or private insurance companies. Practically speaking, that means that the technology must be shown to improve outcomes. The time from discovery and invention to clinical use is a source of great concern and frustration to technology developers, as well as members of the public who eagerly await these advances, none more impatiently than those whose mission is to reduce the toll of breast cancer.

---

[a]"Technology" is used here in the broadest sense and includes biology, drugs, software, devices, and procedures.

188

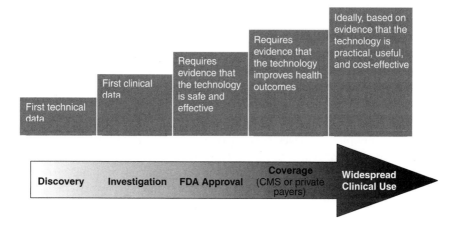

FIGURE 6-1 Pathway of medical technology development.

This chapter describes the stages of technology development and considers the degree to which there are obstacles that cause unreasonable delays and proposals for reducing those obstacles. Avoidable pitfalls, such as clinical studies designed so poorly that they fail to provide clear answers or technologies developed with little understanding of what physicians and patients really need, are also covered. The development of medical technologies is a complex enterprise that requires the integrated expertise of engineers, biologists, physicians, statisticians, and health care administrators. This chapter thus highlights a variety of initiatives that illustrate different approaches to integrate the necessary expertise for innovations that save lives.

SUPPORT FOR DISCOVERY RESEARCH IS ADEQUATE

Fostering the invention and early stage development of medical technology is essential and depends on the nurturing of basic medical research. Due in no small part to the long-standing and tireless efforts of breast cancer activists, breast cancer research has been generously supported over the past few decades. With the possible exception of AIDS, breast cancer research receives more funding than any other disease. The National Cancer Institute (NCI) currently supports more research projects and clinical trials for breast cancer than for any other type of cancer.[51] According to their website, NCI supports 2,932 breast cancer projects and 112 clinical trials. By comparison, the average for all 56 types of cancer (or aspects of cancer) listed by NCI is only 276 projects and 8 clinical trials. In addition to the National Institutes of Health (NIH), breast cancer research is supported by private health charities and the Department of Defense (DoD) Congressionally Directed Medical Research Program, which together provide more than $300 million per year, for a total of roughly $800 million per year (Figure 6-2). By comparison, NCI spent $311 million on prostate cancer and DoD's Medical Research Program spent $85 million for a total of just under $400 million (Figure 6-3). Table 6-1 lists the major funders of breast cancer research.

The Committee believes that current priorities for basic research are appropriate. The investment in basic research over the past few decades has yielded a wealth of knowledge that fuels the invention of a rich array of powerful new technologies from imaging devices that can display the activity of individual cell types to assays that can simultaneously measure the activity of thousands of genes or proteins.

A broad consensus among experts in breast cancer over the last few years supports this view. In 1998, the NCI convened the Breast Cancer Research Progress Group, a panel of 30 prominent members of the scientific, medical, and advocacy communities to identify the most important research needs in breast cancer. The panel's recommendations included research to identify biomarkers, molecular analysis of the transition from pre-invasive to invasive disease, the importance of tissue banks as a critical research resource, the need for biologically based imaging, and the need to develop databases and bioinformatics so that the wealth of data can be

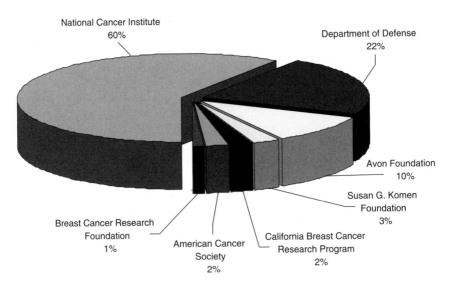

FIGURE 6-2 Distribution of public and charitable funding of breast cancer.

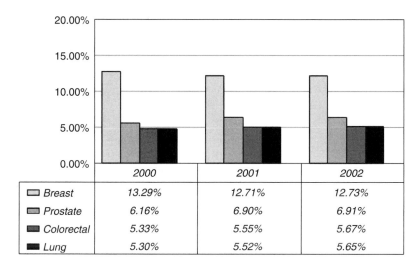

	2000	2001	2002
▢ Breast	13.29%	12.71%	12.73%
▨ Prostate	6.16%	6.90%	6.91%
▨ Colorectal	5.33%	5.55%	5.67%
■ Lung	5.30%	5.52%	5.65%

FIGURE 6-3 Percentage of NCI budget allocated to selected cancer types.

assimilated and exploited for maximum benefit. Three years later, these same areas were recommended for support in the 2001 *Mammography and Beyond* report.[33] The NCI and DoD breast cancer research portfolios reflect these priorities, as do the research portfolios of key private funders. Further, these same themes have been equally emphasized for all types of cancer. The individual technologies in development for detecting breast cancer are proceeding equally or better than in other disease research areas.

Many new technologies hold great promise to improve breast cancer detection. Over the years "breakthroughs" have been announced with great regularity. But there is a long passage between the development of a promising technology and determining whether its promise can be realized. Few of the breakthroughs heralded in past decades have proved their worth in reducing breast cancer mortality. Although the research engine that drives technology advances is well fueled, the validation and implementation of those advances is another matter.

Technology Assessment

The term "technology assessment" is used in different ways by different people. In the narrowest, but also the most widely used, sense, health technology assessment refers to the synthesis of evidence collected from clinical studies and the application of that synthesis to decisions about whether a particular technology should be adopted by a health care pro-

TABLE 6-1 Major Funders of Breast Cancer Research

Organization	Comments	Number of 2001 Grants (grant amount)	Type of Organization
National Cancer Institute	National cancer program that conducts and supports research, training, health information dissemination, and other programs with respect to cancer patients and family members	Overall: 6,397 grants ($2.8 billion) Breast cancer: 2,826 grants ($475.2 million)	Government
Breast Cancer Research Program (DoD)	Promotes research directed toward eradicating breast cancer	378 grants ($175 million)	Government
Avon Foundation	Motivated to benefit women through research, clinical care, support services, education, and early detection, with emphasis on reaching medically underserved women	>200 grants ($83 million)	Nonprofit
Susan G. Komen Foundation	Aims to eradicate breast cancer as a life-threatening disease, by advancing research, education, screening and treatment; 90 percent of money raised goes to research	115 grants ($20.4 million)	Nonprofit
California Breast Cancer Research Program	Seeks to reduce the impact of breast cancer in California by supporting research on breast cancer and facilitating the dissemination of research findings and their translation into public health practice	64 grants ($18 million)	State government
American Cancer Society	Dedicated to eliminating cancer as a major health problem by preventing cancer, saving lives, and diminishing suffering from cancer, through research, education, advocacy, and service	Overall: 84 grants ($46.4 million) Breast Cancer: ($17 million for breast cancer in 2000)	Nonprofit

TABLE 6-1 Continued

Organization	Comments	Number of 2001 Grants (grant amount)	Type of Organization
Breast Cancer Research Foundation	Dedicated to funding clinical and genetic breast cancer research; 85 percent of the money goes to research	48 grants ($8.5 million)	Nonprofit
Susan Love MD Breast Cancer Foundation	Aims to support the eradication of breast cancer through education, research, and advocacy	12 grants ($110,000)	Nonprofit
Friends . . . you can count on	Works to educate, promote awareness, raise funds, evaluate promising new projects, and make grants for research for new and improved methods of earlier detection of breast cancer	3 grants ($100,000)	Nonprofit
Total breast cancer research funding		More than $826 million awarded for more than 3,640 grants	All funding sources

vider or reimbursed by a health care payer, such as a private health insurance company or Medicare. Technology assessment of this sort is conducted by federal and private organizations (Table 6-2). In practice, the initial phase of technology assessment done by health care payers does not usually consider cost, feasibility, or social and ethical issues.

The Institute of Medicine (IOM) Committee for Evaluating Medical Technologies in Clinical Use defined medical technology assessment more broadly as:

> any process of examining and reporting properties of a medical technology used in health care, such as safety, efficacy, feasibility, and indications for use, cost, and cost-effectiveness, as well as social, economic, and ethical consequences, whither intended or unintended.[32]

Assessing Medical Technologies, IOM, 1985, p. 2

This definition includes clinical studies of efficacy, effectiveness, diagnostic accuracy, the impact of a technology on quality of life, FDA review, and assessment for health insurance coverage, and post-market.

TABLE 6-2 Federal and Private Technology Assessors

FEDERAL ORGANIZATIONS

Centers for Medicare & Medicaid Services (CMS)	Responsible for tracking emerging technologies and patterns of care to determine applicability of existing national coverage policy and to assess the need for policy change. (Named changed from Health Care Financing Administration, or HCFA, in June 2001.)
Medicare Coverage Advisory Committee (MCAC)	MCAC advises CMS on whether specific medical items and services are "reasonable and necessary" under Medicare law. MCAC is advisory in nature, with the final decision on all issues resting with CMS.
Agency for Healthcare Research and Quality (AHRQ)	AHRQ's Evidence Practice Centers (EPCs) conduct systematic, comprehensive analyses and syntheses of the scientific literature to develop evidence reports and technology assessments on clinical topics that are common, expensive, and present challenges to decisionmakers.
U.S. Preventive Services Task Force (USPSTF)	Independent panel of preventive health experts, convened by AHRQ, who are charged with evaluating the scientific evidence for the effectiveness of a range of clinical preventive services and producing age-specific and risk factor-specific recommendations for these services.
Office of Medical Applications and Research (OMAR)	Established in 1977 as part of the NIH Consensus Development program. This is the focal point for evidence-based assessments of medical practice and state-of-the-science on behalf of the medical community and the public. More than 120 NIH Consensus Statements and State-of-the-Science Statements have been issued since the program's inception.

PRIVATE ORGANIZATIONS

Blue Cross Blue Shield Association Technology Evaluation Center (BCBSA-TEC)	Evaluates the clinical effectiveness and appropriateness of medical procedures, devices, and drugs. The TEC averages 20 to 25 assessments each year, and provides healthcare decision makers, such as Kaiser Permanente and CMS, with information on clinical effectiveness.

TABLE 6-2 Continued

ECRI	Nonprofit health services research agency that monitors technology-related hazards, disseminates the results of medical product evaluations and technology assessments, and supplies clinical practice guidelines and standards through several membership-based publications and databases.
Hayes, Inc.	For-profit technology assessment company that evaluates and monitors emerging health care technologies. Hayes provides assessment information to providers and payers, such as United HealthCare, WellPoint Health Network, and AHRQ.

NOTE: For the purposes of this table, technology assessment is defined as the synthesis of clinical evidence concerning medical technologies for making coverage decisions and developing clinical guidelines.

Assessments of how well a technology is implemented in clinical practice or how it is most effectively integrated with existing technologies are rarely conducted. (Post-market surveillance studies assess product failures as opposed to optimizing performance.) In other words, how effectively a new technology improves overall health outcomes is rarely studied.

Medical technology assessment in the United States has been described as "a battle that's been fought and lost many times before"[29] (Box 6-1). Although national advisory panels have called for a nationally coordinated system of health technology assessment for decades,[32] no federal agency in the United States has both the mandate and the power to support a comprehensive approach to technology assessment.

The mission statement of the Agency for Healthcare Research and Quality (AHRQ) includes technology assessment, but that agency has never been allocated enough funds to support comprehensive technology assessment. The NIH budget is more than 100 times greater than AHRQ's, but its mandate for technology assessment is limited to clinical trials and NIH has historically resisted further expansion in that direction. In coming years, the gap between technology innovation and assessment might begin to narrow. In May 2002, the NIH director, Elias Zerhouni, laid out the "NIH Roadmap" describing a strategic vision for a more integrated approach to basic research that enables technological innovation and technology development. The Roadmap is discussed later in this chapter.

BOX 6-1
Brief History of Medical Technology Assessment in the U.S. Federal Government[21]

1972   **Office of Technology Assessment (OTA)** was created in 1972 as an analytical arm of Congress and conducted studies in nine areas, one of which was health.

1977   **NIH Consensus Development Program** was established as a mechanism to judge—in an unbiased, impartial manner—controversial topics in medicine and public health. NIH has conducted 115 consensus development conferences, and 22 state-of-the-science (formerly "technology assessment") conferences, addressing a wide range of issues.

1978   **Office of Medical Applications of Research (OMAR)** was established as part of the NIH Consensus Development Program. This is the focal point for evidence-based assessments of medical practice and state-of-the-science on behalf of the medical community and the public. NIH resisted the establishment of this office for many years, but eventually could no longer resist congressional pressure.

1978   **National Center for Healthcare Technology** was established to advise the Health Care Financing Administration (HCFA, now CMS) on coverage decisions for new medical technologies under the Medicare program.

1981   **National Center for Health Care Technology (NCHCT)** was eliminated. The American Medical Association (AMA) and Health Industry Manufacturers Association (HIMA) (now known as AdvaMed), led the move. However, the center paved the way for the AHRQ.

1981   **Office of Health Technology Assessment (OHTA)** of the National Center for Health Services Research assumed the responsibilities of NCHCT following its elimination.

1995   **OTA** was not funded by Congress during a time of budgetary concerns.

1999   **American College of Radiology Network (ACRIN)** is the first large-scale collaborative clinical trials group devoted to the development of technologies for medical imaging. Clinical trials were launched in 1999.

2001   **National Institute of Biomedical Imaging and Bioengineering (NIBIB)** was established. The NIBIB mission statement includes the "translation and assessment of technological capabilities in biomedical imaging..." This is the first NIH institute to include technology assessment in its mission statement.

2003   Intense debate over the value of the **AHRQ**, the only "official" federal medical technology assessment agency. Some lawmakers were in favor of closing the agency. The AHRQ budget, which was already too small to allow anything beyond very limited funding of clinical technology assessment, was reduced. AHRQ was reauthorized only until 2005.

The Role of Cost-Effectiveness Analysis

As noted above, cost-effectiveness is rarely assessed in the initial phase of technology assessment done by health care payers. Nor is it part of FDA's approval criteria. The Committee agrees that this is appropriate, because it makes little sense to assess cost-effectiveness analysis before effectiveness is determined. Likewise, it is premature to be overly concerned about cost-effectiveness during research and development of new technologies. Besides lacking information about the effectiveness of technologies that have not been clinically tested, later generations of a technology are almost always less expensive and often more effective.[60]

Consideration of cost-effectiveness is important during the technology adoption process, but at this stage formal cost-effectiveness analysis is seldom undertaken and generally does not play a role in the decision to adopt a new technology. As technology diffuses, or is poised for diffusion, cost effectiveness, or perceptions of it, influence policymaker's views and the decisions of insurers and health care systems about whether to recommend or use a technology.

Cost-effectiveness analysis has the potential to contribute to rational decision making by providing estimates of the magnitude of costs and health outcomes. When conducted in an unbiased way, it can help with decisions about whether or not to recommend a technology in different subgroups (such as screening of men for breast cancer) and with choices between alternative interventions for the same group (for example, screening women for breast cancer versus recommending the use of a drug that has been shown to prevent breast cancer). Cost-effective analysis also can be used to choose between alternative strategies to achieve some overall societal or population goal; for example, in choosing whether to implement a screening program for breast cancer versus a screening program for ovarian cancer to reduce the burden of cancer in women.

Cost-effectiveness analysis is not and should not be the only consideration in decisions about technology use. Cost-effectiveness analysis does not address value judgments that are key to individuals making decisions about their health. Cost-effectiveness analysis is influenced by perspective—that is, whose benefits, costs, and burdens are "counted" and are thus included in the analysis, and whether to count all benefits, burdens, and cost that accrue to certain individuals or groups.[27] For example, patients, physicians, health plans, and insurers have different perspectives and will likely weigh costs and benefits differently. A decision to adopt a new technology because it is "worth the cost" is an ethical and moral judgment—not an economic one. Opinions about whether something is "worth" a certain amount of money are subject to differences in the perspective and values of those making the judgment.[55]

METHODOLOGICAL ISSUES

Clinical studies are one of the first steps in assessing medical technologies. Unfortunately, far too many clinical studies yield uninformative data and fail to answer the basic question as to whether a new technology improves health outcomes. Too often, the appearance of a positive result is an illusion based on overlooked assumptions and failures to appreciate the many ways that hidden biases can skew results (Box 6-2).

Poor Study Designs Impede Progress

The consequences are disheartening. The developer of a new technology has typically invested millions of dollars in a clinical study—not to mention the time and effort of participating physicians, nurses, and patients. The ability to fund a clinical study is often a limiting factor for a small company hoping to develop a promising medical technology.

From a company's perspective, failure to obtain FDA approval spells disaster, and often signals the end of the project. Small companies whose fortunes are tied to a single technology and who rely on venture capital will find it considerably more difficult—if not impossible—to raise further capital, which often leads to the demise of the company. Ultimately, it is the patients who suffer most from these lost opportunities.

BOX 6-2
Common Failures in Clinical Trial Designs Submitted for Review (See Appendix D for Detailed Descriptions)

- ◆ Poorly Described Patient Populations
- ◆ Too Narrow a Patient Population
- ◆ Failure to Use Appropriate Controls or Comparison Groups
- ◆ Failure to Demonstrate the Comparability of Patients in Treatment and Control Groups
- ◆ Unclear Definition of Study Endpoints
- ◆ Bias
  - • *Confounding*
  - • *Systematic Errors or Differences in Measurement*
  - • *Loss of Patients to Follow-Up*
- ◆ Inappropriate Statistical Analysis and Planning
- ◆ Poorly Described Techniques

Poorly designed studies have impeded the development of more refined models of risk stratification. In an attempt to develop a model for breast cancer risk, in 2001 AHRQ reviewed 500 studies involving more than 30,000 women. Unfortunately, poorly collected data and insufficient evidence prevented the inclusion of all factors except age. Age was the only risk factor that definitively showed clinical significance. Problems with the meta-analysis included a lack of standardization of risk factor reporting, lack of standard reporting formats, and failure to link risk factors to an eventual diagnosis of breast cancer.[6] Because improving the early detection of breast cancer requires the development of better models to assess risk, critical attention must be given to improving the quality of clinical trials.

Population Measure of Cancer Status

There are three major measures of cancer status in a population: *incidence*, *survival*, and *mortality*. Cancer incidence represents the occurrence of cancer in the population and is often reported as a rate. Most cancer registries report cancer incidence in units of number of cases per 100,000 population per year. Calculations of short-term cancer incidence rates can be distorted by the extent to which a population is subjected to tests that might lead to cancer detection. Because studies of cancer screening are designed to do just that, these studies inevitably lead to major perturbations in the "reported" incidence, rendering cancer incidence an invalid endpoint for evaluating the real impact of the screening intervention.

Survival is the term used for the time interval from diagnosis to death from cancer, in patients who contract the disease. Since many patients will not die of their cancer, the survival experience must be calculated actuarially, using methods such as the life table, or the Kaplan-Meier method (Box 6-3). Although such calculations are definitive and unambiguous, the duration of survival is heavily dependent on the time of incidence of the cancer, and, as indicated, this can be strongly influenced in an artifactual way by the intervention under study (for example, screening). Although survival of cancer patients is the critical endpoint for studies of cancer therapies, it has little utility in studies of cancer prevention.

Mortality (or cancer-specific mortality) is the term used to describe the rate at which subjects die of the disease in the population targeted for the cancer prevention intervention; that is, it is the cancer death rate in the population under study. Mortality is the fundamental endpoint for cancer prevention studies, and to the extent that other endpoints—such as detection of cancer—are employed, they are used in lieu of mortality. Mortality is the only endpoint among these three that is valid for studies of cancer screening.

Screening is a form of *secondary prevention*, which is the control of

BOX 6-3
Measuring Breast Cancer Survival: Kaplan-Meier Curves

Kaplan-Meier curves are used to illustrate the effects of different factors on survival. These curves are used to show the results of screening studies, because they can depict survival data even when patients are followed for different lengths of time.

For example, the figure below shows that a woman diagnosed with a 12-mm breast cancer tumor has a 97 percent chance of surviving another 5 years, and an 85 percent chance of surviving 15 years. A women diagnosed with a 30 mm tumor has close to a 75% chance of surviving another 5 years, but only a 50 percent chance of surviving 15 years.

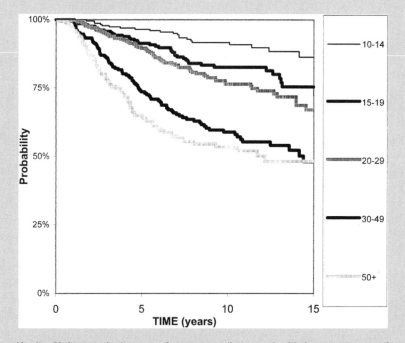

Kaplan-Meier survival curves for women diagnosed with breast tumors of different sizes. The box on the right indicates tumor size in millimeters (mm).[43] The Y-axis indicates survival probability.

cancer by reducing population mortality through early detection and effective treatment. (*Primary prevention* is the control of cancer through reduction in the incidence of the disease.) Screening tests are not intended or expected to affect the underlying cancer incidence rates, but rather to save lives by detecting cancer earlier than in the absence of screening. It is important to recognize that the early diagnosis conferred by screening can only be useful to the patient if there is an effective treatment for the cancer. More specifically, there must be a treatment whose efficacy is enhanced by early diagnosis.

Definitive Evaluation of a Cancer Screening Modality

The evaluation of any screening test can be affected by two profound sampling biases, *length-biased sampling* and *lead-time bias*, and these can only be circumvented by a randomized trial of women at risk of breast cancer, with breast cancer mortality as the endpoint.[37] Length-biased sampling occurs when the survival experience of a group of screen-detected cases is compared with a complete sample of incidence cases or with symptomatically detected cases. Because the growth rates of tumors are generally heterogeneous, patients with slow-growing tumors will enjoy a longer period during which the cancer is potentially screen-detectable but not yet symptomatic than patients with fast-growing tumors. This means that patients with slow-growing tumors have a selective advantage in being screen-detected. Consequently, any series of screen-detected cases will have a preponderance of slow-growing tumors, and so will enjoy a longer average survival regardless of whether the early detection confers a therapeutic advantage. Length-biased sampling is only a problem if the purported benefits of screening are derived from a series of screen-detected cases. The experimental group should be a population of subjects who are screened, and the cases derived from such a population will include both screen-detected cases and cases detected symptomatically. Any population-based series of incident cases will include a random selection of slow-growing and fast-growing tumors, and thus represents a valid series for evaluating the impact of screening.

Lead-time bias, however, affects even a population-based series of incident cases. When an asymptomatic population is screened, the time of diagnosis of every screen-detected case is earlier than if screening had not occurred. This advancement of the time of diagnosis is known as the lead time. Lead-time biases are introduced even if the screening test is extremely inaccurate. However, an accurate test will tend to produce more, longer lead times, and will therefore offer a greater opportunity for more patients to be effectively treated earlier in the course of their disease. Because a screened population will diagnose diseases earlier than a comparable unscreened population, the apparent survival times of the screened cases will be longer than the unscreened cases. Therefore, increased survival times are observed regardless of whether the early treatment of the screened cases actually affects their survival. For this reason, case survival is an invalid endpoint for evaluating screening programs.

As a result of these issues, the only accepted study design using a definitive technique for evaluating a new screening test is a randomized trial of individuals at risk of cancer in which the endpoint is cancer mortality. Patients must be followed to ascertain and compare cancer-specific mortality rates, or total numbers of cancer deaths (if the same numbers of subjects are randomized to the comparison group).

These trials are necessarily large and expensive, and require many years of follow-up. The sample sizes for the breast screening trials have ranged from approximately 25,000 to more than 100,000 women, and the trials generally require in excess of 10 years of follow-up.[1] To date, there have been only about a dozen or so definitive cancer prevention trials completed, several of them trials of mammography and breast cancer. However, these trials have validated the strategy that radiologic screening can reduce breast cancer mortality. The prevailing view among experts in the field of cancer prevention is that a definitive randomized trial of this nature (with cancer mortality as the endpoint) is necessary to validate strategies for any novel screening strategy.

Studies to Improve Screening and Diagnostic Accuracy

Many techniques designed to enhance the accuracy of or complement mammography screening are under active development. These include digital mammography, computer-assisted detection (CAD), magnetic resonance imaging (MRI), and others. Demonstrations that any of these methods are successful in improving screening in a randomized trial of cancer mortality are prohibitively expensive, and so investigations focus on trials to demonstrate improved screening accuracy rather than improvements in mortality compared with mammography. Because we know that mammography saves lives, more accurate technologies must be presumed to save as many or more lives. Evaluating new diagnostic modalities with respect to accuracy is methodologically challenging, and can be affected by numerous biases. Resulting from a good deal of recent research on the appropriate methodological designs of these trials, a comprehensive summary of current thinking on the issue is contained in the recent Standards for Reporting Diagnostic Accuracy (STARD) guidelines for published articles.[3] A related project by a team of experts to develop a quality assessment tool (QUADAS: Quality Assessment of Diagnostic Accuracy Studies) provides a concise tabulation of the key issues that challenge the validity of studies of diagnostic accuracy.[71]

The key issues from the STARD and QUADAS checklists that pertain to the design of studies to evaluate breast cancer screening technologies can be grouped broadly into four general categories:

- Construction of the reference standard diagnosis
- Manner and circumstances in which the various tests are "read"
- Representativeness of study subjects
- Statistical analysis and reporting of the results

In general, studies of diagnostic accuracy should be conducted on samples from the population from which the test will be used. For example, the accuracy of mammography in a group of women with symptoms of breast cancer will differ from the accuracy in an asymptomatic screening population. The former will have a preponderance of cancer patients, in addition to patients with larger tumors. Thus, ideally, studies of new screening technologies are conducted in a population of asymptomatic women. However, determination of accuracy involves evaluation of both sensitivity (proportion of true cases of breast cancer detected) and specificity (proportion of normal women who test negative), and thus to achieve adequate statistical power, the study must identify substantial numbers of both cases and controls. What makes this challenging is that in a general population, only a tiny fraction of people being screened will have cancer, and so very large sample sizes are required to achieve statistical power. This issue is exemplified by the design of the American College of Radiology Imaging Network (ACRIN) Digital Mammography Imaging Screening Trial (DMIST), which is a comparison of digital mammography with film mammography. The trial has recruited approximately 49,500 asymptomatic women in order to identify 150 to 500 women with cancer. The sensitivity of a screening tool cannot be sufficiently estimated with a smaller number of detected cancers because the number of cancer patients directly serves as the basis for quantifying sensitivity. Thus, to satisfy the methodological principle of conducting the study in the appropriate target population, a sample size of nearly 50,000 women is required. (See later section below, ACRIN: Network for Cooperative Development of Imaging Technology.)

Another general methodological issue is the construction of the reference standard diagnosis. For breast cancer, the ideal reference standard is biopsy. However, in a screening study such as DMIST only those patients suspected of cancer, based on mammography (or digital mammography), will receive a biopsy. That is, the decision to obtain a biopsy is heavily dependent on the results of the tests under evaluation, and it is well known that this can lead to serious bias in estimates of accuracy (i.e., sensitivity and specificity). In other words, false-negative tests could not be identified. In order to circumvent this problem, one must conduct follow-up exams of trial participants to discover individuals who are identified with breast cancer subsequent to the original screen. The DMIST design includes a follow-up testing at 10 to 15 months following the initial screen.

Finally, aspects of the statistical analysis and reporting of the results are important for the valid assessment of new technologies, and for their comparison with the current standard, which for breast cancer screening is mammography. Measures such as sensitivity and specificity are arbitrary in the sense that they depend on an arbitrary classification of a test as either positive or negative, when in fact many tests have equivocal findings. To avoid this problem diagnostic or screening tests are compared using a statistical method known as receiver operating characteristic (ROC) analysis, which is described in Appendix C. A large body of research to refine this and related statistical techniques has been conducted in recent years, including refinements of ROC analysis that allow for the measurement of the degree to which patient covariates affect mammographic accuracy, and the use of repeated screening tests on the same individual. An important principle for the evaluation of all medical trials is the commitment to report the results of all patients, and not limit the analysis to a selected subset. Thus it is important, for example, to report the frequency with which the test produces uninterpretable test results, especially if this differs in systematic ways between the different test situations or technologies.

Studies of Biomarkers

A screening tool based on a blood test offers a potentially much cheaper option than radiologic approaches. Efforts to identify individual over-expressed proteins, such as riboflavin carrier protein,[59] or patterns of proteomic over- or underexpression, such as in the study of ovarian cancer by Petricoin and colleagues,[56] are likely to expand in the foreseeable future. The preliminary evaluation of a serum marker is simpler than for a radiologic test, because the serum marker study can be applied retrospectively to stored blood samples. All that is needed are stored blood samples on cases of breast cancer and controls. However, for valid results, it is critical that the cases are representative of incident cases of breast cancer. That is, the serum samples should have been obtained during the workup to diagnose consecutive incident cancers, prior to any treatment. The controls should also be representative of the population at risk of breast cancer. In practice these studies are usually performed on "convenience" samples—samples that are most readily available as opposed to samples that are most relevant. For example, in the study by Rao and his colleagues,[59] the control samples were obtained from clinic patients with fibrocystic breast disease, leukemia, and volunteers. In the study by Petricoin's group,[56] the cases and the preponderance of the controls were obtained from a high-risk clinic, and the remainder had other gynecological conditions.

Even if the study involves valid case and control selection, care must be taken in extrapolating results to the context of screening. If the specificity appears to be high, the vast preponderance of screenees who test positive may still be negative for disease when the test is extrapolated to a screening population. That is, the positive predictive valve cannot be estimated directly from the case-control approach and will appear to be much higher in the case-control sample than it will be in the screening population. When a test rule (conditions required for indicating potential presence of cancer) is derived from a battery of markers, as in a microarray or proteomic study, the statistical analysis of the results becomes more challenging, because there are certain to be markers that appear to be associated with disease by chance alone. In these circumstances one must estimate the sensitivity and specificity of the rule through a two-stage process, where only a portion of the data is used to derive the rule (the "training" data set) and the remainder of the data is used to evaluate the accuracy of the rule (the "test" data set), as in the analysis by Petricoin and his colleagues.

LARGE-SCALE, HIGHER QUALITY
CLINICAL TRIALS ARE NEEDED

Inevitably, more exciting new technologies are announced than are proven useful in clinical practice. While basic research enables the development of early stage technologies, different strategies are needed to identify which technologies are truly feasible and add clinical value by improving people's health or the delivery of health care services. This involves large-scale, well-designed multicenter clinical trials. However, clinical trials have historically received substantially less support from NIH than basic research. In 2000, Congress passed the Clinical Research Enhancement Act, which directed NIH to expand the resources for clinical research. Approximately 10 percent of the total NIH budget goes toward clinical trials, although NCI invests relatively more. Sixteen percent of the 2003 NCI budget went toward clinical trials.[46] Clinical trials account for approximately 30 percent of the spending on clinical research overall.

In clinical practice, physicians usually have several choices and must choose among different technologies or procedures. Unfortunately, they rarely have access to comparative information on which to base those choices, and the lack of such information reflects a common weakness in our ability to identify optimal strategies in medical care. The Antihypertensive and Lipid Lowering Treatment to Prevent Heart Attack Trial (ALLHAT) illustrates the rare clinical trial that generates evidence necessary to choose among options. The DMIST trial comparing digital with screen-film mammography is another groundbreaking comparative clinical trial.

ALLHAT: A Watershed Trial

Most clinical trials are designed to establish the efficacy and safety of a single treatment compared with an alternative, often a placebo. Clinical trials done to meet FDA requirements for approval to market a drug are required to include a placebo comparison group except in rare circumstances. There are few large clinical trials that directly compare the effects of different treatments and even fewer that are comparisons among active, standard interventions. The ALLHAT was a watershed trial, because it was a large-scale trial that directly compared different FDA-approved drugs already in widespread use—in this case, treatments for hypertension and high cholesterol.

ALLHAT had more than 40,000 participants. The hypertension treatment component was a randomized, double-blind study in which hypertensive patients who were at high risk for heart attacks were randomly assigned to one of four treatments routinely used to treat hypertension: doxazosin, lisinopril, amlodipine, and chlorthalidone (Box 6-4). The doxazosin arm of the trial was terminated early because of a higher rate of combined cardiovascular events.[42] Final results from the trial showed that, for preventing major coronary events or increasing survival neither of the newer, more expensive treatments (lisinopril or amlodipine) was superior to the diuretic.[64] The ALLHAT data demonstrated that lowering blood pressure is the most important aspect of hypertension management, and that the three classes of drugs that were tested were similarly effective.[70] Furthermore, the diuretic had other advantages over both drugs, such as better tolerance and fewer cases of heart failure.

BOX 6-4
Treatments for Hypertension Tested in the ALLHAT Comparative Trial

Doxazosin is an alpha-blocker, also used to treat hypertension.

Lisinopril is an angiotensin-converting enzyme (ACE) inhibitor that is marketed under two brand names: Zestril® (Astra Zeneca) and Prinivil® (Merck)

Amlodipine is a calcium channel blocker, marketed under two brand names: Norvasc® (Pfizer) and Lotrel® (Novartis).

Chlorthalidone is a diuretic, marketed under the brand name Hygroton® (Novartis), as well as by several generic drug manufacturers.

An earlier ALLHAT trial reported that chlorthalidone is superior to doxazosin, an alpha-blocker, that is also used to treat hypertension.

Although expensive, the trial cost a fraction of the billions of dollars spent each year on antihypertensive medications. Each year, about $15 billion is spent to treat the 50 to 60 million people in the United States with hypertension.[9] Diuretics can cost as little as 10 cents per pill, whereas generic ACE inhibitors cost 63 cents per pill and calcium channel blockers cost $1.93 per pill.[72] The American Heart Association estimates that $3.1 billion could have been saved if diuretics had been used over the more expensive ACE inhibitors and calcium channel blockers from 1982 to 1992.[64]

The trial was a cooperative effort among clinical centers, the NIH, and the pharmaceutical companies that produce the leading antihypertensive drugs. The study was funded by the National Heart, Lung, and Blood Institute and Pfizer; the drugs for the hypertension were provided by Pfizer (amlodipine and doxazosin) and AstraZeneca (atenolol and lisinopril); Bristol-Myers Squibb (pravastatin) provided the drug for the lipid-lowering treatment arm. It cost $125 million, and was conducted over 8 years in more than 600 "real-life" clinical settings throughout North America. The trial met with many challenges, but was ultimately successful.

The success of ALLHAT serves as a model for future large-scale trials, such as those required for screening.[58] The trial illustrates the willingness of community practitioners to participate in research with long-term follow-up, the willingness of for-profit industry to co-fund well-conceptualized research overseen by an independent group of scientists, and the willingness of subjects to enroll in head-to-head comparisons of standard interventions. All of these are often cited as barriers to large-scale clinical trials.

This trial is also a reminder of the need for definitive clinical data. Prior to the publication of the ALLHAT data, the use of diuretics as initial therapy for hypertension had been reduced by nearly 50 percent in favor of the newer, more expensive calcium channel blockers and ACE inhibitors— despite the absence of definitive evidence for their superiority.[41] Organization of trials along the ALLHAT model has the potential to accelerate the development of the evidence base for making informed choices among the current and emerging options for the early detection of breast cancer.

Engaging the Public in Clinical Studies

Large-scale, well-designed clinical trials are the linchpins for converting the raw potential of new technologies into interventions that improve health and prolong lives. High-quality trials generate high-quality information, but that information accumulates slowly, one person at a time. Indeed, it often takes 3 to 5 years to enroll enough subjects for a scientifically meaningful and statistically valid clinical trial. Subject enrollment is a major roadblock and is the most frequent source of delay in clinical trials.[15]

The problem of adequate accrual is of broad concern in the medical research community and a series of reports points to certain trends:[19,63]

- Fewer than one out of six cancer patients are aware of the opportunity to enroll in a clinical trial, and only 2 to 3 percent of cancer patients participate in a clinical trial.[62]
- The most significant positive influences in participation are a physician's recommendation and a relationship of trust between the physician and the patient or volunteer. However, many physicians are reluctant to encourage their patients to participate.
- There are many reasons why people choose not to participate in clinical trials, including the demands on their time (including traveling to the study site), cumbersome processes for obtaining coverage of their medical expenses associated with participation, and a mistrust of the clinical trials process.[5,19,38]
- Compared to whites, African Americans are more reluctant to participate in clinical trials, although racial and ethnic minorities representation in NCI clinical trials is comparable to their representation in the general population.[44,62]
- Many participants are motivated by the desire to help others and take pride in their involvement.

However, there are different classes of clinical trials and they pose very different challenges for accrual. Trials that evaluate cancer risk or screening strategies in healthy, symptom-free people are fundamentally different from those that evaluate treatment interventions for cancer patients. The commonly perceived advantage of participating in a clinical trial—receiving the most "advanced" treatment for a life-threatening disease—does not apply to screening or detection trials. Cancer detection and screening trials generally require vast numbers of participants—as many as 20,000 to 50,000—because the endpoint (cancer incidence or death) is infrequent. For example, because roughly 5 cases of breast cancer occur per year in every 1,000 women over age 40, a study would require about 10,000 women to achieve a sample size of 50 breast cancers per year.

Cancer detection studies, such as the ongoing DMIST that is comparing digital with screen-film mammography, require thousands of subjects. But they have an advantage in that they can often be integrated into routine practice. Both recruitment of the participants and the study procedures can be conducted within existing organizations (for example, receiving regular breast screening in one's usual health care facility). Women in the DMIST trial also receive a direct benefit from participating, which is that they receive "extra careful" screening, because they are screened with two systems. From this perspective, it is not surprising that enrollment in DMIST has been spectacularly successful.

In contrast, epidemiological studies offer no direct benefit to volunteers, but instead involve the nuisance of filling out long questionnaires and the risks and discomfort of donating DNA samples. Furthermore, the methodology of these studies requires the investigators to solicit representative members of the public who have specific risk factors for breast cancer, as opposed to calling for "volunteers." These subjects are then compared with cases of breast cancer and analyzed with respect to the risk variables under investigation. For these reasons, enrollment in epidemiological studies is particularly challenging. As an example, investigators for the recently completed Long Island Breast Cancer Research Project set out in great detail the steps that were necessary to recruit controls.[25] This involved randomly dialing thousands of telephone numbers to identify suitable control subjects under 65 years of age, and use of CMS rosters to identify older women. The recruitment drive was bolstered by community service announcements and various other strategies to encourage participation. In the end, 63 percent of those identified as eligible agreed to participate and completed a questionnaire, and 46 percent provided a blood sample for genetic analysis. Even with a major, well-orchestrated effort such as this one, it is difficult to persuade the majority of candidates to donate DNA samples and fill out questionnaires.

Many people decline to participate in genetic testing or research because they fear the results of tests could be used by health and life insurance companies and employers to discriminate against them.[16] One study investigated the reasons that relatives of people with hereditary colon cancer would decline an offer of genetic testing, and found nearly 40 percent rated the potential negative effect on their health insurance as the most important reason to not undergo testing.[28] Without protections in place, individuals who do agree to participate will represent a self-selected group that could skew research results and interfere with efforts to find better ways of improving breast cancer screening.[17]

Various strategies for improving enrollment in clinical trials have been tested.[18,36,39,54] Passively distributed information, such as brochures, has little effect, whereas personal discussions are more successful. When the ALLHAT ran into difficulties in meeting its recruitment goals of greater than 20,000 African Americans, the study investigators adopted several strategies to accelerate the lagging accrual phase.[58] One of their most effective strategies was to initiate a field personnel program to assist selected clinics. As a result, those sites achieved more than 90 percent of their goals. Another strategy was to mount a nationwide advertising campaign, which recruited about 1,500 additional participants for an added cost of $1,100 per participant. Other strategies were based on increasing the number of

---

BOX 6-5
Herceptin®

Also known as trastuzumab, Herceptin® is a monoclonal antibody that was engineered to target a specific cancer cell protein, HER2 (also called HER2/neu or c-erbB2), and to inhibit tumor growth.

Herceptin® is the first biologic therapy ever approved for the treatment of breast cancer. Unlike previous treatment protocols (such as chemotherapy) which are toxic to all cells, healthy and malignant, biologic therapies target specific malfunctions in cancer cells and correct those cells alone.

---

participating sites. Finally, the investigators increased the reimbursement for participants' health care to some of the clinics. (Other aspects of ALLHAT will be discussed below.)

Private breast cancer organizations have had a significant impact on the accrual of several critical breast cancer trials. In the mid-1990s, the National Breast Cancer Coalition was instrumental in rescuing the Herceptin® trials (Box 6-5), partly through advising the study investigators on how to redesign the study to make it more acceptable to participants, and partly through campaigning to encourage women to enroll. In contrast, breast cancer advocates were initially a deterring force in trial enrollment for the trials of high-dose chemotherapy with bone marrow transplantation (HDC/BMT). The completion of those trials was delayed for several years because of a widespread, but mistaken belief that the HDC/BMT treatment already had been shown to be effective. When well-designed trials were eventually completed, the treatment was shown to be largely ineffective. Over time, breast cancer advocacy groups rallied to support these trials, and they are clearly an important ally in the success of clinical trials in breast cancer (Table 6-3).

The public has shown tremendous support for breast cancer research. Last year alone, tens of thousands of women ran 26-mile marathons. Thousands more walked 3-day marathons in heroic efforts to reduce the suffering of others from breast cancer. Many more added their support by donating money—millions of dollars altogether.

Major corporations also support breast cancer research. Pink ribbons are everywhere, from stamps to yogurt lids to T-shirts. The Breast Cancer Research Foundation website notes that given two equally matched products, consumers are more likely to choose the one associated with a pink ribbon.

Many of the thousands of women who participate in or donate their support for marathons might also embrace the idea of contributing in other ways, such as participating in clinical research studies. The need for public support in the fight against breast cancer goes beyond dollars, yet much of the public is unaware of the opportunity to contribute through participation in clinical studies.

It could be relatively simple to integrate information about "Other Ways to Help" with publicity about fundraisers. Such campaigns could inform people about the need for tissue samples and for participants in clinical studies. In fact, it is conceivable that organizers of clinical studies could collaborate with race marketers to promote either specific studies, or to conduct a more general campaign to educate the public about the merits of research and the need to donate specimens or time if they are invited to participate in a research study.

Epidemiologic studies needed to identify breast cancer risk factors require carefully selected study populations; self-selected volunteers would not be eligible. Unfortunately, the type of trial for which enrollment is particularly difficult is also the most restrictive in terms of eligible study populations. Nonetheless, there are certain studies for which volunteers could be helpful, such as preliminary trials of novel screening technologies.

Encouraging enrollment in well-designed clinical studies could facilitate the development of more effective approaches to the early detection of breast cancer. Breast cancer advocacy groups, the American Cancer Society, and funders of clinical research studies each bring different areas of expertise and constituencies that could complement each other effectively if they were to collaborate in improving enrollment in clinical studies. Breast cancer advocates are expert in mobilizing support for breast cancer research. They are also attuned to how potential study participants might react to enrollment requirements and could provide time-saving advice on ways that the design of clinical studies might be refined to promote more efficient enrollment, or to identify aspects of a study design that might needlessly deter enrollment. Finally, breast cancer advocacy groups are in an ideal position to promote enrollment through their established outreach programs. Clearly, such collaborations should apply only to studies that are not for financial gain on the part of the researchers or their institutions and that are clearly aligned with the shared goals of researchers and advocates—specifically for reducing mortality from breast cancer.

Will HIPAA Hamper Research?

The Health Insurance Portability and Accountability Act of 1996 (HIPAA) is a complex federal regulatory effort that has many parts and purposes. It was created to streamline industry inefficiencies in data transfer, improve access to health insurance, better detect fraud and abuse, and ensure the privacy and confidentiality of health information.

TABLE 6-3 Participation of Breast Cancer Organizations in Clinical Trial Accrual

Organization	Information Posted on Websites	Active Recruitment	Comments
Breast Cancer Action	X		Writes bimonthly newsletters dedicated to increasing public awareness of breast cancer clinical trials
MAMM	X		Magazine that publishes articles to educate public on the advantages and disadvantages of enrolling in clinical trials; the websites also provides links to clinical trial listings and informative clinical trial websites
National Alliance of Breast Cancer Organizations	X		Writes educational articles and provides links to other websites where women can find out more about enrolling in clinical trials
SusanLoveMD.com	X		Writes articles and provides links to other websites for more information on clinical trials; the clinical trials information is specifically geared towards women diagnosed with breast cancer
Y-Me National Breast Cancer Organization	X		Provides background information on participation and the barriers to clinical trial accrual. The website does not provide direct links to clinical trial listings
National Breast Cancer Coalition (NBCC)	X	X	Provides resources to educate the public on clinical trials via links to clinical trial listings and informational articles. NBCC partners with industry to help recruit

TABLE 6-3 Continued

Organization	Information Posted on Websites	Active Recruitment	Comments
			women for clinical trials, providing that the trials are scientifically rigorous with meaningful outcomes, costs of patients care are adequately compensated, and the trials enroll a diverse population
Susan G. Komen affiliate, Komen Greater New York City	X	X	Raises funds for clinical trials to help increase the percentage of women able to participate, particularly minority women; the project is known as Clinical Research Affiliates Funding Trials

The purpose of the HIPAA Privacy Rule, a component of HIPAA, is to establish minimum federal standards for safeguarding the privacy of individually identifiable health information. Concern about the privacy and confidentiality of health information available in electronic form was and still is a concern of the public. The use of medical information to target people for marketing and some well-publicized breaches of individual privacy based on unauthorized use of medical information fuels concern.

The HIPAA Privacy Rule went into effect on April 14, 2003. Although the Privacy Rule applies only to "covered entities" (health plans, health care providers, and health care clearinghouses[b]), it changes the way hospitals, doctors, and health plans must handle personal health information, and affects how such information can be shared with and among health researchers.[2] The intent of HIPAA was not to impede research. Indeed, before the Rule became final, there were many changes made from a draft rule issued in August 2002 in an attempt to minimize the effect of the rule on conduct of research. The implications and effects on research are still unfolding.

---

[b]Health care clearinghouses include public or private billing services, health management information systems, and networks or switches that process health information.

BOX 6-6
Personal Health Information Identifiers Under HIPAA

1. Names

2. All geographic subdivisions smaller than a state, such as street address, city, county, precinct, or ZIP code

3. All elements of dates (except year) for dates directly related to an individual, including birth date, admission date, discharge date, date of death; and all ages over 89 and all elements of dates (including year) indicative of such age, except that such ages and elements may be aggregated into a single category of age 90 or older

4. Telephone numbers

5. Facsimile numbers

6. Electronic mail addresses

7. Social Security numbers

8. Medical record numbers

9. Health plan beneficiary numbers

10. Account Numbers

11. Certificate/license numbers

12. Vehicle identifiers and serial numbers, including license plate numbers

13. Device identifiers and serial numbers

14. Web universal resource locators (URLs)

15. Internet protocol address numbers

16. Biometric identifiers, including fingerprints and voiceprints

17. Full-face photographic images and any comparable images

18. Any other unique identifying number, characteristic, or code, unless otherwise permitted by the Privacy Rule for reidentification

SOURCE: NIH. 2003. Protecting Personal Heath Information in Research: Understanding the HIPAA Privacy Rule52.

How Researchers Can Obtain Protected Health Information

Central to understanding the Privacy Rule is an understanding of what it defines as "protected health information" (PHI). PHI is information about the health of an identifiable individual. PHI is protected by HIPAA; information that is not PHI is not protected. The Rule describes what can be done with information about persons with health and illness that would make it unprotected (i.e., not PHI), namely deidentification. Health information is considered deidentified if all of 18 specified identifiers (Box 6-6) have been removed. Statistical methods can also be used to establish de-identification instead of removing all 18 identifiers, and HIPAA describes the process for establishing this in detail.[52]

HIPAA describes several procedures for obtaining access to PHI (Table 6-4). In general, a researcher will be required either to obtain consent from the person whose information is needed or obtain a waiver of authorization from an Institutional Review Board (IRB) or Privacy Board.

Impact of HIPAA on Medical Research

The potential effects of the HIPAA Privacy Rule on research are far-reaching.[13] Researchers in medical and health-related disciplines rely on access to many sources of health information, from medical records and epidemiological databases to disease registries, hospital discharge records, and government documents reporting vital and health statistics. For this reason, the Privacy Rule is likely to affect numerous areas of research, including clinical research, repositories and databases, and health services research. Population-based research that requires broad and unbiased access to medical records of community health providers is of special concern. This would include epidemiological, health services, environmental and occupational health research, as well as post-marketing studies of drugs and medical devices.

Research that involves the establishment of information repositories, including tissue and data repositories, is also of concern. Several of the data resources that are described in this report (for example, large databanks of breast images aggregated across institutions) would be more difficult to establish under HIPAA rules and might not be able to take full advantage of the potential to link data and do longitudinal follow-up. If data or tissue provided to a repository are completely deidentified, it is impossible to identify duplicates or to conduct follow-up of individuals.

> *The debate over the content and effect of the HIPAA regulations has been fierce over the past four years. . . . Whatever one's view of the HIPAA regulations, they will form the starting point for future national regulation of medical privacy. In this sense, they are akin to movie contracts, about which one Hollywood executive is reported to have said, "we have to have a contract so we have a basis for renegotiation."*[10]

George Annas, 2003
New England Journal of Medicine

TABLE 6-4 Options for Obtaining Protected Health Information for Research Under HIPAA Privacy Rule

Option	Requirement	Comment
Deidentification	Deidentified health information is not PHI and thus is not protected by the Privacy Rule. To qualify as deidentified health information, all 18 identifying elements enumerated in the Privacy Rule must be removed.	Limited research value. Not useful for research that needs to link records, including many longitudinal or epidemiologic studies. Can result in duplication of cases in various files.
Limited Data Set	Limited Data Sets refers to PHI that excludes 16 categories of direct identifiers and may be used or disclosed for research purposes without obtaining either an individual's authorization or waiver of authorization. A covered entity may use and disclose a Limited Data Set for research activities if the disclosing covered entity and the Limited Data Set recipient enter into a Data Use Agreement. Requires adequate assurance that data will be safeguarded and not used for unauthorized purposes.	Data Use Agreement must establish the ways in which the information in the Limited Data Set will be used and how it will be protected.
Individual authorization	An individual may authorize a covered entity to use and disclose his/her PHI for research purposes. This requirement may be in addition to the informed consent to participate in research required under federal regulations for protection of human subjects in research.	Impracticable for database research or research that uses data collected in routine practice.
Waiver of authorization	Researchers may obtain PHI from covered entities if they document that an IRB or Privacy Board (PB) has waived the requirements for individual patient authorization. The documentation must include a set of specified statements describing the IRB or PB process and the need for a waiver.	IRBs vary in their willingness to approve waivers of consent. Privacy Boards are new and it is uncertain how they will apply the rules.

TABLE 6-4 Continued

Option	Requirement	Comment
Preparation for research	Researchers may obtain PHI from covered entities without authorization in order to conduct a review in preparation for research. This requires a formal declaration that the use is solely to prepare a research protocol, no PHI will be physically removed from the covered entity during the course of review; and the PHI is necessary for research purposes.	Of very limited scope.

Variations in interpreting the HIPAA Privacy Rule are contributing to high levels of uncertainty and confusion that have already resulted in delays in research. The variations are partly because of the extreme complexity of the Rule, the details of which encompass more than 350 pages.[14] The parts of the Rule that relate to research are not easy to either identify or understand. For example, although the Rule's definition of "covered entity" clearly encompasses most, if not all, insurance companies and all hospitals and health plans, researchers working in settings that seem similar do not apply the definition consistently. In a multisite study of diabetes in youth, for example, the Department of Preventive Medicine at the University of Colorado School of Medicine did not define itself as a covered entity whereas the Department of Public Health Services at Wake Forest School of Medicine did.

Review of grants and contracts may also be affected. NIH has indicated that it may require applicants to provide plans for acquiring or accessing data under the Privacy Rule Program Announcements and Requests for Applications. Membership on review committees would need to be augmented to include expertise to evaluate those plans.

For radiology in general and clinical imaging research, HIPAA will be a hurdle to web-based access to images. Despite the advantages of having web-based images that physicians can view from any place at any time, many institutions might not allow image distribution beyond their controlled premises before they can address the security and privacy issues raised by HIPAA.

The Privacy Rule Has Far-Reaching Tentacles

Although the bioscience industry might at first seem to be beyond the reach of HIPAA, it is "an electronic nightmare expected to surpass many firms' Y2K preparations in both the scope and cost of the required systems changes."[12] Many bioscience companies such as those doing protein or gene diagnostics will end up being classified as business associates or vendors to a covered entity. The bioscience industry has developed much of its software in-house, in an environment where a high level of documented security has not been a concern. Indeed, software engineers made it their goal to develop systems open enough for scientists to collaborate on projects, encourage open communication, and extend the scope of research developments.

AAMC Initiative to Gather Data on HIPAA and Research

The Association of American Medical Colleges (AAMC) has been deeply concerned about the effect of HIPAA on biomedical and health research and lobbied vigorously for modifications to earlier versions of the Privacy Rule. After intense lobbying by the AAMC and numerous other groups, the AAMC decided the most effective approach to further mitigation, either by regulatory change or legislation, will depend on credible evidence of adverse effects of the HIPAA Privacy Rule on ongoing or future research. Thus the AAMC has begun a project to monitor and document the effects of HIPAA on research. The association has developed a network across the various disciplines of medical and health research to build a database and provide an effective mechanism for receiving and recording credible data on HIPAA's impact.[10] The AAMC will serve as the lead organization in this network and has asked members to forward specific cases illustrating the detrimental effects of HIPAA. The AAMC will thus ensure that "credible data are obtained to provide an accurate picture of the effects of HIPAA on medical and health research and inform further advocacy efforts."

This database should provide an important benchmark to determine whether the new approach to protecting patient privacy does, in fact, have a chilling effect on the "pace and volume of research." If it does, then it will be important to develop other approaches to protecting patient privacy.

FDA ASSESSES SAFETY AND EFFICACY

Over the years, many new cancer detection technologies have been proposed and even developed. Unfortunately, many of them were of no value to patients. The role of the FDA is to evaluate manufacturers' claims, so that the public has some assurance that products on the market indicated as FDA-approved at least meet the claims of their manufacturers. In particular, FDA review is designed to safeguard the public against false and exaggerated medical claims—although, unfortunately some of those claims are beyond the reach of the FDA. The basic requirement for FDA approval is that a product is both "safe and effective" for a specified use. Products that clear the hurdles of FDA review are thus cleared for entry into the medical marketplace, although as discussed below some detection and diagnostic tools can be used even without FDA approval.

Although FDA approval grants permission to enter the marketplace, it is no guarantee of success. For example, the T-Scan™ device that measures electrical impedance in breast tissue was approved as an adjunct to mammography by the FDA in 1999, but 4 years later the manufacturer had not sold a single machine in the United States.

The following section provides an overview of the FDA approval process for medical devices, how medical devices can be utilized without FDA approval, FDA efforts at collaborating and fostering communication with industry, and the unique regulatory problems posed by novel in vitro diagnostics, such as genetic tests that might be used in breast cancer diagnosis or risk prediction.

Classification of Devices Determines Their Regulatory Pathway[c]

Potential Safety Risk

Medical devices are as varied in type and purpose as Band-aids® and pacemakers, so claims that the FDA is inconsistent in how it regulates medical devices should not be surprising. The degree of regulatory scrutiny a device receives from the FDA depends on three factors:

1. How much risk it poses to users;
2. How different it is from other devices currently on the market; and
3. The intended use of the device.

How a device "scores" on these three factors determines how much evidence of safety and effectiveness the FDA will require for the device to enter the market or be used for a new medical purpose.

The first step in the FDA approval process for medical devices is to classify a device into one of three categories which then determines how much regulatory control is needed to ensure its safety and effectiveness (Table 6-5). Class I devices pose the least amount of risk of harm to the user and thus require the least amount of FDA oversight. Putting a Class I device

---

[c]This section is based on presentations at the March 25, 2003 workshop by David Feigal and Joseph Hackett of the FDA.

TABLE 6-5 Device Classification and Application Requirements for FDA Review

Device Class	Product Examples	Level of Control	Exempt/ Substantially Equivalent*	Type of Application
Class I Low risk	Crutches, Band-aids®, tongue depressors	General controls	Exempt	None
			Without exemption	510(k)
Class II Medium risk	Syringes, wheelchairs, CAD	General and special controls	Exempt	None
			Without exemption	510(k)
Class III High risk	Mammography devices, pacemakers, breast implants	General controls with premarket approval	New device	Premarket approval
			Substantially equivalent to device already approved before 1976**	510(k)

*Class I/II devices are exempt from the 510(k) application process if they have not been significantly modified or changed since before the passage of the medical device amendments in 1976 or they are specifically exempted by FDA regulations. For Class III devices, a 510(k), instead of a premarket approval, can be used to show substantial equivalence in safety and efficacy to a predicate device, having the same intended use and technological characteristics.
**For all Class III devices a premarket approval application is required unless the device was on the market prior to the passage of the medical device amendments in 1976, or substantially equivalent to such a device. The 510(k) application will be required for "substantially equivalent" Class III devices.

on the market is relatively simple. Class II devices pose more safety risks. Prior to marketing, manufacturers of these devices must meet all the requirements of Class I devices, as well as any existing standards for their product. Those standards can be physical (if a physically similar device already exists) or written (descriptions of the physical attributes of the device). In addition to analytical data demonstrating that the device measures what is claimed—for example, that a genetic test actually measures the gene it claims to measure—the FDA may also require clinical safety and efficacy studies of some Class II devices before considering approval for the market.

Class III devices pose the greatest degree of safety risk and thus require the most regulatory scrutiny by the FDA. Manufacturers of Class III devices must submit a "premarket approval application" (PMA) that requires them to provide clinical data showing their devices are safe and effective for the intended uses.

Intended Use

The FDA also considers the intended use of a medical device. A Class II device can be boosted to Class III status if a manufacturer wants to advertise a new claim for how the device can be used, and the FDA decides there is insufficient data on the safety and effectiveness of the device when used for this purpose.

The scope of claim that the manufacturer is going to make influences the level of evidence for safety and effectiveness that will be required by the FDA. For example, manufacturers of the endoscopes that physicians commonly use to detect abnormal masses in the gastrointestinal tract never had to show clinical data for the safety and effectiveness of these devices in detecting tumors because they do not advertise that claim. Instead, they claimed these devices are tools for providing images of features within the colon or stomach.

But if a device is likely to be used for a specific clinical purpose as opposed to a general indication covering a variety of purposes, then the FDA is likely to require clinical studies to prove the safety and effectiveness of the medical indication for the device. When digital mammography came under FDA scrutiny, "We were not willing, and we have not been willing with breast cancer detection to say, these are just tools [that provide images]," noted David Feigal, Director of the FDA's Center for Devices and Radiological Health.[22]

Only about 10 percent of devices are approved on the basis of clinical evidence of safety and effectiveness. The rest are approved on the basis of engineering, and other kinds of performance specifications that are used to show that the devices are substantially similar to those already on the market, per the 510(k) requirement. Feigal also noted that every business day about 50 new medical devices are brought to market, but about half of them are not reviewed for safety and efficacy by the FDA.

Table 6-6 lists the devices that have been approved by the FDA for breast cancer detection since 1995.

FDA Expands Interactions with Industry

To avoid "surprises" to manufacturers during the FDA review process of medical devices, the FDA offers many avenues through which industry can communicate or collaborate with the agency in a nonadversarial way.

TABLE 6-6 FDA Device Approvals for Breast Cancer Detection from 1995-2004*

Device Type	Device Name	Company	Approval Date	Approved Use
Digital mammography system	Lorad Digital Breast Imager SensoScan FFDM Senographe 2000D FFDM	Hololgic, Inc. Fischer Imaging Corp. GE Medical Systems	03/15/2002 09/25/2001 01/28/2000	Screening and diagnosis of breast cancer
CAD system	Second Look™ MammoReader M1000 Image Checker	Qualia Computing, Inc. iCAD, Inc. R2 Technology, Inc.	01/31/2002 01/15/2002 06/26/1998	Identify areas on mammogram that may warrant a second review
Ductal lavage DucPrep™ Breast	ProDuct Catheter Windy Hill Technology, Inc. Aspirator	ProDuct Health, Inc.	04/10/2000 12/23/1999	Collection of breast duct fluid for subsequent cytological evaluation
Infrared imaging	BreastScanIR™ BioScanIR® Technologies, Inc.	Infrared Sciences Corp. OmniCorder	2/20/2004 12/23/1999	Adjunct to mammography for breast cancer diagnosis and for detecting diseases that affect blood flow
Electrical impedance scanner	T-Scan 2000	TransScan Medical, Inc.	04/16/1999	Adjunct to mammography in patients with BI-RADS® 3 or 4
Pulsed doppler ultrasound system	Ultramark 9 HDI Ultrasound System	Advanced Technology Laboratories, Inc.	04/11/1996	Determine whether biopsy is needed in breast lumps over 1 cm in diameter
Diagnostic test (radioimmunoassay)	Truquant® BR™ RIA	Biomira, Inc.	03/29/1996	Blood test used in conjunction with other procedures to monitor the recurrence of Stage II or Stage III breast cancer

Device	Device Name	Manufacturer	Date	Use
Breast self-exam device	My Best Friend Breast Self-exam Pad	MBF Sales LLC	11/26/2002	Pad to aid in breast self-examination by reducing friction between fingers and skin of the breast
	Aware™ Pad	AAC Consulting Group, Inc	7/20/1999	
	Sensor Pad	Inventive Products, Inc.	12/22/1995	
Screen-Film Mammography System	Modified 650 Mammography System	Lorad, A Hologic Co.	07/11/2001	Screening and diagnosis of breast cancer
	Modified M-IV Mammography System	Lorad, A Hologic Co.	07/11/2001	
	Bennett Contour 2000 Mammography System	Trex Medical Corp.	02/05/1999	
	Bennett Profile 2000 Mammography System	Trex Medical Corp.	02/05/1999	
	Alpha Model Mammography Systems	Instrumentarium Corp.	07/17/1998	
	OPDIMA Mammographic X-ray System	Siemens Medical Systems	05/08/1997	
	Bennett Profile Mammography System	Trex Medical Corp.	01/10/1997	
	Aurora Imaging Sytem	Advanced Mammography Systems, Inc.	02/26/1996	
	Preference Mammography System	Phillips Medical Systems, Inc.	03/31/1995	
	Mam-Ch22s Mammography System	Elscint, Inc.	03/31/1995	

*Biopsy devices not included in this table. Scintimammography is not listed because it is FDA approved for breast cancer detection as a drug (99-Technetium Sestimibi).

Companies can meet with FDA officials to get advice and feedback about clinical studies they are planning to conduct on their new devices before submitting either an official "investigational device exemption" (IDE) application, 510(k), or PMA. An approved IDE application is required to conduct clinical studies on experimental devices prior to seeking marketing approval of the devices. Pre-IDE and pre-510(K) or PMA submission meetings can help manufacturers assess whether their studies will meet FDA criteria for safety and effectiveness.

One frustration cited by device manufacturers is that on occasion the FDA has suggested a specific protocol in these meetings, only to require changes at a later date.[57] To prevent such developments from occurring, the FDA Modernization Act of 1997 requires the agency to make a written record of meetings with manufacturers. Agreements made during those meetings are binding and not subject to change unless there is a written agreement with the manufacturer or unless the FDA discovers, after the meeting, a new scientific issue that might compromise the safety or effectiveness of the device. In this case, the FDA must give a device sponsor a chance to meet with the agency staff to discuss the new science affecting the sponsor's study protocols.[66]

Manufacturers of in vitro diagnostic tests also have the opportunity to give the FDA a mock 510(k) application for the agency's comments prior to submitting an official one. Companies can also provide the FDA with basic information about devices they have in the development stage to further discussion with the agency about what they need to do to garner FDA approval of the devices and/or to educate the agency about the new technology they are developing.

To support innovation in medical technology, the FDA also invites companies to offer suggestions on how to develop the appropriate standards, guidance documents, or policies for devices under the agency's purview. In 1995 the agency began offering roundtables on topics such as pharmacogenomics and in vitro diagnostics. Representatives from both industry and the FDA attend these roundtables, which are designed to foster communication and collaboration between these two entities.

Finally, on its website, the FDA offers numerous guidance documents, device advice, and other information to clarify what manufacturers need to do to legally put their devices on the market.

Some Medical Devices Do Not Require FDA Approval

There are a surprisingly large number of ways that medical devices used for cancer screening purposes can enter the market without FDA approval for those indications.

Many devices used for screening were actually approved for other indications. The prostate-specific antigen (PSA) test, for example, was initially approved only as an indicator of prostate cancer progression, but it was widely used "off-label" for many years to screen healthy men for the cancer. Eventually a manufacturer did provide the FDA with a submission for this claim, and since then it has become a commonly reviewed claim and a widely used device. Such "off-label" use of a medical device is legal as long as its manufacturer does not advertise that the device can be used for such a purpose. The manufacturer of the PSA test, for example, cannot advertise that it is a good screening tool for prostate cancer, although clinics and doctors using the test can make such claims.

Although many in industry believe that in order to get the FDA to approve their new medical products for marketing, the agency requires them to study off-label uses of the products, this is not the case. The FDA Modernization Act of 1997 stipulated that the agency cannot impose such requirements.[22]

Many genetic and other diagnostic tests come on the market without undergoing FDA review for safety and efficacy because they are considered "analyte-specific reagents" or "home brew in vitro diagnostics." *Analyte-specific reagents* are monoclonal antibodies, receptor proteins. and other compounds that are used for diagnostic purposes to detect and quantify individual substances (such as a specific genetic sequence) in biological specimens. *Home-brew in vitro diagnostics* are diagnostic tests that are custom-made in individual laboratories combining several devices or reagents. Home-brew in vitro diagnostics are common in university settings. The university provides a test result, rather than a diagnostic kit for sale, and the makers of the test are not permitted to market it.

Analyte-specific reagent tests or home-brew in vitro diagnostics used clinically must be performed by a laboratory that meets the highest quality standards set by the Clinical Laboratory Improvement Amendment (CLIA) of 1988. But these tests do not have to be shown to be safe and effective prior to their clinical use. Genbank, an NIH-contracted resource for genetic tests, offers more than 1,000 genetic tests, and as of 2003, only 6 of them have been brought to the FDA for approval. None of the tests for mutations in the BRCA1 and BRCA2 genes has been approved by the FDA, and none require approval for use by law.

One of the first-ever proteomics diagnostic tests, OvaCheck, which tests for ovarian cancer in blood samples, is scheduled to be released early in 2004. As required, the tests will be CLIA-certified but will not require FDA approval under existing regulations. However, the FDA has begun to increase its scrutiny of such tests and in February 2004 asked to meet with the company that makes the test to discuss the appropriate regulatory status of the technology.[69] Another early application of applied genomics is OncotypeDX, which claims to predict breast cancer recurrence, appeared on the market in early 2004. The test is CLIA-certified, but not FDA-approved.

Devices or the medical procedures using them may bypass a great deal of FDA regulatory scrutiny if they are customized by the doctors or clinics that use them. An example of this is Laser-Assisted In Situ Keratomileusis (LASIK) surgery to improve vision. This surgery is done with a multipurpose FDA-approved laser that is then modified by ophthalmologists to perform the specific surgery needed to correct for nearsightedness or other visual flaws. The LASIK procedure, however, was never shown to be safe and effective prior to its use by ophthalmologists.

The FDA also grants "humanitarian device exemptions" to devices designed to aid the diagnosis or treatment of rare conditions. Manufacturers of these devices must show that they are safe, but are not required to conduct tests of their effectiveness. Costs of such tests are not balanced by the revenues from a small market and requiring them would inhibit development of devices for rare conditions.

Accelerating Medical Technology Development at the FDA

Medical technology developers have long expressed frustration at the rising costs of product development and the uncertainty of the FDA review process. In January 2003, the FDA launched an initiative designed to accelerate the development of new technologies. The initiative has been enthusiastically welcomed by the medical technology community, which predicts that this effort to make FDA reviews more efficient will help to get lifesaving and life-improving technologies to patients faster and reduce the costs associated with bringing innovations to market.[3,4]

Three primary areas of improvement have been targeted: reducing review delays, improving the quality and efficiency of the review process, and facilitating new product development. These FDA goals are being sought through improving biomedical science, risk-management science, and economic science within the FDA.[40] The major changes, some of which the FDA has already begun implementing, are outlined below.[67]

- Reducing time delays and overall costs of development
  - ☐ Avoiding cycling of application process
  - ☐ Increasing communication between the FDA and industry

- Quality systems approach to the review process
  - ☐ Education and training of FDA review staff in latest developments in science and technology
  - ☐ Development of review templates to improve consistency
  - ☐ Common Technical Document to harmonize application processes of the United States, European Union, and Japan

- Collaborative clinical guidance development (input from work-

shops, advisory committee meetings, developers, and scientific community)
  □ Guidance development priority areas include oncology, diabetes, and obesity
- Priority areas of emerging technologies identified
  □ Cell and gene therapy
  □ Pharmacogenomics
  □ Novel drug delivery system

Many of the companies that are generating genomic or proteinomic technology are small start-up firms that lack experience in interacting with the FDA, are unfamiliar with the manufacturing quality controls the agency requires of them, and lack expertise in running clinical trials. There are 14,000 device companies in the United States, but only 10 percent of them would meet the definition of a large business. In fact, 5,000 are very small with revenues of $1 million or less and five or fewer employees.

David Feigal has commented that one of the challenges for the FDA is, "How do you reach all of those different firms and entities?" He noted that few device companies take advantage of the meetings they can have with the FDA to discuss research protocols or their data prior to making official submissions. Many, however, do utilize the FDA's Device Advice group, which answers 45,000 telephone inquiries a year and posts information on the agency's website.[22]

FDA's detailed guidance documents on what is needed for FDA approval of various types of devices expedite the approval process. When a guidance document exists for a Class II product, the manufacturer of such a device has about an 85 percent chance of getting it approved after the first cycle of FDA's review of the company's submission (as opposed to having to gather more data and undergo additional FDA review cycles before approval). When there is no guidance, the review process takes, on average, 5 months longer with only a 45 percent chance of approval on the first cycle.

HEALTH CARE PAYERS ASSESS CLINICAL VALUE

Overcoming the regulatory hurdles required to get a new cancer detection technology into the market is no guarantee that the new technique will be readily used. Widespread implementation of new breast cancer detection procedures will depend, in part, on whether federal (Medicare[d]) and private

---

[d]Everyone age 65 and older and those with certain disabilities are eligible for Medicare. Approximately 94 percent of women over 65 are covered through Medicare[20]; Medicaid covers low-income people. Some people are eligible for health insurance coverage under both programs.

health insurers will pay for these procedures. Reimbursement depends, in turn, on whether the new procedure or device results in improvement of clinical outcomes, whether such improved outcomes are relevant to the covered population, and whether they are legally mandated to cover the new technique.

Coverage Depends on Proven Clinical Utility

FDA approval of a new technology is not enough to ensure that insurers will pay for it. Health insurers also require proof that use of the new technology will improve the net clinical outcomes of patients, including reductions in morbidity and mortality, changes in management decisions, and improvements in quality of life (Box 6-7, Box 6-8).

The use of positron emission tomography (PET) in evaluating palpable breast masses illustrates the importance of changes in patient management. Once such masses are discovered, a biopsy is inevitable, and therefore PET adds nothing to the management approach. CMS has therefore decided not to reimburse for this application of PET. On the other hand, they do reimburse when PET is used to monitor response to treatment for breast cancer because the results of such scans will alter how these women are treated. Currently, there are no other imaging modalities that serve this purpose. "The magnitude of an improvement has to be clinically meaningful as opposed to quantitatively described," according to Sean Tunis, director of the Office of Clinical Standards and Quality at CMS.[65]

Medicare, as well as many private payers, also requires that a new technology be shown to be effective outside the research setting in which it is originally tested. Medicare is particularly interested in knowing whether the new technique will be useful to its older beneficiaries. Because most clinical trials exclude participants older than 65 years, most trials do not have adequate numbers of elderly patients. In some cases, it is reasonable to assume that older patients will benefit as much as younger patients. In other cases, however, if there is reason to think its performance will differ in the elderly, Medicare will not cover the new technique. According to Alan Rosenberg of WellPoint Health Networks, the effectiveness of a technology "has to be reproduced in a variety of clinical settings" and WellPoint will not normally pay for it unless it has been shown "effective outside investigational settings."[61] What insurers will pay for also depends on legal statutes. When it was first created, screening and preventive services were not covered by Medicare. Since then, Congress added screening mammography, PSA screening for prostate cancer, and colorectal cancer screening to Medicare's benefit package. Although the Blue Cross Blue Shield Association Technology Evaluation Center could not determine whether digital

---

BOX 6-7
Blue Cross Blue Shield Association Technology Evaluation
Committee Requirements for National Coverage

- FDA approval
- Data must permit conclusions about effectiveness
- Technology must improve net health outcomes
- Technology must be as good as others
- Outcomes must be attainable outside investigational settings

---

BOX 6-8
Medicare Requirements for Coverage:
Steps to Obtaining Medicare Coverage

- Regulatory approval
- Benefit determination
- Coverage (reasonable and necessary)
- Safe and effective (approved by the FDA)
- Improved health outcome verified using evidence-based medicine framework
- Equivalent to or better than current intervention
- Outcomes can be generalized to Medicare population
- Coding
- Payment
- MCAC Guidelines for Diagnostic Tests
- Adequate evidence to determine whether test provides more accurate diagnostic information
- Evidence to determine how accuracy affects health outcomes

---

mammography detects breast cancer better or even with the same accuracy as film mammography, Congress has mandated higher reimbursements for digital mammography.[11] The higher reimbursement levels have encouraged increased adoption of the technology before the results of the definitive digital mammography trial, DMIST, are released. Various states have passed laws that require private insurers such as WellPoint to cover specific procedures or treatments.[35]

The Catch in Determining Clinical Value

Although insurers are reluctant to pay for a new medical procedure until enough clinical experience shows that it improves net clinical outcomes, acquiring such clinical information can be difficult. Companies developing and marketing the new technology often do not have the resources to conduct the well-designed, definitive studies needed to document a technique's clinical effectiveness.

Research on preventive services often is unable to determine outcomes within the desired timeline of a technology producer's desire to bring a product to market. As Sean Tunis from CMS noted, there is a clinical research "Catch-22" in that insurance coverage of the new technology would increase its use, providing both some of the resources needed for its developers to study its clinical value and more clinical experience with the new technology. Yet, once coverage is granted there is little incentive (and more likely a disincentive) for companies to gather data and formally evaluate the clinical effectiveness of their new technology.

According to WellPoint's Rosenberg, gathering such information is critical, because research indicates that, nationwide, our health care resources are not spent wisely. A 2003 study that examined Medicare spending found that even though there was as much as a 30 percent difference in spending by state, such regional differences in spending were not associated with significant differences in health outcomes.[23,24] But as Tunis pointed out, "There really isn't a place right now in the public or private sector that makes evaluative clinical research a high priority." Such research would include conducting head-to-head trials of two or more comparable technologies or treatments to see which is more effective. It is not within the NIH mission to do a large number of this sort of studies and they are not a priority of industry, he said. "So there is a big hole in the funding streams of the evaluations of the appropriate clinical uses of new and emerging technologies, particularly as they relate to existing technological alternatives," Tunis concluded. Rosenberg added, "How do we prioritize spending large sums of money in terms of these new technologies? There is very little opportunity to systematically, as a country, go forward and analyze this."

Tunis referred to a recent paper on the findings of the IOM Roundtable on Clinical Research that suggested collaborative efforts between public and private organizations involved in the clinical research enterprise should focus on streamlining the overall process.[63] CMS is currently participating in a committee composed of private and government health insurers that is trying to prioritize clinical research from the perspective of those who foot most of the health care bills in this country. The committee plans to publish findings with the hope that others will pursue conducting the studies they deem necessary.

Conditional Coverage

Another way around the clinical research Catch-22 is to have "conditional coverage" of new promising technology prior to firm evidence that it improves clinical outcomes. Insurance reimbursements would be conditional on the requirement that coverage of the new technology would be reevaluated in a few years, during which time studies of the technology's effectiveness would be done. If those studies indicate the technology did NOT improve clinical outcomes, then insurance companies would stop reimbursing its costs.

However, once coverage has been granted for a medical procedure or treatment, it may be very difficult to rescind it. Historically, Medicare has had problems withdrawing or limiting coverage for any medical procedure or treatment in the absence of definitive evidence that it is truly useless or harmful.

Another problem with conditional coverage is that companies may not do the studies needed to document clinical utility of their new medical product. The proposed process for conditional coverage of new procedures is akin to that already in operation for the FDA's "accelerated approval" process of new drugs. Accelerated approval, which was initiated in 1987, is based on surrogate endpoint data on the condition that the sponsor confirms actual clinical benefit through well-controlled studies. The effectiveness of this process has varied.

During the post-approval period, nearly all AIDS drugs that received accelerated approval underwent the expanded clinical tests needed to confirm preliminary clinical findings. Those tests revealed clinical benefits, so no drugs needed to be withdrawn from the market. This experience is in stark contrast to that of the agency's accelerated approval of oncology treatments. Almost no confirmatory clinical studies have been completed on these drugs.[49] But for accelerated approval, the FDA does not specifically require that confirmatory studies be under way at the time of approval. Such a specification might give the agency the added muscle it needs to make accelerated approval work the way it was designed.[22]

An important prerequisite for conditional coverage is that the decision to cover a new entity must be linked to high-quality studies whose funding is assured. The Committee does not recommend conditional coverage without careful analysis of feasible mechanisms for implementation. Such an analysis would require a separate study, ideally one that focused specifically on the issue of conditional coverage, as opposed to consideration in the context of a study focused on a specific health issue, such as the current study.

Evidence-Based Evaluations Done by Insurers

In the absence of definitive studies of a new technology's clinical utility, WellPoint considers other information when evaluating the technology. This information includes input from clinical experts throughout the country, as well as the degree of acceptance of the product or service in the national organized medical community. For example, WellPoint puts a lot of weight on recommendations by well-respected organizations such as the USPSTF, the American Heart Association, and the American Cancer Society. If any of these organizations recommend a screening procedure, WellPoint will likely reimburse its costs.

Rosenberg noted that a WellPoint committee meets annually to evaluate new medical technology. The committee relies on a number of inputs to determine which medical products should be evaluated, such as reviews of recent FDA-approved medical products, requests from WellPoint's claims and medical review units, and information supplied by device manufacturers. Medicare's evidence-based reviews are done in an ad hoc fashion, rather than at regularly scheduled intervals. The agency is currently trying to rectify this ad hoc approach by establishing a medical technology council to determine which products or procedures should be evaluated.

Neither WellPoint nor the BCBSA-TEC consider cost when deciding whether to cover a new medical product or procedure. "We go by our legal contract which does not include cost effectiveness," said Rosenberg. "Dollars and cents are never presented [during our evaluations]." Cost-effectiveness also does not enter into Medicare's evaluations of new medical technology, although they tend to focus their internal evidence-based reviews of new technology on those that are particularly expensive. Medicare will also conduct evaluations at the request of people or organizations outside the agency when they want a new medical product or procedure to be approved for coverage. But Medicare has only recently started to do extensive evidence-based reviews of medical products. Consequently, many well-used techniques, such as MRI, never underwent Medicare scrutiny for clinical utility.

Other technologies bypass such scrutiny by falling under existing coding categories that Medicare has already determined are reimbursable. Digital mammography, for example, falls under the same payment code as standard mammography. "The whole process of developing new codes for new technologies is actually incredibly more important and influential in what technologies become available in the Medicare program than one would think," said Tunis. He added that "incremental improvements in technology are fairly seamlessly handled in the Medicare program," because they don't require a new payment code.

Most New Technologies Cannot Be Reimbursed Without New Payment Codes

Current Procedural Terminology (CPT) codes are used by Medicare and Medicaid to reimburse doctors. The development of new CPT codes is critical to new technologies, because without the code, health care providers cannot bill for reimbursement. The CPT code is thus a key step toward facilitating market penetration and broad clinical use of new technology. The assigning of Medicare payment codes is under the control of the AMA and various partner organizations, such as the American College of Radiology and the American Society of Clinical Oncology.

Delays in assigning CPT codes to new medical technologies have long been a source of frustration to technology developers. CPT codes were historically updated once each year and CMS often took 1 to 2 years to issue the codes, creating barriers to patient access. In the past few years, Medicare reform laws called for changes to streamline Medicare coding for new technologies and procedures. Under the Balanced Budget Refinement Act of 1999, Congress called on CMS to reduce coding delays and respond more promptly to advances in medical technology. As a result, codes for the outpatient prospective payment system are now updated quarterly. (Codes for other payment system are still updated annually.)

In 2001, the AMA's CPT Editorial Panel established a new category of CPT codes called Category III codes, which are a set of temporary codes intended for tracking emerging technologies. For laboratory tests, these codes represent emerging technologies that may not be performed by many laboratories and may not yet have been approved by the FDA. Review of emerging technology codes is done by the CPT Editorial Panel as part of its procedures to annually update CPT codes. The CPT Editorial Panel determines if a temporary emerging technology code should be converted to a permanent existing technology Category I CPT code or if a new emerging technology code should be established.

Reimbursement Can Be Out of Sync with Real Costs

Once a medical procedure or technology has been approved for coverage, the next step is a determination of the appropriate payment amount for reimbursement. Although mammography has long been covered by Medicaid and private payers, there has been much discussion about the fact that the reimbursement that health care providers receive for mammography services is less than the cost of providing the services. Indeed, mammography is widely considered a money-losing service that is in effect supported by other radiology services.

Mammography rates were raised in 2002, but they are still estimated by most radiology services to be below real costs (see Chapter 2).

RESEARCH AND DEVELOPMENT SHOULD BE INTEGRATED

The need to develop stronger links between basic and clinical research has become increasingly clear. In addition, the cost and complexity of clinical research has expanded over the years, making it increasingly important to capture the economies of scale that come from establishing multi-institutional collaborative networks. Initiatives to achieve these goals have been established at all levels of the research enterprise, from interagency projects such as the Interagency Council on Biomedical Imaging in Oncology (ICBIO) to specific projects such as the National Digital Mammography Archive (NDMA). Six of these initiatives are described below. They are not a comprehensive summary of all such initiatives, but rather a set of examples that are particularly relevant to breast cancer detection.

AHRQ Initiative for Research Networks

Since 1999, the AHRQ has issued a series of research funding announcements that support projects on the translation of research findings into "sustainable improvement in clinical practice and patient outcomes." In 2002, the NCI articulated that a key part of its mission was the rapid movement of research discoveries through program development into service delivery, which included projects designed to "identify and overcome infrastructure barriers to the adoption of evidence-based interventions in clinical and public health systems that serve the American public, with a particular emphasis on reaching those who bear the greatest burden of cancer." In 2003, AHRQ and NCI issued a joint request for applications, for research projects that assess the use of intervention to translate research into practice in the primary care setting and measure the impact of those interventions.

Although there is broad agreement about the urgent need to accelerate the rate of uptake of evidence-based findings and tools into practice, considerable uncertainty persists about the best strategies for doing this and the setting(s) in which each strategy is most effective. The majority of strategies that have been studied focus on changing clinical behavior. From these trials, it is known that passive diffusion of information (such as distribution of educational materials or lectures) is generally ineffective as a method of promoting behavioral change. Studies of the multidimensional challenges of translating research into everyday practice are hampered by the current concentration of clinical research in academic settings.

Cancer Biomedical Informatics Grid (caBIG)

The pilot project for the Cancer Biomedical Informatics Grid (caBIG)—launched in July 2003 by the National Cancer Institute Center for Bioinformatics (NCICB)—is an attempt to create an open-source, open-access, cancer information network. With the rapid evolution of biomedical research technology, various disciplines of cancer research have been generating enormous amounts of data. However, discrete fields of cancer research, such as radiology, molecular biology, and epidemiology, have no direct means of communicating and sharing information. Thus the main goals of the caBIG project are to enable researchers to internationally share tools, standards, data, application, and technologies according to agreed-upon standards.

In its pilot phase, which is scheduled to be completed in 2006, the NCICB will work with selected cancer centers to join their expertise and infrastructure into a common web of communications, data, and applications.[50] Currently, there is no common mechanism for individuals, institutions, or private companies to easily share data and there is no common standard that researchers use. Yet, caBIG will attempt to overcome obstacles to collaboration by implementing several streamlining initiatives. Most importantly, in order to facilitate data sharing, the network will attempt to unify terminology, data sets, and deployment among all the cancer centers and the NCI.[50] Another major goal of caBIG, a standardized repository, may facilitate additional insight from previously published datasets. The infrastructure was also established to facilitate sharing of data among consortium groups prior to publication or public release. Finally, caBIG will attempt to integrate several isolated disciplines, potentially resulting in increased efficiency and cost-effectiveness of most aspects of cancer research.

Ultimately, the development of this unique data-sharing platform is intended to allow research groups to tap into the rich collection of emerging cancer research data while supporting their individual investigations in an attempt to accelerate the pace of cancer research. For example, a comprehensive and standardized infrastructure could facilitate collaborations among centers and may result in quicker, less expensive, and more easily coordinated multi-institutional trials. If successful, this project may have a significant positive impact on translating basic research into better patient outcomes.

ACRIN:
Network for Cooperative Development of Imaging Technology

ACRIN is an organization of institutions, funded by the NCI, which manages clinical trials of cancer-related imaging technologies. The first large-scale cooperative imaging trials group was the Radiology Diagnostic Oncology Group, established by the NCI with Harvard Medical School, the American College of Radiology, and 45 institutions throughout the country. During its existence from 1987 to 1997 it evaluated nine cancers in terms of staging and follow-up, and resulted in approximately 100 articles and abstracts. It was followed by ACRIN, which has been in operation since March 1999 and is funded by NCI, at least through 2007.

ACRIN offers a unique opportunity to assess emerging technologies and determine their optimal use by providing both funds and an infrastructure for multi-institutional clinical trials. This arrangement allows for both extremely large and smaller trials, to recruit outstanding researchers, gain access to new technologies, and produce high-quality results. More specifically, ACRIN facilitates the standardization, development, and implementation of trials, including data acquisition and management, protocol design and biostatistical analysis, monitoring and quality assurance, financial management, and reporting of trial results. In addition all ACRIN trials include measures of cost-effectiveness and quality of life, except for individual trials where investigators present compelling reasons for why such measures would not be useful.

As of March 2004, ACRIN is conducting seven trials with two others conditionally approved for development. Several of the trials are dedicated to breast cancer imaging. One approved trial that will begin enrollment is for the study of ultrasound as a screening tool for breast cancer, and two other trials are analyzing the role of MRI in breast cancer—one for monitoring breast cancer treatment results and another for screening of the contralateral breast. One of the largest ACRIN studies is the DMIST, which is comparing digital with screen-film mammography. The trial reached its accrual goal of 49,520 participants in November 2003, but the 1-year follow-up results and data analysis will not be complete until 2005.[8]

As new technologies emerge, trials like ACRIN will be at the forefront. Although the trials are designed to answer specific questions regarding screening, the data collected will also be useful in developing mathematical models that evaluate the incorporation of new techniques, such as risk stratification and nonimaging screening methods.[30] (Several of the ACRIN trials involve the collection of both biological and imaging data.) As technology evolves over the next 20 years, from gross anatomic and pathologic imaging to molecular imaging of physiology and metabolism, ACRIN is poised to be involved in the clinical validation of these future technologies.

Overall, ACRIN has the potential to improve clinical practice and patient outcomes by identifying the appropriate use of imaging technologies through rigorous, large-scale clinical studies that otherwise would not be possible for small-scale organizations to conduct. ACRIN also provides a unique opportunity for imaging professionals to participate in rigorous, multicenter clinical trials and learn about how high-quality research is conducted.[7]

NIH Roadmap for Medical Research

In September 2003, NIH director Elias Zerhouni announced a 5-year plan, known as the NIH Roadmap for Medical Research. The goal of the Roadmap is to reduce the time it takes to turn basic knowledge into tangible benefits—for example, better technologies for breast cancer detection. It is based on a collection of NIH-wide initiatives designed to transform the way research is done at the agency, and is organized around three broad themes:

1. New pathways to discovery,
2. Research teams of the future, and
3. Reengineering the clinical research enterprise.

The strategic initiatives to be funded under the NIH Roadmap will address critical roadblocks and knowledge gaps that currently constrain rapid progress in biomedical research.

Radiology and the emerging field of molecular imaging play prominent roles in the Roadmap. They factor into each of three major initiatives listed above. The theme of reengineering the clinical research enterprise is particularly relevant to what the Committee believes is especially needed to promote the development of more effective approaches to the early detection of breast cancer, and is described on the NIH website as "undoubtedly the most difficult but most important challenge identified by the NIH Roadmap process."[53] This theme is further subdivided into three initiatives—translational research, clinical workforce training, and enhancement of clinical research networks—all of which address the Committee's conclusion that basic research should be integrated with technology development and assessment (see Box 6-9).

At present, the Roadmap does not specifically address the need to incorporate research intended to optimize the value of new technologies in clinical practice, which the committee believes is also important.

Interagency Council Counsels Technology Developers

The ICBIO was established in 1999 to bring together technology developers and representatives from the federal government to expedite the process of bringing new products to market. The multiagency group includes the NCI, FDA, and the CMS. The group is another example of federal agencies working proactively with early stage technology developers—many

BOX 6-9
Reengineering the Clinical Research Enterprise

Over the years, clinical research has become more difficult to conduct. However, the exciting basic science discoveries currently being made demand that clinical research continue and even expand. This is undoubtedly the most difficult but most important challenge identified by the NIH Roadmap process. The United States must recast its entire system of clinical research if efforts to fight disease are to remain as successful as they have been in the past.

The NIH Roadmap will promote the creation of better integrated networks of academic centers that work jointly on clinical trials and that include community-based physicians who care for sufficiently large groups of well-characterized patients. Implementing this vision will require new ways to organize the way clinical research information is recorded, new standards for clinical research protocols, modern information technology, new models of cooperation between NIH and patient advocacy alliances, and new strategies to reenergize the clinical research workforce.

Translational research. Scientists have become increasingly aware that the bench-to-bedside approach to translational research is really a two-way street. Not only do basic scientists deliver to clinicians new tools to examine patients, but clinical researchers also make novel observations about the nature and progression of disease that can stimulate basic investigations. Translational research is a powerful process that primes the entire clinical research engine, but this component of the clinical research enterprise should be optimized and accelerated through a stronger infrastructure.

NIH is exploring development of regional translational research centers. These centers would provide sophisticated advice and resources to better enable scientists to master the many steps involved in bringing a new product from the bench to clinical use.

Clinical workforce training. Our nation's ability to fully explore the ever-expanding opportunities for medical advances is limited only by our resources, the most important of which is the scientific workforce. To fulfill the promise of 21st century medicine and to make further progress in controlling major human diseases, we must cultivate and train a cadre of clinical researchers with skills commensurate with the increasing complexity and needs of the research enterprise.

The NIH Roadmap effort envisions two major programs to expand, enhance, and empower the clinical research workforce: the establishment of an agency-

of whom have little experience with regulatory processes and often founder as a result—to help avoid wasting time and money in what is normally a long and expensive process.

The Council provides advice to medical technology developers on the spectrum of scientific, regulatory, and reimbursement issues related to developing an imaging device or technology. Any business or academic investigator developing a device or technology relevant to biomedical imaging in wide Multidisciplinary Clinical Research Workforce Training Program and a cadre of NIH Clinical Research Associates.

Clinical research networks. An enriched pipeline of biomedical discoveries, an infrastructure to facilitate their translation from the lab to the clinic, and a robust force of clinical investigators will make it possible to test new detection and diagnostic strategies in larger numbers of patients far sooner than at present. These large studies are often best conducted through networks of investigators who are equipped with tools to facilitate collaboration and information sharing.

Because of the vast number of procedures and technologies that must be evaluated through clinical trials, many clinical research networks operate simultaneously, but independently of each other. As a result, researchers must sometimes duplicate already existing data because they are unaware the data exist or they cannot access them. Standardizing data reporting would enable seamless data and sample sharing across studies. Reduced duplication of studies will leave more time and funds to address additional research questions. A blueprint for a national informatics network using standardized data, software tools, and network infrastructure will evolve from an inventory of existing clinical research networks.

Other impediments to efficient clinical research to be addressed through this set of initiatives are the multiple requirements of diverse regulatory and policy agencies. Researchers face a tremendous diversity of requirements in reporting adverse events to NIH, the FDA, the Office of Human Research Protections, and institutional review boards, among others. Clinical researchers must understand and fulfill these varying requirements that often overlap and might even contradict one another.

NIH aims to take a leadership role in working with other agencies to develop better processes and to standardize requirements for reporting adverse events, human subjects protections, privacy and conflict-of-interest policies, and standards for electronic data submission. Harmonizing policies and reporting requirements will help minimize unnecessary burdens that slow research, while at the same time enhancing patient protections.

By standardizing the regulatory requirements of clinical research networks and enhancing their interoperability, clinical research will advance more swiftly, and more and better therapies will reach patients nationwide. By creating a partnership with patients and physicians—true "communities of research"—this ambitious set of NIH Roadmap initiatives promises to enhance the scope, resilience, efficiency, and impact of the nation's clinical research workforce, ultimately improving the health of all Americans.

SOURCE: See http://nihroadmap.nih.gov/clinicalresearch. Accessed March 1, 2004.[47]

cancer may submit a request to make a presentation, and small businesses are particularly encouraged to apply. A presenter typically meets with the Council for an informal, confidential discussion with emphasis on helping the presenter develop an effective approach for FDA approval and streamlining the process of coverage and reimbursement decisions from CMS.

The Council hosts an annual conference on biomedical imaging in oncology, designed to identify areas of new biomedical opportunity and address challenges in the cancer imaging community, focusing on the regulatory, coverage, and reimbursement issues associated with more developed and established technologies.

FDA and CMS coordination of their discussions of new technologies is another value of ICBIO, with the potential of easing an oft-cited bottleneck to technology development.

Developers of early stage medical technology have long commented that the process of FDA and CMS review are so unpredictable and burdensome that they unduly impede the development of innovation technologies.[33] ICBIO is one example of the series of proactive strategies that federal agencies have taken in recent years to address these problems.

National Digital Mammography Archive

As digital imaging technology becomes increasingly cost-effective, mammography is expected to move away from a film-based format. This transition will also increase opportunities for electronic sharing of images, data, and other information among a wide network of clinicians and researchers. To this end, researchers at the Universiy of Pennsylvania, along with collaborators at the Universities of Chicago, North Carolina, and Toronto and contractors at Oak Ridge National Laboratory in Tennessee, have assembled and tested a prototype for a national database, the NDMA.[1]

Mammography services could be greatly streamlined if breast imagers were able to examine mammographic images stored at multiple sites from their own facility. This would eliminate the need to physically transfer mammograms from site to site, and would go a long way toward ending the all too common frustration and delays caused by lost mammograms. This project tests the computer's ability to store and instantly retrieve vast numbers of high-quality digital mammograms from distant sites. Medical image data is different from other types of data because the file sizes are large (hundreds of megabytes per exam) and the required turn-around time is short. The NDMA system exploits the speedy content-delivery capabilities of Internet2, which has made it feasible to transfer large quantities of medical image data over low-cost and high-speed wide-area networks. Cumbersome files will no longer have to be mailed in hard-copy format. The NDMA can also facilitate consultation and collaboration among physicians on difficult cases, particularly when they occur in underserved areas. For example, researchers at the University of Toronto are using a mobile van to download mammograms in remote locations.[45] These functions may be further enhanced by the planned development of the NDMA as a central resource for computer-aided diagnosis. InfoWorld, a media group that specializes in information technologies, recognized the NDMA in 2002 as the #1 project that best exemplifies the implementation of innovative technology.

Initiated in 2000 with a 3-year grant from the National Library of Medicine's Next Generation Internet initiative, the NDMA project went live in 2002 at the four participating institutions (Figure 6-4). The pilot archive, comprising digital images and information, can be accessed through web portals at each of the four institutions. With continued funding, the network is expected to expand gradually to connect approximately 2,000 mammography facilities.[45] This will be accomplished through the construction of a few large regional archives distributed across the country, linked to smaller, more local archives that store data collected within 2 to 3 years, which in turn serve individual hospitals, universities, and other health care institutions through secure portals that can both send and receive information. Currently, a single area archive connects all of the participating institutions.

During the first 3 years of the project, researchers enrolled about 10 patients per day, uploading their mammography data to the NDMA.[68] Archived images are primarily derived from digital mammograms; films also have been digitally scanned for inclusion in the archive, but produced

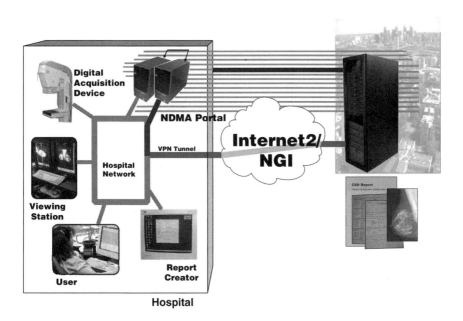

FIGURE 6-4 Architecture of the National Digital Mammography Archive (NDMA). Courtesy of Dr. Mitchell Schnall and Pat Payne.

lower-quality images.[45] Mammography reports, conforming to BI-RADS®
guidelines, are also posted to the archive. In additional to digital mammography, the NDMA can store MRI, ultrasound, and other imaging formats
that conform to the binary standard known as Digital Imaging and Communications in Medicine.

The expanded capabilities of the Internet2, also known as Next Generation Internet, are essential to the efficient storage, retrieval, and security
of mammography information. Indeed, devising a means of storing enormous quantities of data was one of the most significant challenges. Unlike
the standard Internet, the bandwidth and technology of Internet2 can accommodate the storage of very large digital image files—which are predicted to exceed capacity for management and storage by breast center
sites—and enable their instant transfer across the network.[1] The use of
grid-computing addresses is "the trick of making use of digital images,
indexing them, and delivering them to hospital locations on demand," says
Robert Hollebeek, chief architect of the NDMA. The Internet2 "grid"
framework is also key to ensuring patient privacy and confidentiality, as
required by the HIPAA Privacy Rule. Multiple levels of system security
include access control, encryption, and the use of virtual private networks,
as well as confidentiality safeguards for research purposes that strip personal information that could be used to identify individual patients.

With these safeguards in place, the NDMA constitutes a rich reserve of
data that can be "mined" for research and education. Epidemiologists could,
for example, use the database to compare breast cancer incidence and
prevalence among women of various ages or ethnicities, or in different
areas of the country. A national teaching file is being developed as part of
the NDMA project to provide teaching and testing material for mammography training programs.[1,68] Currently, teaching cases for the training of
radiologists and mammographers tend to be developed separately at individual institutions, and this limits students' exposure to cases that occur in
that medical center. Some day, radiologists may be able to annotate mammogram images with specific location data and upload them to the NDMA
for inclusion in cases file for teaching, testing, and advanced training.[48]

In the future, the NDMA could link to similar databases under development in the United Kingdom, France, Germany, and Japan to create an
international mammography archive.[31] The U.K. project, which is jointly
funded by that nation's government and IBM, resembles the NDMA in size,
scope, and design. These expanded, global networks offer the potential of
even greater opportunities for research, education, and the efficient ex-
change of patient information.

Technology Assessment Centers for Breast Cancer Detection

In contrast to the relative wealth of resources for discovery research, there are very limited resources devoted to the clinical testing of new technologies for breast cancer detection. Companies developing new technologies often hire academic investigators to run their FDA trials. These trials tend to have limited aims—to prove the safety and efficacy of the new products for purpose of marketing and selling the new product. FDA approval does not require assessment of utility of a new technology in clinical practice. The real clinical utility of a new technology depends on how it will be used or co-used with other tests and on which population of women at risk for breast cancer. The specificity, sensitivity, and diagnostic accuracy all vary with the clinical question being addressed and the population being tested. So, while a device may meet FDA's requirements for marketing, deciding whether the device adds value to their decision-making process or merely adds cost is a more complicated question to physicians and their patients. Unfortunately, because little clinical testing of devices is done after the FDA approval process, the adoption of new technologies by users such as radiologists too often depends more on marketing hype and the need to be perceived as having the latest and greatest new products than by clear evidence as to whether those products are really useful to patients.

Currently, very few clinical trials are funded annually to determine whether new technologies might improve the detection and/or diagnosis of breast cancer. Such trials require access to patient populations willing to undergo extra experimental tests, as well as a cadre of investigators who are skilled in trial design and execution. As a rule, academic medical centers do not consider the clinical testing of new technologies to be part of their mission. Multicenter, collaborative studies offer an effective way to meet the need for timely and generalizable clinical evaluations of imaging technologies.[26]

The NIH uses many criteria in determining the need to establish specific research center programs, but certain criteria are applied across the board, each of which applies to centers for research on developing, assessing, and implementing new technologies for breast cancer detection (Box 6-10).[34]

The model of Comprehensive Cancer Centers and their utility in testing new drug therapies could be applied to the testing of new technologies. Centralized resources where imaging experts, including scientists who can adapt a technology to a new clinical problem, patients willing to participate in clinical trials, and an institution whose mission includes the application and testing of new technologies would provide an infrastructure that would allow new devices to become tested and available to those who need them much more systematically (and quickly) than the system that is currently

---

BOX 6-10
NIH Criteria for Establishing Center Programs

- The scientific opportunities and/or public health needs that the program would address have high priority.

- The center would provide an organizational environment that would facilitate activities that are most effectively undertaken by teams of investigators working in close proximity. The activities include:

- Multidisciplinary collaborations for problems that require diverse scientific backgrounds.

- Multi-investigator teams capable of a scope of activities not possible with other funding mechanisms.

- Translating the results of basic research into clinical practice.

- Complementing existing and stimulating new investigator-initiated applications for research project grants.

- Training of graduate students, postdoctoral fellows, physician-scientists, nurses, and other health professionals in cross-disciplinary or translational research.

- Attracting experienced researchers into a new area of research.

- Networking with other centers in the program to conduct coordinated research beyond the capacity of any single center.

- The centers would provide critical research resources needed for productive research that are difficult or too expensive to develop in most individual laboratories.

- The centers would build the infrastructure to promote the institutional development of a field of research.

---

available. In addition, other endpoints besides diagnostic accuracy, such as cost effectiveness and quality of life, could also be centrally and more uniformly studied in such centers.

REFERENCES

1. National Digital Mammography Archive. 2001, May 1. Web Page. Available at: http://nscp01.physics.upenn.edu/NDMA/ndma.html.

2. AcademyHealth. 2003. *Playing by New Rules: Privacy and Health Services Research*. Background paper for the April 29, 2003. Workshop Playing by New Rules: Privacy and Health Services Research.

3. AdvaMed. 2003, August 5. AdvaMed Commends FDA Commisioner's Plan to Speed Review Times; Effort to Complement MDUFMA Performance Goals. Web Page. Available at: http://www.advamed.org/publicdocs/PR-188.htm.

4. AdvaMed. 2004, February 20. AdvaMed Welcomes President Bush's Announcement to Nominate Mark McClellan as New CMS Administrator. Web Page. Available at: http://www.advamed.org/publicdocs/PR-203.htm.

5. Advani AS, Atkeson B, Brown CL, Peterson BL, Fish L, Johnson JL, Gockerman JP, Gautier M. 2003. Barriers to the participation of African-American patients with cancer in clinical trials: a pilot study. *Cancer* 97(6):1499-1506.

6. Agency for Healthcare Research and Quality. 2001. Diagnosis and Management of Specific Breast Abnormalities. *Summary, Evidence Report/Technology Assessment.* AHRQ Publication No. 01-E045. Rockville, MD: Agency for Healthcare Research and Quality.

7. American College of Radiology Imaging Network (ACRIN). 2004. ACRIN—Frequently Asked Questions. Accessed March 4, 2004. Web Page. Available at: http://www.acrin.org/faq.html#current.

8. American College of Radiology Imaging Network (ACRIN). 2004. Digital Mammographic Imaging Screening Trial (DMIST). Accessed March 4, 2004. Web Page. Available at: http://www.dmist.org.

9. American Heart Association. 2001. *Heart Disease and Stroke Statistics—2002 Update.* Dallas, TX: American Heart Association.

10. Association of American Medical Colleges. 2003. Group on Institutional Advancement. Accessed April 4, 2003. Web Page. Available at: http://www.aamc.org/members/gia/start.htm.

11. Blue Cross Blue Shield Association Technology Evaluation Center. 2003. Full Field Digital Mammography. *Tec Assessment Program* 17(7):1-22.

12. Bole K, Bio-IT World. 2003. Decoding HIPAA: Are You Ready? Accessed February 2003. Web Page. Available at: http://www.bio-itworld.com/archive/030702/hippa.html.

13. Bonetta L, Dove A, Watanabe M. 2003. The road to research is paved with restrictions. *Nat Med* 9(6):630.

14. CenterWatch. 2003. Projecting HIPAA's Impact. *CenterWatch Newsletter* 10(5).

15. CenterWatch. 2002. Breaking the development speed barrier. *CenterWatch Newsletter* 9(6).

16. Cho MK, Sankar P, Wolpe PR, Godmilow L. 1999. Commercialization of BRCA1/2 testing: practitioner awareness and use of a new genetic test. *Am J Med Genet* 83(3):157-163.

17. Collins FS, Watson JD. 2003. Genetic discrimination: time to act. *Science* 302(5646):745.

18. Corbie-Smith G, Ammerman AS, Katz ML, St Georg DM, Blumenthal C, Washington C, Weathers B, Keyserling TC, Switzer B. 2003. Trust, benefit, satisfaction, and burden: a randomized controlled trial to reduce cancer risk through African-American churches. *J Gen Intern Med* 18(7):531-541.

19. Cox K, McGarry J. 2003. Why patients don't take part in cancer clinical trials: an overview of the literature. *Eur J Cancer Care (Engl)* 12(2):114-122.

20. Division of Adult and Community Health, National Center for Chronic Disease Prevention and Health Promotion Centers for Disease Control and Prevention Behavioral Risk Factor Surveillance System Online Prevalence Data. 1995. Accessed June 1, 2004. Web Page. Available at: http://apps.nccd.cdc.gov/brfss/age.asp?cat=HC&yr=2000&qkey=4341&state=US.

21. Eisenberg J, Zarin D. 2002. Health technology assessment in the United States: Past, present, and future. *Int J Technol Assess Health Care* 18(2):192-198.

22. Feigal D. 2003. Challenges in Assessing the Safety and Efficacy of Cancer Detection Devices. *Institute of Medicine Workshop: From Development to Adoption of New Approaches to Breast Cancer Detection and Diagnosis.* Washington, DC: The Institute of Medicine of the National Academies.

23. Fisher ES, Wennberg DE, Stukel TA, Gottlieb DJ, Lucas FL, Pinder EL. 2003. The implications of regional variations in Medicare spending. Part 2: health outcomes and satisfaction with care. *Ann Intern Med* 138(4):288-298.

24. Fisher ES, Wennberg DE, Stukel TA, Gottlieb DJ, Lucas FL, Pinder EL. 2003. The implications of regional variations in Medicare spending. Part 1: the content, quality, and accessibility of care. *Ann Intern Med* 138(4):273-287.

25. Gammon MD, Neugut AI, Santella RM, Teitelbaum SL, Britton JA, Terry MB, Eng SM, Wolff MS, Stellman SD, Kabat GC, Levin B, Bradlow HL, Hatch M, Beyea J, Camann D, Trent M, Senie RT, Garbowski GC, Maffeo C, Montalvan P, Berkowitz GS, Kemeny M, Citron M, Schnabe F, Schuss A, Hajdu S, Vincguerra V, Collman GW, Obrams GI. 2002. The Long Island Breast Cancer Study Project: description of a multi-institutional collaboration to identify environmental risk factors for breast cancer. *Breast Cancer Res Treat* 74(3):235-254.

26. Gatsonis C, McNeil BJ. 1990. Collaborative evaluations of diagnostic tests: experience of the Radiology Diagnostic Oncology Group. *Radiology* 175(2):571-575.

27. Goold SD, Vijan S. 1998. Normative issues in cost effectiveness analysis. *J Lab Clin Med* 132(5):376-382.

28. Hadley DW, Jenkins J, Dimond E, Nakahara K, Grogan L, Liewehr DJ, Steinberg SM, Kirsch I. 2003. Genetic counseling and testing in families with hereditary nonpolyposis colorectal cancer. *Arch Intern Med* 163(5):573-582.

29. Health Care Information Center. 2002. *Medicine and Health* 58(38).

30. Hillman BJ, Schnall MD. 2003. American College of Radiology Imaging Network: future clinical trials. *Radiology* 227(3):631-632.

31. IBM News-Australia. 2002, October 14. Oxford University, IBM and UK Government to build massive computing grid for breast cancer screening and diagnosis. Accessed August 21, 2003. Web Page. Available at: http://www.ibm.com/news/au/2002/10/2002102201.html.

32. Institute of Medicine. 1985. *Assessing Medical Technologies*. Washington, DC: National Academy Press.

33. Institute of Medicine. 2001. *Mammography and Beyond: Developing Technologies for the Early Detection of Breast Cancer*. Washington, DC: National Academy Press.

34. Institute of Medicine. 2004. *NIH Extramural Center Programs: Criteria for Initiation and Evaluation*. Washington, DC: The National Academies Press.

35. Kaiser Family Foundation. 2002. State Mandated Benefits: Contraceptives. Accessed July 27, 2003. Web Page. Available at: http://www.statehealthfacts.kff.org/cgi-bin/healthfacts.cgi?action=compare&category=Women%27s+Health&subcategory=Mandated+Benefits%3a+Private+Insurers&topic=Contraceptives.

36. Klabunde C, Kaluzny A, Ford L. 1995. Community Clinical Oncology Program participation in the Breast Cancer Prevention Trial: factors affecting accrual. *Cancer Epidemiol Biomarkers Prev* 4(7):783-799.

37. Kramer BS, Gohagan JK, Prorok PC. 1990. *Cancer Screening: Theory and Practice*. New York: Marcel Dekker.

38. Lara PN Jr, Higdon R, Lim N, Kwan K, Tanaka M, Lau DH, Wun T, Welborn J, Meyers FJ, Christensen S, O'Donnell R, Richman C, Scudder SA, Tuscano J, Gandara DR, Lam KS. 2001. Prospective evaluation of cancer clinical trial accrual patterns: identifying potential barriers to enrollment. *J Clin Oncol* 19(6):1728-1733.

39. Marsden J, Bradburn J. 2004. Patient and clinician collaboration in the design of a national randomized breast cancer trial. *Health Expect* 7(1):6-17.

40. McClellan MB, Commissioner of Food and Drugs. 2003. Technology and innovation: their effects on cost growth of healthcare. Joint Economic Committee.

41. McCormack J. 2003. ALLHAT—so what? *J Inform Pharmacother* (12).

42. Messerli FH. 2001. Doxazosin and congestive heart failure. *J Am Coll Cardiol* 38(5):1295-1296.
43. Michaelson JS, Silverstein M, Wyatt J, Weber G, Moore R, Halpern E, Kopans DB, Hughes K. 2002. Predicting the survival of patients with breast carcinoma using tumor size. *Cancer* 9(4):713-723.
44. Mouton CP, Harris S, Rovi S, Solorzano P, Johnson MS. 1997. Barriers to black women's participation in cancer clinical trials. *J Natl Med Assoc* 89(11):721-727.
45. Murray W. 2002. Cancer's new enemy. *New Architect* 7:10-12.
46. National Cancer Institute. FY2003 Bypass Budget. 2001. *Plans & Priorities for Cancer Research: The Nation's Investment in Cancer Research for Fiscal Year 2003.* Bethesda, MD: National Cancer Institute.
47. National Cancer Institute. 2003. Summary, Fourth National Forum on Biomedical Imaging in Oncology. Accessed August 21, 2003. Web Page. Available at: http://cancer. gov/dctd/forum/summary03.pdf.
48. National Cancer Institute. 2003. *Fourth National Forum on Biomedical Imaging in Oncology Meeting Summary.* Bethesda, MD: National Cancer Institute.
49. National Cancer Institute. 2003. Understanding the Approval Process of New Cancer Treatments: A Short History. Accessed July 27, 2003. Web Page. Available at: http://www.nci.nih.gov/clinicaltrials/understanding/approval-process-for-cancer-drugs/page6.
50. National Cancer Institute. 2003. caBIG at a Glance: Overview of Activities and Accomplishments to Date. Accessed August 27, 2003. Web Page. Available at: http://cabig.nci.nih. gov/overview.
51. National Cancer Institute. 2004. Cancer Research Portfolio. Accessed February 23, 2004. Web Page. Available at: http://researchportfolio.cancer.gov/cgi-bin/search.pl?Search=cancer&x=47&y=13.
52. National Institutes of Health. 2003. *Protecting Personal Health Information in Research: Understanding the HIPAA Privacy Rule.* Bethesda, MD: National Institutes of Health, Department of Health and Human Services.
53. National Institutes of Health. 2004. Re-engineering the Clinical Research Enterprise. Accessed February 20, 2004. Web Page. Available at: http://nihroadmap.nih.gov/clinicalresearch.
54. Paskett ED, Cooper MR, Stark N, Ricketts TC, Tropman S, Hatzell T, Aldrich T, Atkins J. 2002. Clinical trial enrollment of rural patients with cancer. *Cancer Practice* 10(1):28-35.
55. Petitti DB. 2000. *Meta-Analysis, Decision Analysis, and Cost-Effectiveness Analysis.* 2nd ed. New York: Oxford University Press.
56. Petricoin EF, Ardekani AM, Hitt BA, Levine PJ, Fusaro VA, Steinberg SM, Mills GB, Simone C, Fishman DA, Kohn EC, Liotta LA. 2002. Use of proteomic patterns in serum to identify ovarian cancer. *Lancet* 359(9306):572-577.
57. Pisano ED. 2000. Current status of full-field digital mammography. *Radiology* 214(1):26-28.
58. Pressel S, Davis BR, Louis GT, Whelton P, Adrogue H, Egan D, Farber M, Payne G, Probstfield J, Ward H. 2001. Participant recruitment in the Antihypertensive and Lipid-Lowering Treatment to Prevent Heart Attack Trial (ALLHAT). *Control Clin Trials* 22(6):674-686.
59. Rao PN, Levine E, Myers MO, Prakash V, Watson J, Stolier A, Kopicko JJ, Kissinger P, Raj SG, Raj MH. 1999. Elevation of serum riboflavin carrier protein in breast cancer. *Cancer Epidemiol Biomarkers Prev* 8(11):985-990.
60. Rogers EM. 1995. *Diffusion of Innovations.* 4th ed. New York: Free Press.

61. Rosenberg A. 2003. Private Payers' Perspectives on Adoption of New Breast Cancer Detection Technologies. *Institute of Medicine Workshop: From Development to Adoption of New Approaches to Breast Cancer Detection and Diagnosis.*

62. Sateren WB, Trimble EL, Abrams J, Brawley O, Breen N, Ford L, McCabe M, Kaplan R, Smith M, Ungerleider R, Christian MC. 2002. How sociodemographics, presence of oncology specialists, and hospital cancer programs affect accrual to cancer treatment trials. *J Clin Oncol* 20(8):2109-2117.

63. Sung NS, Crowley WF Jr, Genel M, Salber P, Sandy L, Sherwood LM, Johnson SB, Catanese V, Tilson H, Getz K, Larson EL, Scheinberg D, Reece EA, Slavkin H, Dobs A, Grebb J, Martinez RA, Korn A, Rimoin D. 2003. Central challenges facing the national clinical research enterprise. *JAMA* 289(10):1278-1287.

64. The ALLHAT Officers and Coordinators for the ALLHAT Collaborative Research Group. 2002. Major outcomes in high-risk hypertensive patients randomized to angiotensin-converting enzyme inhibitor or calcium channel blocker vs diuretic: the Antihypertensive and Lipid-Lowering Treatment to Prevent Heart Attack Trial (ALLHAT). *JAMA* 288(23):2981-2997.

65. Tunis S. 2003. CMS Perspectives on Adoption of New Breast Cancer Detection Technologies. *Institute of Medicine Workshop: From Development to Adoption of New Approaches to Breast Cancer Detection and Diagnosis.* Washington DC: Institute of Medicine.

66. U.S. Food and Drug Administration. 1998. Overview—FDA Modernization Act of 1997. Web Page. Available at: http://www.fda.gov/cdrh/devadvice/371.html. P. 4.

67. U.S. Food and Drug Administration. 2003. *Improving Innovation in Medical Technology: Beyond 2002.* Rockville, MD: U.S. Food and Drug Administration.

68. UNC Lineberger Comprehensive Cancer Center. 2003. Research Resources: Etta D. Pisano, MD. Web Page. Available at: http://cancer.med.unc.edu/researchers/DisplayByList.asp?ID=142.

69. Wagner L. 2004. A test before its time? FDA stalls distribution process of proteomic test. *J Natl Cancer Inst* 96(7):500-501.

70. Wang JG, Staessen JA, Heagerty AM. 2003. Ongoing trials: what should we expect after ALLHAT? *Curr Hypertens Rep* 5(4):340-345.

71. Whiting P, Rutjes AW, Reitsma JB, Bossuyt PM, Kleijnen J. 2003. The development of QUADAS: a tool for the quality assessment of studies of diagnostic accuracy included in systematic reviews. *BMC Med Res Methodol* 3(1):25.

72. Winslow R, Hensley S. 2002, December 18. Dose of reality: study questions high cost of drugs for hypertension. *The Wall Street Journal.*

7

Translating New Technologies into Improved Patient Outcomes

In health care, invention is hard, but dissemination is even harder.

Donald Berwick
JAMA 2003

The development of new technologies for breast cancer detection and diagnosis is important in improving patient outcomes, but is not sufficient on its own.[a] In fact, the translation of a new technology into improved patient outcomes involves at least three overlapping processes: (1) decisions by healthcare delivery organizations to adopt these new technologies that are based on assessment of the efficacy and cost-effectiveness of the technologies, (2) deployment of these technologies within the complex organizational structure of healthcare providers, and (3) monitoring the use of these new technologies. Clearly, new technologies must be adopted by healthcare providers in order to affect patient outcomes. However, it may be less obvious that these technologies must be deployed in a manner that takes into account the frequent need for healthcare delivery organizations to adapt their organizational structures to deliver the full benefit of the new technologies. Furthermore, the use of new technologies by healthcare practitioners must be monitored to ensure and improve the quality of care. All too often, in the view of this Committee, analyses of healthcare technology have emphasized the development and assessment of new technologies and paid less attention to the process by which clinicians deploy new technologies into routine medical practice. The distance between efficacy and effectiveness is long and not always bridged (Box 7-1).

---

[a]As is the case throughout the report, "technology" is used in its broadest sense to include imaging devices, biologically based approaches (such as gene or protein biomarkers), detection software, and new procedures.

BOX 7-1
Efficacy and Effectiveness

Efficacy refers to the likelihood that a particular intervention will benefit patients when used under *optimal or ideal experimental* conditions. Such conditions are rarely met except in controlled clinical studies. An efficacious treatment is one whose effects have been shown to have a statistically significant improvement in health or well-being, typically in a randomized controlled trial (RCT).

Effectiveness refers to the likelihood that a particular intervention will benefit patients when used under *usual and routine clinical practice* conditions. Such conditions are generally more complex than those used in RCTs. For example, many people have coexisting conditions that alter the effect of interventions; they may not consistently follow treatment instructions; or they might be much older or younger or of different ethnicity than the people with whom the RCT was conducted.

The Committee believes that because technologies that completely replace mammography are unlikely to reach the market—at least within the next 10 years—organizations will be faced with the challenge of adopting technologies that will be used in conjunction with existing modalities. These new technologies will have to be integrated into current practice and will require the creation of new organizational routines for screening and diagnosis.

Mammography creates a high standard for any new technology. The value of any new breast cancer detection technology will be determined largely in reference to mammography. If any new technology were shown to outperform mammography for any specific groups—for example, for women whose breast density exceeds a certain threshold—then it might be adopted.

Our discussion in this chapter distinguishes among the activities of (1) technology assessment and adoption, (2) technology deployment, and (3) monitoring of technologies in use. This tripartite schema, however, is a description of best practice. Technology assessment leading up to the decision to adopt, or purchase and use, is covered in Chapter 6. In fact, many health care delivery organizations undertake technology assessment and adoption. But far fewer plan systematically for the organizational, technological, and other complementary requirements for the deployment of these technologies. Even fewer healthcare delivery organizations, in the judgment of this Committee, invest sufficiently in the monitoring of the use and effectiveness of these technologies as employed by healthcare practitioners. One of the central arguments of this chapter is the need for greater attention to these second and third activities in order to improve patient outcomes.

PROCESS OF TECHNOLOGY ADOPTION

The foregoing implies that following Food and Drug Administration (FDA) approval, the successful introduction into routine clinical practice of any new technology relies on three phases: assessment, deployment, and monitoring (Table 7-1). Although many discussions of technology adoption focus only on the *decision* to adopt technology, this report refers to these phases together as the adoption *process*, in which the decision to adopt is just one element.

The **assessment** of a new technology relies on an evaluation of its efficacy and effectiveness, based on the results of clinical studies that often are carried out in academic medical centers or other centers of research. This activity is typically undertaken by regulators (such as the FDA), technology developers, academic clinicians, delivery organizations and insurers (for example, Blue Cross Blue Shield). Without assessment, patients are subject to ineffective, or even harmful, medical treatments. Medical history is rich with examples of technologies that were applied only on the basis of what seemed plausible at the time, but were later proven to be inappropriate. Even today, an estimated 80,000 unnecessary hysterectomies and 500,000 unnecessary cesarean deliveries are performed in this country every year.[3,9]

The clinical settings where the assessments of effectiveness and efficacy are conducted may differ in significant ways from the typical health delivery environment within many health care organizations. Practitioner exper-

TABLE 7-1 The Three Phases of Technology Adoption

Phase	Definition/ Examples
Technology assessment	Evaluation of the results of scientific testing of a technology: • Cost-benefit analysis* • Efficacy • Specification of the target population
Technology deployment	Putting technology into practice: • Early experience and learning • Development of new work routines • Integration with existing technologies and work routines
Technology monitoring	Post-application monitoring: • Evaluation of outcomes • Detection of anomalies

*In practice, cost is rarely considered at this stage.

tise may be less highly developed, patients not involved in a clinical trial or evaluation may be less committed to following the guidelines for specific procedures, and equipment may be less well maintained or operated by less highly qualified practitioners. Therefore, some evaluation of the scope of the task of technology deployment is an important step in successful introduction of a new medical technology. **Technology deployment** includes the activities of implementing the technology in routine use, gaining early experience in using it, and then making its use routine. In other industries this phase often includes a review by technology users of their capacity to apply the technology in routine work and evaluates the system and organizational requirements needed to support the use of the technology, such as the number and types of staff, their training needs, and the facilities needed. In health care, few parties undertake such reviews of the technology prior to actual use.

Not all technologies are the same. Some are easily integrated into clinical practice because they can be substituted for existing technologies without requiring significant changes in work routines. Others require substantial changes in order to fully realize their potential. In the latter case, patient outcomes are not only a function of the technology itself (efficacy), but of the way it is applied by users; therefore the success of the technology depends on the organizational and clinical skill of individual users and user organizations (effectiveness).

Finally, **technology monitoring** is the surveillance of patient outcomes after the introduction of new technology, with the intent of identifying opportunities for improvement or failures of the technology or its use.

Ideally, issues related to technology use, such as "ease of use," are integrated into technology design, and user experience with a technology is an important piece of feedback for designers. But formal evaluations of technologies by practitioners and delivery organizations focus more on technology assessment than application, and therefore a highly desirable "feedback loop" is less effective than it should be. In addition, the organizational adaptations necessary to exploit new technologies effectively (especially those based on digital technologies that create high potential for greater cross-functional integration and interaction within the delivery system) are rarely codified or incorporated with new technologies for breast cancer detection and diagnosis.

All but the first phases of technology adoption are typically undertaken by healthcare delivery organizations that are planning widespread use of a technology (although some provider organizations also conduct their own technology assessment in addition to those undertaken by the FDA and Centers for Medicare & Medicaid Services [CMS]). In conducting the assessment, however, users may not have access to well described models of service delivery and operational processes, or strategies for staff training.

Nor may users have the capability to experiment with different service models for placing a new technology into routine practice. These deficiencies will impede technology adoption and may produce less successful outcomes for those technologies that are adopted.

Many of the technological possibilities for improving detection and diagnostic outcomes in the relatively near future will involve integrated "portfolios" of technologies or technologies spanning different functions within the health care delivery organization. Adoption of such technologies is likely to be a complex process and one for which evaluation of effectiveness and outcomes in the clinical setting, rather than in an academic research center, will be particularly important. The complexity of technology adoption is likely to be further increased by the reduction in size of patient populations as smaller risk groups are successfully identified, each possibly requiring a different screening strategy and suite of screening technologies. This approach could be less complicated when used by an integrated health care team that provides all aspects of a breast cancer diagnosis. Thus, the responsibility will remain with the physician, and not the patient, to ask the right questions and obtain the appropriate information to determine the most effective approach for each woman.

The tasks of technology deployment and monitoring have become more complex and demanding. Multiple risk and morphology identification technologies need to be integrated with each other in a way that helps to guide clinicians in their selections of evaluation strategies for each individual patient. Head-to-head comparisons of the performance of technologies under both research conditions and conditions of routine use will be an essential component of the development of clinical strategies for screening subgroups of at-risk patients. Two excellent, but unfortunately rare, examples of head-to-head comparison trials are discussed in Chapter 6: the Antihypertensive and Lipid Lowering Treatment to Prevent Heart Attack Trial comparing different medications for hypertension and the Digital Mammography Imaging Screening Trial (DMIST) comparing digital with screen-film mammography.

New technologies or portfolios of technologies also need to be integrated into practice through training, change in organizational structure, and the design of appropriate incentives. Research on the organizational determinants of an individual technology's performance and the collation and dissemination of organizational "best practices" are needed to aid individual clinicians, delivery organizations, and systems of care in planning for the implementation of new screening technologies or portfolios of technology.

The thesis of this chapter is that the scope of technology assessment must be expanded to include considerations of "value in use," or whether the technology will deliver its promise of improving health outcomes. The first stage of technology assessment, clinical trials, was addressed in Chapter 6. This chapter continues with consideration of the subsequent stages through which new technologies are incorporated into clinical practice, and how their potential value can be delivered once they are adopted.

THE MANY DRIVERS OF TECHNOLOGY ADOPTION

The study of diffusion of innovation has a long history in social science, although much of that history focuses on the decision to adopt innovations. Individuals who adopt specific innovations have been classified into five groups based on their rates of adoption of new technologies and students of innovation have identified distinctive personalities and social roles that are linked to adoption (Box 7-2).[20]

In addition to the characteristics of the people who adopt innovations, perceptions of an innovation are a major determinant of how quickly and extensively that innovation will be adopted. The belief that an innovation is both beneficial and compatible with the values and needs of individuals is particularly influential—as it should be. Another important factor that is particularly relevant to breast cancer detection technologies is complexity.

BOX 7-2
Typology of Technology Adopters

The fastest individuals or groups to adopt new technologies are the **innovators** who tend to be wealthier than average or otherwise able to accept the risks and costs inherent in innovation. They are not opinion leaders; in fact, they may be thought of as mavericks or may appear to be heavily invested personally in a specialized topic. The next group is the **early adopters**. They are opinion leaders who do not tend to search as widely as the innovators, but do seek out the innovators. Such people are generally testing several innovations at once. Early adopters are often elected as leaders of professional groups, and they are the likeliest targets of pharmaceutical or device company detailing. The next third of the distribution is the **early majority**, who tend to learn mainly from people they know well. They tend to travel less and interact less with the innovators than do the early adopters. The next group, another third of the population, is more conservative: the **late majority**. They will adopt an innovation when it appears to be the new standard of practice, but not before. Members of the final group are termed "laggards," although **traditionalists** is perhaps a better term. They are the physicians who swear by the tried and true.

SOURCE: Text quoted from Donald Berwick. Disseminating Innovations in Health Care (*JAMA* 2004) based on typology developed by Everett Rogers (*Diffusion of Innovations*).

Generally, simple technologies are adopted faster than complicated ones.[4] Complicated technologies almost always change as they spread, and local adaptation is nearly always necessary for successful adoption.

Approval from both the FDA and health care payers is usually a necessary step for technology adoption, but neither can ensure that the "right" technologies will find their way into widespread clinical use. There is no guarantee that a technology that receives a favorable review during the technology assessment process will be used in routine practice.

In addition to the general patterns that drive technology adoption, idiosyncratic aspects of particular technologies can influence the likelihood that they will be adopted into clinical practices. Finally, clear evidence of efficacy and effectiveness should be, but is not always, the basis for a decision to adopt a new technology.

FDA Approval Only Partly Predicts the Adoption of Technology

FDA approval is a critical step in the development of most new medical technologies. When a fledgling company obtains FDA approval for its product, its ability to raise capital soars, which in turn enables the company to continue developing the product. Likewise, the label "FDA approved" is commonly used as a marketing tool.

Although FDA approval enables a new technology to enter the marketplace, it does not guarantee success. For example, the T-Scan™ device that measures electrical impedance in breast tissue was approved by the FDA in 1999 as an adjunct to mammography, but 4 years later the manufacturer had not sold a single machine in the United States (see Box 7-3). Another example is the case of thermography, first approved by the FDA in 1982 for use as an adjunct to mammography. Definitive clinical trials of thermography have never been conducted to determine its effectiveness in detection breast cancer and no thermographic devices have gained widespread clinical acceptance. Therefore, it should not be surprising that FDA approval is no guarantee that a technology will be widely adopted. Even so, thermography service centers are currently open for business and promoting the use of thermography for breast cancer detection.

The FDA approval process focuses primarily on assessing whether the technology is safe and effective and uses data drawn exclusively from highly structured experimental settings in order to make this determination. FDA approval implies nothing about the likelihood of realizing these optimal outcomes in the setting of routine practice, nor does the FDA provide guidance on what structures or activities might be necessary in order to realize optimal outcomes. Importantly, FDA approval says nothing about how a new technology might be practically used in concert with other technologies already in use, which is an especially important issue when a

---

BOX 7-3
T-Scan: FDA Approval, but No Market

In 1999, the FDA approved the T-Scan˜ 2000, which is based on a technique known as electrical impedance scanning, as an adjunct to mammography. The T-Scan, developed by TransScan Medical, Inc., works by creating a map of the breast using a small electrical current.

Unlike mammography, electrical impedance spectroscopy measures do not require compression of the breast. Images are made at the time of testing and are simple to interpret, which reduces the waiting time for results. It is also much less expensive than magnetic resonance imaging (MRI) or ultrasound. The first models cost about $70,000; the second generation models are expected to cost about $30,000. Individual exams could cost as little as $10 to $20. Comparatively, screen-film mammography devices cost approximately $70,000 and individual exams are reimbursed approximately $80 by CMS.

Limitations. Although a website sponsored by Siemens (the international distributor of T-Scan) describes T-Scan as "diagnostically accurate" and "cost-effective to own and operate," there are limitations to the device in breast cancer detection. The accuracy, as defined by sensitivity and specificity, is lower than either mammography or current biopsy techniques. It is also less sensitive than any of the current technologies used to investigate the results of suspicious mammograms—either ultrasound or surgical biopsy—and it cannot detect microcalcifications, often associated with early stage breast cancers. In the event of a suspicious mammogram, the premium on specificity is very high.

No Sales in the United States. As of January 2003, 125 devices had been sold outside the United States. Sixty-five of them had been sold in Europe, 50 in Asia, and 10 in Latin America. However, no units have been sold in the United States. The company decided not to market in the United States because they did not think it would be accepted, and they were probably right, because the fear of malpractice litigation exerts strong pressure to avoid false negatives. In addition, some cancers detectable by mammography will be missed if this technology is used in its place.

---

new technology complements existing technologies, as opposed to replacing them.

In certain cases, such as for BRCA testing or other "home-brew" tests, FDA approval is not even necessary. The FDA does not regulate the BRCA test, because the test kits are not marketed to consumers and do not claim to produce a beneficial clinical outcome. The test is certified only by the CMS under the Clinical Laboratory Improvement Amendments (CLIA) of 1988 and lacks any other regulation within the United States. CLIA requires only that the laboratories demonstrate accuracy and reliability in measuring the substances that they claim to be assaying.

BRCA testing also illustrates another issue that crops up regularly, which is the potential for patents to impede the development and dissemi-

BOX 7-4
Myriad Problems in International Gene Patenting

Through several patents, Myriad Genetics, Inc., legally owns a DNA sequence associated with an increased risk of developing breast cancer. The Salt Lake City, Utah-based company was awarded "composition of matter" and "method-of-use" patents on the BRCA1 and BRCA2 breast cancer susceptibility genes from the U.S., European, and Canadian Patent Offices. However, as of this writing, Myriad has granted only a few limited licenses to other companies, effectively making Myriad the only legal source for BRCA testing in Europe and North America. This business strategy has created international controversy, because it restricts others from testing for BRCA mutations even with superior methods. For example, several cheaper tests with similar effectiveness have been developed, yet the broad scope of Myriad's patent prevents health care systems worldwide from adopting other technologies.[21] For instance, a faster and cheaper genetic test cannot be offered locally within a system of care that is linked to genetic counseling services and the other testing services offered by the system, thus restricting access to care.[25]

Testing begun in the Canadian province of Ontario for a third of the cost of Myriad's test and with results available eight weeks sooner, was threatened with legal action by Myriad against the province of Ontario in late 2002. However, under the direction of Ontario's Health Minister Tony Clement, regional hospitals have disregarded the patent and continue to offer BRCA gene testing services. Clement opposes Myriad's patent saying, "We do not accept their claim and we are disregarding that claim." In response to threats from Myriad Genetics to enforce their patent, Clement stated that he was willing to take the issue to the highest court.[16]

However, care may be affected by the cost of the test, the length of time it takes for samples to be mailed and processed, and the inability of Myriad to test for every possible breast cancer mutation, resulting in false negatives. Only 10 to 20 percent of the potential BRCA1 mutations are tested by Myriad, and their testing has missed mutations.[11]

nation of new technologies. Although the patent system was designed to "promote the useful arts," the ability of patent holders to restrict access to their technologies can create obstacles, as has been the case for BRCA testing[7] (Box 7-4).

Coverage Matters More for Some Technologies Than Others

As with FDA approval, the decision by health care payers (insurance companies, health maintenance organizations, and Medicare) to reimburse health care providers is usually an important driver of technology adoption. Gaining coverage is still no guarantee of adoption, nor is it required for the successful adoption of an innovative technology into routine practice. For example, testing for BRCA mutations was widely done even in the absence of coverage. Most insurance companies now cover BRCA testing. Even though MRI is not covered for screening, it has nonetheless been marketed for screening and is requested by consumers on a daily basis (see Box 1-3 in Chapter 1).

Reimbursement policies will have their greatest effect on the adoption of more expensive technologies. Positron emission tomography (PET), computer-aided detection (CAD), and digital mammography all experienced a surge in usage after health care payers decided to cover them.

Reimbursement procedures also influence technology adoption. Since CAD is a technology to improve interpretation of mammography, its reimbursement could have been bundled into a single payment for mammography. Instead, CAD is covered as a separate add-on payment, and that clarifies the economic implications of employing this technology and is more likely to encourage its diffusion. Frost & Sullivan, a leading market analyst firm for medical technology, reports "skyrocketing" sales for CAD, with 18 and 8 percent growth in 2002 and 2003, propelled by the increased reimbursement rates for mammography CAD screening.[10] They also report that use of CAD has "boosted the confidence levels of both radiologist and patients." As discussed in Chapter 3, the evidence that the use of CAD improves breast cancer detection is promising, but not definitive.

Digital mammography is a different story. Although CMS will reimburse health care providers for the use of digital mammography for screening mammograms, many insurance companies will not. The Blue Cross Blue Shield Technology Evaluation Center and the Kaiser Foundation Health Plan have both decided not to cover digital mammography, because it has not been demonstrated that:[5]

- It improves net health outcomes,
- It is as beneficial as screen-film mammography, and
- It improves outcomes outside investigational settings (i.e., in routine clinical practice).

This conclusion was reached in July 2002 and was based on the data available up to that point, but could be revised if new evidence indicates clear advantages of digital over screen-film mammography, such as the results from the DMIST trial expected in 2005 (see Chapter 6). In the meantime, lack of reimbursement will limit the adoption of digital mammography. Digital mammography is an expensive technology when compared with conventional screen film, with digital systems ranging from $350,000 to $500,000 versus $80,000 to $90,000 for screen-film units.[2] In general, decisions by healthcare payers to deny reimbursement puts a brake on the adoption of expensive and unproven technologies (at least for screening), including PET, MRI, laser tomography, and thermography.[1] Although lack of validation and lack of coverage are strong deterrents, as noted

BOX 7-5
Drug-Eluting Stents

Coronary stents are metallic mesh devices that are often placed at the site of angioplasty to keep the artery open. In some patients, scar tissue grows at the site of the stent, thereby creating a new blockage or narrowing in the artery. Drug-eluting stents are coated with a polymer containing a drug that is released into the surrounding tissue to prevent scar tissue formation.

earlier, there are many drivers to technology adoption, including patients who pay out of pocket for new technologies. Indeed, leading market analysts predict that digital mammography will slowly replace traditional screen-film mammography—anticipating, in part, that evidence will eventually shift in favor of digital mammography. (Other factors such as increased efficiency in processing and handling of images are also likely to influence the rate of adoption.)

Even without clear evidence and without widespread coverage, digital mammography generated about $70 million in revenues, and is predicted to be 70 percent of overall mammography revenues.[19] (By comparison, the mammography market in North America generated $203 million in 2002.)

Delays in coverage decisions are frequently cited as a major source of delay in the diffusion of medical innovations. In 2001 the Lewin Group reported that Medicare can take 15 months to 5 years or more to make policy decisions on new blood tests like those for colon cancer, breast cancer, and prostate cancer.[13] But in some cases, such as the use of drug-eluting stents in cardiac surgery, the superiority of the technology is so immediately clear that coverage decisions are made quickly (Box 7-5). The use of drug-eluting stents in cardiac surgery spread more rapidly than any recent innovation in medical technology and in that sense represents the extremely rare "magic bullet." Perhaps even more important to the rapid dissemination of drug-eluting stents was that effective use of them required minimal learning on the part of surgical teams and did not require significant adaptation of conventional procedures.

Consumer Demand Can Override Lack of Data

In many cases, widespread technology adoption occurs in the absence of strong evidence that it delivers any measurable benefit to consumer health. Sometimes this adds up only to wasted time and money, but other times the outcomes—as in the treatment of breast cancer patients with high-dose chemotherapy—can be fatal.

Such cases are generally propelled by consumer demand, sometimes to the point of being enshrined in legal mandates. In 1997, Congress passed a law mandating reimbursement of bone densitometry for osteoporosis screening and for prostate serum antigen testing for prostate cancer, despite the lack of data indicating that those tests reduced mortality for either condition. The case of treatment of breast cancer with high-dose chemotherapy combined with bone marrow transplants (HDC/BMT) is a particularly grim example, because the treatment itself carried a significant risk of mortality, about 20 percent in the early years. In the mid-1980s a few preliminary studies indicated that HDC/BMT might be beneficial, and belief in the treatment spread like wildfire. Health care payers initially denied coverage on the grounds that the treatment was unproven, but patients took their insurers to court and won.[23,b] Ten states passed laws mandating coverage for HDC/BMT. The Office of Personnel Management, which provides health insurance coverage for more than 9 million federal employees through the Federal Employees Benefits Program, required all participating health insurers to cover HDC/BMT. Most private insurers followed their lead. In spite of the lack of evidence for the procedure, insurers were strongly influenced by the threat of litigation (in which the insurers were usually unsuccessful), public relations concerns, and the government mandates.[24]

Definitive clinical trials that eventually showed the treatment to be generally ineffective were delayed for many years because so many women believed the treatment had already been proven and were not willing to enroll in trials. Many patients with advanced disease had been told at cancer centers that this treatment had shown promise.[23] In the meantime, more than 15,000 women with invasive breast cancer had been treated with HDC/BMT, a grueling treatment that involved weeks of isolation in extreme pain.[15]

Void-Filling Technologies Are Adopted More Readily

When mammography was introduced, it was a "void-filling" technology and thus had no competition during the adoption process. New imaging technologies for breast cancer detection face a different scenario. Not only must they be as effective as mammography, but they must offer enough added value to justify the cost of substituting the new technology for the old.

---

[b]The precedent-setting case was Fox v. Health Net of California in 1993, a highly publicized case in which a jury awarded $89 million in damages to the family of Nelene Fox whose insurance company had denied coverage of HDC/BMT. (Fox's local community raised the money for treatment, but she died soon after it; Case no. 219692 California Supreme Court.)

As a rule, technologies that fill a void are adopted more rapidly than those that perform the same functions as technologies already in use. If history had been reversed and electrical impedance scanning (EIS) had been well established as a life-saving technology before the advent of mammography, it likely would have found a strong market in the United States. But if mammography had come along with better sensitivity and specificity than EIS, it is likely that EIS would have been replaced. Furthermore, if mammography had followed EIS, then it might have been welcomed more skeptically in the face of an existing technology that did not carry with it the discomfort and exposure to radiation associated with mammography.

For now, the combination of sensitivity, specificity, and relatively low cost of mammography set a high bar for the entry of new breast cancer detection technologies. In general, anatomically based technologies that rely on nonspecific aspects of cancer-associated changes (such as temperature, water content, or conductivity) are unlikely to be widely adopted because mammography already occupies that niche. For widespread adoption, new technologies will have to be demonstrably superior to mammography. This would include technologies where increased efficiency or reduced costs permit increased access or treatment quality. In contrast, other technologies such as blood tests that could reliably and accurately identify breast cancer risk or that could distinguish among potentially invasive and noninvasive cancer would be void-filling technologies and would be expected to be readily adopted. BRCA testing and protein profiling based on microarray analysis are both examples of void-filling technologies.

TECHNOLOGY AND ORGANIZATIONAL CHANGE

In innovation, new concepts usually must come from outside the current system, but new processes—the things that make the concepts live—must come from inside or they will not work.

Donald Berwick, *JAMA* 2003

One of the most robust findings of more than two decades of research on the adoption of new technologies, especially technologies that rely heavily on digital transmission or storage of information, is the need for complementary organizational changes to fully realize the economic, efficiency, or productivity benefits of these technologies. For example, an analysis of 1,000 drug approvals since 1987 revealed that several drug development companies consistently outperformed the others in drug development times, developing their drugs as much as 50 percent faster than other companies. The top performers tended to be those that invested in new technologies to speed the routing of documents—a seemingly small aspect of a complex scientific process that was nonetheless identified as a critical strategic step.[6]

Technologies that affect the transmission or storage of information have particularly significant implications for organizational structure, precisely because organizational hierarchies often are based on differential access to various types of data or information. But when a new technology involves a significant change in procedures or the costs of those procedures, the most efficient roles for different team members are likely to change. This may also require changing organizational hierarchies, which is, by definition, disruptive.

Many of the important new technologies in breast cancer detection and diagnosis rely on improvements in information handling, and therefore have significant implications for organizational structure. Moreover, as Maanen and Barley[14] and Edmondson and colleagues[8] have shown, the adoption of many other types of new medical technologies has followed this pattern. Significant organizational change is necessary in order to exploit the potential of these technologies for improvements in patient care and patient outcomes.

An important part of the "technology deployment" task, therefore, is the instigation and management of the organizational changes necessary to accommodate new medical technologies. Organizational capabilities are what determine the difference between technology potential and technology yield. Adopting new technology requires a high degree of organizational adaptation.[12] As a rule, once research has established the efficacy and safety of a device and it has obtained regulatory approval (if needed), the factors that should be considered in the decision to acquire a particular technology include:

- How it fits into the culture or operational style of a health organization or practices,
- How it affects workflow and work processes,
- What other technologies it displaces or changes,
- How easy it is to master and set up,
- How easy it is to maintain,
- Whether it is reimbursable (more important for relatively expensive technologies),
- Whether there is recognition or demand for it, and
- Promotional initiatives.

For example, a study that compared the ability of different surgical teams to adopt minimally invasive procedure for cardiac surgery found that their proficiency was linked to their ability to adopt new work routines and relationships among surgical team members (Box 7-6).[8,18]

BOX 7-6
Minimally Invasive Cardiac Surgery:
A Case Study in Technology Deployment

The effective adoption of most new medical technologies, including those described in this report, is likely to require changes in clinical practice. A study of the adoption of minimally invasive cardiac surgery indicates that the success of this procedure depends as much on organizational factors as on the efficacy of the technology in question.

When first introduced, minimally invasive cardiac surgery was expected to be a significant improvement over conventional cardiac surgery, because it was so much less traumatic for patients. Recovery from the surgery was much faster and less painful. The most obvious difference between the two approaches is that a surgeon performing a minimally invasive procedure accessed the heart through a small incision between the ribs, rather than by splitting the breastbone apart. But minimally invasive cardiac surgery also differs from conventional cardiac surgery in a number of more subtle ways that affect how efficiently the procedure is implemented. During minimally invasive surgery, heart function cannot be gauged by seeing and touching the organ, as in conventional surgery, but instead is indicated by sensors that measure blood pressure and other vital signs. This information is displayed on monitors that hang from the ceiling of the operating room and are monitored not by the surgeon, but by other surgical team members: the anesthesiologist, the perfusionist (the technician who controls the pump that substitutes for the heart during the procedure), and the nurse.

Although the equipment or techniques used to perform minimally invasive cardiac surgery were not novel, the organization of the procedure represented a major departure from convention. The successful adoption of this approach required members of the surgical team to learn new tasks, establish new routines, and—most importantly—develop ways of working together that differed considerably from their experience in performing conventional cardiac surgery.

A Harvard research team compared the adoption of the minimally invasive procedure among 16 different cardiac surgical units, using the amount of time taken to complete a coronary artery bypass graft (CABG) as an indicator of efficiency. All of the surgical teams received the same standardized training in this procedure, and all performed it in their early cases with much the same efficiency, taking about 3 times as long as the typical 3- to 6-hour conventional CABG. As the surgical teams gained experience, their procedure times decreased. However, the rate by which different teams achieved improvement varied significantly.

Several factors were associated with the rapid learning and successful adoption of the minimally invasive procedure: careful selection of the team members, preparations such as practice sessions before the first case; choosing uncomplicated early cases, and holding debriefing sessions after every early case to review what went well and what could be done better. The teams that were most successful were those that fostered an environment where team members were willing to acknowledge errors, received criticism, or were warned of an impending error by another team member. Interestingly, neither the type of hospital (academic or community) nor the surgeon's seniority appeared to influence success in adopting the new procedure. The worst performing teams tended to be those that followed entrenched clinical routines and status relationships among professional disciplines.

Conventional wisdom holds that institutions with the same amount of experience with a new technology will be similarly successful in applying it (the so-called "volume-outcome hypothesis"). By contrast, the results of the study on adoption of minimally invasive surgery suggest that experience with a new technology is necessary but not sufficient to ensure its successful adoption. To fully realize a new technology's potential, the adopting team needs to develop and optimize work routines and relationships. In fact, although many studies have found a positive association between hospitals' volume of cardiac artery bypass surgery (CABG) and patient outcome, the effect is modest.[17] Most low-volume hospitals achieve excellent outcomes, suggesting that superior processes rather than volume *per se* is important in high performance.[22] However, variation in outcomes is higher among small-volume hospitals. After adjusting for case variation among hospitals, rates of operative mortality decrease only 0.07 percent for every additional CABG procedure conducted.

Organizational changes are as important in improving the application of current technology as they are for the integration of new technologies into existing systems. Technology monitoring is integral to recognizing the need for improvement, as well as for achieving improvement.

Benefits of Organizational Change: The Colorado Mammography Project

The mammography project at the Colorado Permanente Medical Group (CPMG) illustrates the value of attention to organizational design, quality improvement, and performance management, as well as the benefit to patients. The project was started in 1996 in response to quality assessments indicating that detectable breast cancers were being misdiagnosed by several radiologists. It incorporated many innovations in healthcare delivery, including patient safety, continuous quality improvement, and development of practice focus within the specialty of radiology specific to mammography.

The project entailed a series of fundamental changes in the radiology department:

- In 1996, a comprehensive quality assessment program for mammography interpretation was established, with multiple continuous monitors of quality (Table 7-2).

- In 1998, the radiology department consolidated multiple medical office practices into a single central reading facility and instituted standardized practices with respect to every facet of the interpretation of mammograms.

TABLE 7-2 Quality Measures Used in Colorado Mammography Project

Indicator	Project Goals	Benchmarks Established in Other Studies or by Law
Proportion of stage 0 or 1 diagnosed by mammography	80% in 1998 85% by 2003	80%
Sensitivity	80%	73%
Cancers per 1,000 mammograms	> 6	6
Recall rate for screening mammograms	≤ 7%	8.3%
Number of mammograms read per radiologist	4,000/year	480/year

- Prior to 1998, each of the 21 radiologists in the region interpreted mammograms, some as few as 40 per month, the minimum requirement of the Mammography Quality Standards Act. By the end of 1998, the radiologists had specialized, limiting the interpretation of mammograms to a subgroup with proven high performance, and who read, on average, 6,000 to 7,000 studies annually.

- From the inception of the comprehensive quality monitoring process, individual and group results have been fed back to the radiologists. Data are compared to published benchmarks, goals of group performance and individual variation are defined, performance gaps analyzed, specific interventions applied, and the results of interventions measured. Where persistent gaps exist, additional improvement activities are instituted.

- In 1998, project leaders established a mammography self-assessment exercise that is mandatory for each of the subspecialists. This exercise consists of a blinded evaluation of a mix of normal and known, subtle breast cancers. The exercise challenges the radiologist to continually assess and improve his/her mammography interpretation skills.

- Although the quality improvement activities have concentrated on systems improvement and self-learning, certain intractable performance issues have been encountered, necessitating withdrawal of privileges for four radiologists over 8 years.

The project involves a comprehensive performance improvement process, the identification of opportunities at the system and the individual radiologist level, the implementation of plans, and significant and sustainable improvement in patient outcomes. Moreover, the catalyst for this process was a complete reorganization of the radiology department and a commitment to develop mammography as a legitimate subspecialty. Small improvements, such as a 4 percent improvement in sensitivity for detection of breast cancer, resulted from isolated performance interventions, but overall reorganization had much greater impact—for example, raising sensitivity by 11 percent.

Because this process was oriented toward self-assessment and learning, there was little emphasis on applying the information to individual performance management. For example, the information was not used in the radiologist's annual performance appraisal. Each set of cases was certified for $2^1/_2$ hours of American Medical Association Category 1 Continuing Medical Education (CME), and the exercise was available to radiologists from local private practice groups with intermittent participation. Radiologist satisfaction averaged 92 percent for the overall measures included on the CPMG survey.

With the completion of mammography specialization by 1998, however, a sustained level of nearly 90 percent early stage cancer has been achieved. This represents statistically significant improvement and exceeds published benchmarks by 10 percent.

Patients are commonly recalled for additional views when the screening mammogram is inconclusive or demonstrates findings potentially indicative of cancer. Such callbacks produce great patient anxiety, consume limited resources, and expose the patient to additional radiation. In Colorado, both group and individual performance are monitored relative to a goal of 7 percent. When a radiologist exceeds two standard deviations for any quarter, he or she must gain the concurrence of another physician for any proposed recall. Using this simple intervention, the group has experienced rapid normalization in every case.

In addition, as a result of the improved "process efficiency" of mammogram interpretation, the program has generated net savings of greater than $3 million over the past seven years. During the study period the cost of the professional component relative value unit for each mammogram declined 45 percent, and is now approximately $28, which is 77 percent of the Medicare benchmark.

Technology monitoring was integral to this project: first, in the recognition that there was room for improvement, and then throughout the project by establishing monitoring as a routine part of the organization. Finaly, the benefits for the women of Colorado are made clear through the results of monitoring.

SUMMARY

Most approaches to technology assessment imply that it is only the technology that needs assessing and do not address the capabilities of the provider in using the technology—that is, that the technology's performance capabilities are a function of the technology, not the skill of the user.

The Committee believes technology assessment should include more than an assessment of the efficacy of a new technology under ideal circumstances; assessment should also weigh the benefits and costs of the technology in relation to existing interventions and should include a review of the organizational capabilities (skills, resources, and processes) required to successfully utilize the technology in daily practice. This is critical to realizing the full potential the technology has to offer.

Multiple technologies with utility for smaller subgroups of women will need to be integrated (1) with each other, and (2) into existing organization and clinical routines.

In essence, the scope of technology assessment should be expanded to consider "value in use" in much the same way that nonmedical technologies are assessed. This entails the development of implementation plans and assessment of how it works in practice, with opportunities to make improvements.

Technology assessment should thus take "adoptability" into account. The experiences of early adopters should be used to assess necessary adaptations for use of the technology.

REFERENCES

1. Bankhead C. PET tests the waters of breast cancer monitoring. December 2002. Web Page. Available at: http://www.diagnosticimaging.com/communitypet/3.shtml.
2. Batchelor JS. 2003, November 21. Detours mark the road to U.S. adoption of digital mammo. Accessed December 1, 2003. Web Page. Available at: http://www.auntminnie.com/default.asp?Sec=sup&Sub=wom&Pag=dis&ItemId=60067.
3. Bernstein SJ, Fiske ME, McGlynn EA, Gifford DS. 1998. *Hysterectomy: A Review of the Literature on Indications, Effectivenes, and Risks.* Santa Monica, CA: RAND.
4. Berwick DM. 2003. Disseminating innovations in health care. *JAMA* 289(15):1969-1975.
5. Blue Cross Blue Shield Association. 2004. TEC Assessment Program Vol. 17(7) Full Field Digital Mammography. Accessed March 26, 2004. Web Page. Available at: http://www.bcbs.com/tec.
6. CenterWatch Clinical Trials Listing Service. 2002. Web Page. Available at: http://www.centerwatch.com.
7. Cho MK, Illangasekare S, Weaver MA, Leonard DG, Merz JF. 2003. Effects of patents and licenses on the provision of clinical genetic testing services. *J Mol Diagn* 5(1):3-8.
8. Edmondson AC, Bohmer R, Pisano G. 2001. Disrupted routines: team learning and new technology adoption. *Admin Sci Quart* 46:685-716.

9. Flamm BL. 1997. Once a cesarean, always a controversy. *Obstet Gynecol* 90(2):312-315.

10. Frost & Sullivan. 2003. *U.S. Computer Aided Detection (CAD) Markets—An Analysis of an Emerging Market.* MC897194. New York: Frost & Sullivan.

11. Gad S, Scheuner MT, Pages-Berhouet S, Caux-Moncoutier V, Bensimon A, Aurias A, Pinto M, Stoppa-Lyonnet D. 2001. Identification of a large rearrangement of the BRCA1 gene using colour bar code on combed DNA in an American breast/ovarian cancer family previously studied by direct sequencing. *J Med Genet* 38(6):388-392.

12. Leonard-Barton DA. 1995. *Wellsprings of Knowledge: Building and Sustaining the Sources of Innovation.* Boston, MA: Harvard Business School Press.

13. Lewin Group. 2001. *Outlook for Medical Technology: Will Patients Get the Care They Need?* Falls Church, VA: Lewin Group.

14. Maanen JV, Barley S, Frost P, Moore L, Louis M, Lundberg C, Martin J. 1985. *Organizational Culture.* Beverly Hills, CA: Sage. Pp. 31-53.

15. National Cancer Institute. 2001, April 6. High Dose Chemotherapy for Breast Cancer: History. Accessed June 21, 2003. Web Page. Available at: http://www.nci.nih.gov/clinicaltrials/developments/high-dose-chemo-history0501.

16. Palmer K. 2003, January 7. Battle over gene test. *Toronto Star.*

17. Peterson ED, Coombs LP, DeLong ER, Haan CK, Ferguson TB. 2004. Procedural volume as a marker of quality for CABG surgery. *JAMA* 291(2):195-201.

18. Pisano GP, Bohmer RJM, Edmunson AC. 2001. Organizational differences in rates of learning: evidence from the adoption of minimally invasive cardiac surgery. *Manag Sci* 47(6):752-768.

19. Ridley EL. 2003, April 30. Shift to full-field digital units will spur mammography market. Accessed December 20, 2003. Web Page. Available at: http://www.auntminnie.com/default.asp?Sec=sup&Sub=wom&Pag=dis&ItemId=58036.

20. Rogers EM. 1995. *Diffusion of Innovations.* 4th ed. New York: Free Press.

21. Sevilla C, Julian-Reynier C, Eisinger F, Stoppa-Lyonnet D, Bressac-de Paillerets B, Sobol H, Moatti JP. 2003. Impact of gene patents on the cost-effective delivery of care: the case of BRCA1 genetic testing. *Int J Technol Assess Health Care* 19(2):287-300.

22. Shahian DM. 2004. Improving cardiac surgery quality—volume, outcome, process? *JAMA* 291(2):246-248.

23. Sharf BF. 2001. Out of the closet and into the legislature: breast cancer stories. *Health Aff (Millwood)* 20(1):213-218.

24. U.S. General Accounting Office. 1996. *Health Insurance: Coverage of Autologous Bone Marrow Transplantation for Breast Cancer.* Washington, DC: GAO.

25. Walpole IR, Dawkins HJ, Sinden PD, O'Leary PC. 2003. Human gene patents: the possible impacts on genetic services healthcare. *Med J Aust* 179(4):203.

8

Recommendations

The committee's recommendations for strategies to reduce the toll of breast cancer fall into four categories: improve current technology and its application; develop new screening strategies that integrate biology, technology, and risk models; ensure that promising innovative technologies are adequately tested; and improve the implementation and use of new technologies. The committee expects that many of the new detection technologies currently being tested in clinical studies, as well as those in earlier stages of development, will eventually lead to an understanding of the biology and mechanisms of breast cancer and, therefore, will improve all aspects of the continuum from diagnosis to management.

One strategy that should be mentioned, but that is not included in the committee recommendations, would be to increase the use of screening mammography. The committee believes the importance of this should not be overlooked, but the focus of this report is on ways to improve technologies and systems for early detection, rather than ways to improve the utilization of those services. The two are clearly linked, but tackling the problems of service utilization would require another study.

The committee recognizes that they have set a broad and ambitious agenda—one that will require support and cooperation from a spectrum of participants, from Congress and federal agencies and regulatory agencies to physician organizations, the research community, and health care payers and providers. Perhaps most essential will be support from breast cancer and women's health advocacy groups and from women themselves. Without the unwavering support of this vital community, little progress will be

269

possible. Their input must provide the impetus for change, as it has so effectively in the past.

Even with this broad base support, this effort demands strong leadership and coordination. Therefore, for practical reasons, lead responsibility for implementing many of the recommendations is assigned to the National Cancer Institute and to the relevant professional groups, who should, in turn, enlist other groups most able and qualified to assist. Where additional funding or policy changes are required, that responsibility is also designated.

A. IMPROVE CURRENT APPLICATION OF SCREENING MAMMOGRAPHY

Evidence from randomized clinical trials and from community breast cancer screening programs documents the ability of mammographic screening to reduce mortality from breast cancer. However, mammography is not a perfect technology, nor is it always applied perfectly. Wide variations in the quality of mammographic services need to be addressed, as does the serious and growing shortage of qualified mammographers.

The committee identified several key challenges to providing high-quality breast screening services to all women who would benefit: organizing breast screening services to increase their quality and efficiency (Recommendation A1), improving the overall quality of mammography interpretation and encouraging the development and dissemination of adjunct technologies that would further improve mammography (Recommendation A2), and conserving the workforce of breast imagers and support personnel and making optimal use of their skills (Recommendation A3).

A1. **Health care providers and payers should consider adopting elements of successful breast cancer screening programs from other countries. Such programs involve centralized expert interpretation in regionalized programs, outcome analysis, and benchmarking.**

International differences in breast cancer detection patterns and mortality are influenced by the organization of breast cancer screening programs. Comparative studies of screening programs indicate that programs with high rates of abnormal mammograms tend to have low positive predictive value for biopsies. Although these studies cannot determine the underlying causes of this trend, they highlight several characteristics of successful breast cancer screening programs in other countries that are not fully realized in the United States.

Aspects of foreign screening programs can provide models to guide the improvement of domestic programs, including the incorporation of quality assurance measures, the integration of breast cancer screening services with treatment and support, and the organization of regionalized services in which mammograms are read by breast imaging specialists at a central location. In The Netherlands and Sweden, for example, breast cancer screening is performed at outlying facilities, while diagnosis and workup of mammograms occurs at a few dedicated centers. These countries have low rates of false-positive mammograms.

Experience with the Mammography Quality Standards Act (MQSA), which led to nationwide improvements in the technical quality of mammography, demonstrates that a national quality assurance program could be successful in the United States. Evidence indicates that high callback rates cannot be reduced by targeting individual performance, but must be addressed through the establishment of overall standards for program performance and outcomes.

A2. **Breast imagers and technology developers should work in collaboration with health care providers and payers to improve the overall quality of mammographic interpretation by:**

- **Adopting and further developing practices that promote self-improvement of breast imagers, but that do not jeopardize the workforce.**

- **Developing technologies, such as computer-aided detection (CAD), that have the potential to improve quality, and expanding their use once they have been validated.**

The key to improving mammographic interpretation is to reduce known and controllable sources of variability in quality without adding to the burden of an already overextended workforce. Although better training will significantly improve radiologists' performance, merely increasing the amount of mandated training for breast imagers is not likely to improve mammography services. Continuing medical education is required for radiologists in the United States, but course content is not uniformly organized and few programs target recall or cancer detection rates. In the United Kingdom, however, a voluntary self-assessment program is used by more than 90 percent of radiologists who practice mammography.

Benchmarking could include setting ranges for callback rates, sensitivity measures, or predictive values for biopsies and would be adjusted for factors such as case variation that are known to influence such measures.

CAD could also be employed to provide a second reading of mammograms, following interpretation by an experienced radiologist. Although CAD is not necessarily the equivalent of double-reading by two radiologists, it can highlight areas of concern in a mammogram for further interpretation. The addition of CAD is unlikely to improve the accuracy of *all* breast imagers, but it has the potential to raise the performance level of general radiologists to that of breast imaging specialists.

New approaches for quality improvement should be developed in collaboration with the breast imaging community and with experts in human performance, including performance measurement. No technology has proven superior to mammography in its combination of sensitivity and specificity, nor—most importantly—in its ability to reduce breast cancer deaths. Because mammography will continue to play a central role in breast cancer detection for the foreseeable future:

A3. Mammography facilities should enlist specially trained nonphysician personnel to prescreen mammograms for abnormalities or double-read mammomograms to expand the capacity of breast imaging specialists.

The supply of radiologists (and therefore of breast imagers) is unlikely to grow as quickly as demand for their expertise, and many in the breast imaging field contend that the availability of mammography services is undergoing stagnant growth, if not decline. Significant barriers hamper the expansion of training programs for breast imaging and the immigration of well-trained radiologists to the United States.

The judicious use of physician extenders could raise the productivity of the limited number of radiologists who interpret screening mammograms. Evidence suggests that radiological technologists (RTs) can be specially trained to prescreen mammograms for abnormalities[1] or double-read mammograms along with a radiologist. The committee does not suggest that RTs should interpret diagnostic mammograms or that screening mammograms should be interpreted solely by an RT; rather, the RT would expand the capacity of radiologists. Challenges to this proposal include the acceptance of the radiology profession and malpractice coverage.

The MQSA stipulates that mammograms are to be interpreted only by a physician specifically certified in mammography. The Act does not, however, preclude other personnel from examining the mammograms that are *also* interpreted by certified physicians. Although not widely appreciated and rarely practiced, it would in fact be permissible within the provisions of the MQSA to have nonphysician personnel examine mammograms—as long as a certified physician signed the mammogram report indicating that he or she had interpreted it. This suggestion that physician extenders could be enlisted to help read mammograms could thus offer women a more thorough examination than is currently typical of most mammography facilities where mammograms are viewed only by a single breast imager.

Physician extenders could potentially improve the overall accuracy of mammographic interpretation through double-reading, as well as alleviate the burden on the breast imaging physicians by prescreening the mammograms to allow the interpreting physician to spend more time on the more problematic mammograms.

B. INTEGRATE BIOLOGY, TECHNOLOGY, AND RISK MODELS TO DEVELOP NEW SCREENING STRATEGIES FOR BREAST CANCER

The degree of risk for breast cancer varies widely among women. A variety of breast cancer risk factors have been identified, and they continue to be discovered, but it is still not possible to predict who will develop lethal breast cancer, and who will not. This imperfect knowledge informs a spectrum of important medical decisions along the pathway from breast cancer detection to treatment, in some cases involving extreme preventive measures such as bilateral mastectomy.

B1. Researchers and technology developers should focus their efforts on developing tools to identify those women who would benefit most from breast cancer screening. Such tools should be based on individually tailored risk prediction techniques that integrate biologic and other risk factors.

The awareness that women do not have uniform risk for breast cancer suggests the possibility of identifying women who are most likely to benefit from more intensive screening for breast cancer, as well as those who could safely be screened less frequently. Risk-based screening strategies, the committee believes, are essential to improving the early detection of breast cancer. Developing such strategies will require well-designed, large-scale epidemiological studies to gain a better understanding of risk assessment in individuals.

Mammography screening guidelines already take into account two of the most significant breast cancer risk factors: gender and age. A far more comprehensive approach could be obtained through an integration of epidemiologic factors (such as those identified in the widely used Gail model of breast cancer risk prediction), genetic risk factors (of which there is only rudimentary understanding), and the consequences of adverse events such as false-positive and -negative findings. However, until sufficient knowledge and evidence accumulates to enable the individual assessment of breast cancer risk, the committee urges adherence to consensus guidelines for the minimum recommended use of mammography screening.

In addition to research needed to refine and expand knowledge of risk factors for breast cancer, mathematical models must be developed that can reliably integrate the spectrum of risk factors and predict their collective influence. Ultimately, mathematical models will relate genetic predictors, biological expression, natural course of disease, and responses to treatment. Such models will permit researchers to:

- Elucidate the natural course of disease progression

- Identify disease subgroups with distinctive risk profiles and treatment susceptibilities.

- Identify aspects of the models where further research and data collection are needed.

- Provide guidance to technology developers as to what types of technologies will be most useful, including the performance characteristics that are required for them to be useful, and the analytic techniques that would be most appropriate for evaluation.

B2. Technology innovators, including basic scientists, should work with clinicians, health systems experts, and epidemiologists from the earliest stages of development in order to increase the likelihood of creating clinically useful tools for the early detection of breast cancer.

Fulfilling the immense potential of molecular medicine for breast and other cancers will require collaboration between molecular biologists and scientists from a broad spectrum of disciplines. It will fall to epidemiologists and biostatisticians to guide the rational design of biologically based cancer diagnostics, to establish their significance and reproducibility, and, in the case of clinical epidemiologists, to adapt them for routine clinical use.[2] Once these new biologically based detection and diagnostic tools have been developed, they must be tested for safety and effectiveness beyond the research setting in multicenter clinical trials. Finally, these tools will not be used in isolation, but will become part of an arsenal of tools—each with distinctive capacities and caveats. Developing evidence-based systems for integrating this new technology will require attention at all levels of our health care system—physicians, payers, and purchasers (patients).

The research engine that drives technology advances is well fueled, but the validation of those advances is another matter. Although basic research enables the development of early stage technologies, different strategies are needed to identify which technologies are truly feasible and add clinical value by improving health or the delivery of health care services. Large-scale well-designed multicenter clinical trials provide the most definitive answers about the clinical value of new technologies.

The theme of reengineering the clinical research enterprise is particularly relevant to what the committee believes is especially needed to promote the development of more effective approaches to the early detection of breast cancer. This theme is further subdivided into three initiatives—translational research, clinical workforce training, and enhancement of clinical research networks—all of which address the committee's conclusion that basic research should be integrated with technology development and assessment.

Scientists have become increasingly aware that the bench-to-bedside approach to translational research is really a two-way street. Not only do basic scientists provide clinicians with new tools to examine patients, but clinical researchers also make novel observations about the nature and progression of disease that can stimulate basic investigations.

There is no argument that the development of new tools and strategies for breast cancer detection is a multidisciplinary endeavor. But the truth is that research tends to be herded into disciplinary silos, not because researchers do not appreciate the value of multidisciplinary work, but because the reward systems favor this tendency in so many ways. The specialized languages and standards of different research traditions, the composition of grant review committees, and the organization of promotion and tenure within research institutions all promote disciplinary specialization. The result is that few molecular biologists—those who might be developing genomic profiles of breast cancer—understand the methodology necessary to test the validity of a new screening test. Conversely, few epidemiologists—those who might evaluate breast cancer risk factors—appreciate the uncertainties inherent in gene expression analysis. Likewise, few of the physicists or engineers who might develop advanced imaging technology understand the extent and design of clinical studies that are needed to test the technologies, or in some cases, what types of technologies would be most useful in breast cancer detection.

At every disciplinary juncture, there are pioneers who cross the divide. Nearly every report like this one calls for more multidisciplinary research and development. But this is easier said than done. This committee, like so many others before it, was impressed by how often early stage developers fail to engage the appropriate range of expertise in their endeavors.

B3.   Research funders, including the National Cancer Institute and private foundations, should develop tools that facilitate communication regarding breast cancer risk to the public and to health care providers.

The likelihood that a woman will adhere to screening recommendations depends, in part, on her perceived risk of developing breast cancer. Unfortunately, women's perception of their risk of getting breast cancer or dying from it is often distorted. Most women also misunderstand or overestimate the benefits of mammography. Thus, for example, participation in screening programs tends to decline with age, despite women's rising risk of developing breast cancer. Women who develop breast cancer often have distorted perceptions about prognosis; for example, they may not understand that a diagnosis of ductal carcinoma in situ is far less grave than a diagnosis of invasive breast cancer.

If women are to make well-informed decisions regarding breast cancer detection, diagnosis, and treatment, they need a firm understanding of the risks they face. Not only are better methods needed to assess a woman's risk of breast cancer, but more effective means are needed to communicate those risks.

C. IMPROVE THE ENVIRONMENT FOR RESEARCH AND DEVELOPMENT OF NEW TECHNOLOGIES FOR BREAST CANCER DETECTION

C1. The National Institutes of Health, Agency for Healthcare Research and Quality, and Centers for Medicaid and Medicare Services should collaborate to establish programs and centers (which may be virtual) that bring together expertise and funding to enable a more comprehensive approach to technology assessment and adoption.

- These efforts should involve collaboration with technology developers, not-for-profit organizations (including professional societies), advocacy groups, private health care payers, and provider organizations.

- Experimentation with innovative organizational structures for the centers should be encouraged.

- Adoption of standards for collecting and sharing data should be a priority.

The National Institutes of Health is exploring development of regional translational research centers. These centers would provide sophisticated advice and resources to better enable scientists to master the many steps involved in bringing a new product from the bench to clinical use.

Despite the promise of technological advances that might significantly impact breast cancer mortality, the committee is concerned that limited resources and outdated infrastructure will increasingly limit the pace of progress. Thus, to ensure that the promise of these advances is fulfilled, the committee believes that both research and the clinical infrastructure must be adapted in order to overcome existing barriers to research and the adoption of effective technologies.

C2. Professional societies should work together with women's health organizations to identify barriers to participation in studies (especially those that require provision of biologic specimens) and ways in which those barriers might be overcome.

- A public education campaign should be undertaken to inform the public, particularly underrepresented groups, of the merit of participation in research studies that require the involvement of healthy volunteers and the donation of biologic specimens for genetic analysis.

- Advocacy groups and women's health organizations should participate in design and execution of public education about clinical trials. This could be a collaborative effort, and might include the National Cancer Institute and the American Cancer Society.

- The Department of Health and Human Services should join with private entities in monitoring the effect of the Health Insurance Portability and Accountability Act Privacy Rule on the pace of research progress.

Of particular concern are the barriers to public participation in clinical trials that have been raised as the unintended consequences of privacy concerns and other initiatives. Because the development of better and evidence-based methods for the early detection of breast cancer will require large-scale clinical trials and those trials depend on public participation, the committee recommends seeking ways to overcome barriers to public participation. The same barriers threaten to impede essential epidemiological research because the identification of markers depends on the availability of blood and other biologic specimens from healthy volunteers.

Another roadblock to improving the current situation is the tendency of many women to either over- or underestimate their own breast cancer risk, which can affect their decision about whether to participate in a screening program.

D. IMPROVE THE IMPLEMENTATION AND USE
OF NEW TECHNOLOGIES

D1. Breast cancer research funders, such as the National Institutes of Health, Department of Defense, and private foundations, should support research on screening and detection technologies that encompasses each aspect of technology adoption from deployment to application, and should include monitoring of use in practice.

- This will involve identification of optimal combinations and sequencing of breast cancer detection technologies.

- Research funders and private foundations should model and assess changes in practice and organization change that would optimize the benefit of new technology (including risk assessment).

D2. The National Institutes of Health, the Agency for Healthcare Research and Quality, and other public and private research sponsors should collaborate with health systems, providers, and payers to support research that would monitor clinical use of technologies to identify potential failures, as well as opportunities for improvement, with particular attention to:

- How appropriately the technologies are being utilized,

- Their impact on clinical decision making, and

- Their impact on health outcomes.

REFERENCES

1. Casey B. 2003, March 11. Breast Center Enlists Radiographers for First Look at Mammograms. Accessed February 19, 2004. Web Page. Available at: http://www.auntminnie.com/default.asp?Sec=sup&Sub=wom&Pag=dis&ItemId=57614&stm=radiographers.
2. Ransohoff DF. 2002. Challenges and opportunities in evaluating diagnostic tests. *J Clin Epidemiol* 55(12):1178-1182.

Appendix A

Breast Cancer Technology Overview

Many new technologies are being developed for the detection and diagnosis of breast cancer, and many of them have been described as "breakthrough" technologies in the media. For a public eager for definitive results, the summary below will be disappointing. Of the 23 technologies described below, only 10 have been approved by the Food and Drug Administration (FDA). And only 3 (screen-film mammography, digital mammography, and computer-aided detection [CAD]) have been approved for use in breast screening. Other technologies are approved only as adjuncts to mammography or for other uses. For example, positron emission tomography (PET) is approved for monitoring response to treatment for breast cancer, but not for screening or diagnosis. As discussed in Chapter 6, FDA approval does not certify that a particular technology improves health outcomes, only that it is safe and meets the manufacturer's claims for efficacy. As with magnetic resonance imaging (MRI), claims made by groups other than the manufacturer are beyond the purview of FDA.

Over time and with the results of well-designed studies, some of the technologies listed below may earn the title of "breakthrough technology," but without evidence they remain "promising." It is not possible to anticipate which of the many promising technologies will realize their expected potation and which will not.

ANATOMICAL TECHNOLOGIES

Mammography and Its Improvements

Technology	Description	Developmental Stage	First FDA Approval
Screen-Film Mammography	X-rays are sent through the breast tissue. Denser tissue, which is often associated with cancer, absorbs the x-rays and appears as a white region on the film.	Routine clinical use for screening	1969
Computer Aided Detection	Uses computer algorithms to highlight suspicious areas on mammograms for the radiologist to review.	Clinical use for screening	1998
Digital Mammography	Similar to screen-film mammography except x-rays are recorded in digital format instead of on x-ray film.	Clinical use for screening	2000
Tomosynthesis	A computer assembles information from mammograms taken at several different angles to provide high-resolution cross-sections and three-dimensional images.	Experimental use (clinical prototype)	—
Diffraction Enhanced Imaging	A synchrotron-based x-ray machine. Integrates two images, one image based on x-ray absorption (e.g., conventional image from an x-ray) and the other based on refraction.	Experimental use	—

Screen-Film Mammography (Conventional X-Ray Mammography)

The current standard of care for breast cancer screening is x-ray mammography for women over the age of 40. A technician that compresses the breast and takes pictures from different angles, creating a set of images of each breast, usually performs this technique. In the set of images, called a mammogram, breast tissue appears white and opaque, while fatty tissue appears darker and translucent. X-rays travel unimpeded through soft tissues; however, cancerous tissue absorbs x-rays and can show up on the film as white areas. In a screening mammogram, the breast is x-rayed from center to side.

However, a diagnostic mammogram focuses in on a particular lump or area of abnormal tissue. This examination usually takes about 30 minutes. Yearly screening mammography results in sensitivity (proportion tests that correctly indicate a woman has cancer) ranging from 71 to 96 percent and specificity (proportion of tests that correctly indicate that a woman does not have cancer) ranging from 94 to 97 percent.[18] However, several factors influence the correct detection of breast cancer, such as age, breast density, hormone replacement therapy, image quality, and experience of the radiologist.[18]

Computer Aided Detection (CAD)

CAD involves the use of computers to identify suspicious areas on a mammogram after the radiologist's initial review of the mammogram. CAD double-checks the work of the radiologist to help avoid possible oversights. In 1998, the FDA approved the first CAD system, ImageChecker™ (R2 Technology, Inc., Los Altos, CA). This device can either scan a mammographic film with a laser beam and convert it into a digital image, or obtain images directly from a digital mammography system. The radiologist can see if any of the highlighted areas were missed on the initial review and require further evaluation.

Initial studies show CAD technology may improve the accuracy of screening mammography by reducing the number of missed cancers.[3,13] A 2004 study reported that the use of CAD was not associated with statistically significant changes in recall or breast cancer detection rates.[15] However, all radiologists in that study were considered breast imaging specialists, and the results of this study should not be extrapolated to use by community radiologists who vary widely in their proficiency.[11] The greatest clinical value of CAD probably does not lie in its ability to raise the performance level of *all* breast imagers, but rather in its potential to bring the performance level of general radiologists to that of breast imaging specialists.[35]

Digital Mammography

Digital mammography, also known as full-field digital mammography (FFDM), is a technique for recording x-ray images in digital format instead of on x-ray film. The images are displayed on a computer monitor and can be adjusted before they are printed on film. Images can be lightened, darkened, and magnified to zoom in on an area of interest. The first digital mammography system, General Electric Medical Systems' Senographe 2000D, received FDA approval in 2000. From the patient's perspective, the procedure for a mammogram with a digital system is the same as for conventional mammography. However, the utility of the digital images may provide advantages over conventional mammography. For example, FFDM images can be stored and retrieved electronically, making remote consultations with other mammography specialists easier and lost mammogram films less likely. Despite the benefits of a digital medium, studies have not yet shown that digital mammography is more effective in finding cancer than conventional mammography. Digital mammography systems offer better contrast and lower spatial resolution at a lower radiation dose than traditional screen film mammography.[20] However, the relative diagnostic accuracy of digital mammography as compared to traditional mammography has not yet been determined. The results of the Digital Mammographic Imaging Screening Trial, a large trial designed to determine if digital mammography provides any benefit in breast cancer detection over screen-film mammography, are currently being analyzed, and initial results should be available in 2005.

Digital Tomosynthesis Mammography

Digital tomosynthesis mammography, another modification of x-ray mammography, involves moving the x-ray machinery in an arc around the breast while taking several low-dose images (typically 7-12) at the same overall dose as conventional two-view mammography. The procedure reduces the possibility that overlapping structures from a specific angle will obscure a cancer, potentially making abnormalities more visible.[38] With the advent of digital mammography, tomosynthesis to produce a three-dimensional image of the breast tissue became possible. A computer is used to assemble the information to provide high-resolution cross-sectional and three-dimensional images that can be reviewed by the radiologist at a computer workstation.

This technique may improve the specificity of mammography with improved lesion margin visibility and may improve early breast cancer detection, especially in women with radiographically dense breasts, by avoiding the limitation of standard mammography, which attempts to project the three-dimensional anatomical information of the breast into a two-dimensional image.[38] These three-dimensional image views can bring structures into relief, and the image can be rotated in space for more careful examination. Dr. Daniel Kopans, at Massachusetts General Hospital, and his colleagues are currently conducting clinical trials using a prototype machine derived from the commercially available Senographe 2000D digital mammography system.[a] Another system, produced by Hologic, Inc., is expected to be available for clinical testing late in 2004.

Currently, the most significant barrier to the adoption of the tomographic technology is the amount of time that it takes to reconstruct the image. Multiple images are necessary to reconstruct an adequate three-dimensional image of the breast tissue. Approximately 8 to 10 images are required to maximize contrast and detail. The current computer processing time of two hours will have to be shortened to several minutes to make use of this system feasible in a clinical setting.[53]

Diffraction Enhanced Imaging

Diffraction enhanced imaging (DEI), a modification of the current practice of mammography in very early stages of development, may produce better images of breast tissue.[42] Increased radiographic contrast could make this type of mammography more effective in revealing tumors.[16] In DEI, a silicon crystal is placed between the object being studied and the x-ray film or digital detector where the image is recorded. The crystal diffracts a particular wavelength of x-ray producing two images. One image is based on x-ray absorption (conventional image from an x-ray) and the other image is based on refraction. Refraction is a process where light, including x-rays, deviates in angle slightly because of differences in the density of the material it passes through.[4] Thus, the integration of these two images may provide more detail in the tissue.

Researchers used a synchrotron housed at Brookhaven National Laboratory to image seven breast cancer tissue specimens using the DEI technique. The same seven specimens were imaged using conventional x-ray methods at the University of North Carolina at Chapel Hill. Early results indicated that tumor visibility might be superior with DEI in six of the seven specimens.[42] Despite increased imaging capabilities, the large task of developing a prototype that can be used in the clinic still remains before clinical investigation can begin. In addition, training of radiologists to interpret the unique image characteristics may not be effective. For example, it will have to be demonstrated that interpretation will not be negatively affected by specific image features, such as microcalcifications. However, DEI is at a much earlier stage of development than the other technologies described in this overview and is not ready for clinical testing.

---

[a]Mass Gen news release. Dec 10, 2002. http://www.massgeneral.org/news/releases/121002tomosnythesis.htm.

ANATOMICAL TECHNOLOGIES

Approaches Based on Physical Properties

Technology	Description	Developmental Stage	First FDA Approval
Sonography	Noninvasive modality that uses a handheld probe to reflect sound waves, not radiation, off of breast tissues, constructing an image of the breast based upon the physical properties (e.g., reflection of sound waves) of the underlying anatomy. This technique is FDA approved for adjunctive use in the clinic to clarify abnormalities initially detected by screening mammography.	Routine adjunctive clinical use for diagnosis	1977
Electronic Palpation	Electronic version of the clinical breast exam performed by a physician that measures the resistance of breast tissue, providing a quantitative characterization of breast "lumps."	Experimental use (clinical prototype)	—
Elastography	Measures stiffness of breast tissue in response to a mechanical stimulus, developing a map of the mechanical properties of the tissue; thus, assisting the identification of abnormal tissue (e.g., hardened lesions).	Experimental use	—

Technology	Description	Developmental Stage	First FDA Approval
Infrared Thermography	Heat radiating from breast tissue can be imaged using infrared sensors. Regions of increased surface temperature are often associated with increased vascular activity supplying tumors with sufficient nutrients for sustained growth.	Rare adjunctive clinical use	1982
Thermo-rhythmometry	Uses several heat sensing probes to measure the surface temperature of the breast tissue over a 24-hour period to identify suspicious areas of the breast.	Experimental use (clinical prototype)	—

Sonography (Ultrasound)

Sonography, also known as ultrasound, is an imaging technique in which high-frequency sound waves are reflected from tissues and internal organs. Their echoes produce a picture called a sonogram based upon the properties of the tissue. Ultrasound can be used as an adjunct to mammography to evaluate suspicious areas on a mammogram, increasing the accuracy of the combined technologies.[17] It can be of particular use in distinguishing between solid tumors and fluid-filled cysts because differences in reflective characteristics between the tissues are discernable on the sonograph.

Ultrasound does not use any radiation and is usually pain-free. The exam may take between 15 and 30 minutes to complete depending on how difficult it is for the operator to find the breast abnormalities being examined, such as a lesion deep within the breast. Ultrasound is not currently used for routine breast cancer screening because it does not consistently detect certain early signs of cancer such as microcalcifications, which are deposits of calcium in the breast that cannot be felt but can be seen on a conventional mammogram, and are the most common indicator of ductal carcinoma in situ (DCIS). However, the technique is quite useful in conducting image-guided biopsy.[26,33] Many techniques are being developed to enhance the capability of ultrasound to detect cancer single-handedly; however, they are still under clinical investigation and will require further study to determine their utility.[49]

Electronic Palpation

Sensors that record the resistance of tissues to applied pressure can be used to develop density maps of the breast that can be used to detect lumps in the breast. This technique is essentially an electronic version of the manual clinical breast exam, in which the physician applies pressure in a circular pattern over the breast to detect lumps, possibly indicating cancer. The electronic palpation device provides quantitative measurement of the hardness and size of lesions, opposed to the subjective manual breast exam. Several companies have developed palpation devices and received FDA approval. This technique is promising because it does not use radiation or require uncomfortable breast compression, yet its accuracy will have to be proven in clinical trials for widespread clinical adoption. In addition, it is relatively inexpensive.

Elastography

Mapping the mechanical properties (such as stiffness or elasticity) of breast tissue can identify abnormal tissue properties that are often associated with cancer growth.[30] This method of cancer detection is known as elastography. Elastography couples mechanical stimulus (vibrations) with imaging modalities, such as ultrasound or magnetic resonance. Thus, imaging the behavior of the breast tissue in response to mechanical vibrations can discover abnormalities in the elasticity of the breast tissue (e.g., hard tumors) that may not be detected by mammography or are too deep in the tissue to be palpated. Such lesions hidden deep within breasts may not be palpable until they are quite large and difficult to treat.[37] Magnetic resonance elastographic imaging of biopsy-proven breast tumors has demonstrated stiffness two to three times greater than the surrounding fibrous tissue.[46,50] Although the proof of concept for this technology has been established, extensive clinical trials will be required to determine whether application in the clinic will be possible.

Infrared Thermography (Digital Infrared Imaging)

Infrared thermography is based on the principle that chemical and blood vessel activity in both precancerous tissue and the areas surrounding a developing breast cancer is often higher than in the normal breast. Precancerous and cancerous masses have high metabolic rates, and they need an abundant supply of nutrients to grow. In order to do this they increase circulation to their cells by sending out chemical signals to keep existing blood vessels open, recruit dormant vessels, and create new ones (neoangiogenesis).[b] The increased vascular activity often results in an increase in surface temperatures of the breast near the location of tumor, which can be imaged through thermographic devices. In 1982, the FDA approved the first breast thermography device as an adjunctive breast cancer screening procedure.[c] Since then, several devices have been approved under the FDA's 510(k) equivalent device review. However, to date, no thermographic device has gained clinical acceptance. Definitive clinical trials of this technology have never been conducted to determine its effectiveness in detecting breast cancer.

Thermorhythmometry

Although thermorhythmometry relies upon similar principles as infrared thermography to help identify breast cancer, the technique uses a different approach. Instead of imaging the breast, probes are placed on the breast that monitor the skin temperature over a 24-hour period (known as a circadian rhythm) to identify variances which may correspond to neoangiogenesis and cancer.[24,44] This approach aims to identify abnormalities that could be missed with tests that only examine the breast for a brief period of time, potentially missing warning signs that are only evident by analyzing the daily temperature cycles of patients.[52]

---

[b]International Academy of Clinical Thermography What is Breast Thermography. http://www.iact-org.org/patients/breastthermography/what-is-breast-therm.html [Accessed April 29, 2003].

[c]A Review of Breast Thermography. International Academy of Clinical Thermography. http://www.iact-org.org/articles/articles-review-btherm.html [Accessed April 29, 2003].

ANATOMICAL TECHNOLOGIES

Approaches Based on Electrical Properties

Technology	Description	Developmental Stage	First FDA Approval
Electrical Potential Measurement	Electrodes placed on the breast measure the small amount of natural electric charge at various locations on the breast. The abnormal growth of cancer cells may produce imbalances in the ionic gradients of cells that can theoretically be detected by the electrodes.	Experimental use (clinical prototype)	—
Electrical Impedance Scanning	Uses the electrical conducting properties of the breast tissue to identify tumors. A small amount of current is introduced into the body using a handheld probe; the breast tissue is then imaged using a technician-held device.	Approved for clinical use No units sold in the United States	1999
Microwave Imaging	Microwave pulses are used to image the conductivity of the breast. Since the water content of tissue largely determines the conductivity, researchers may be able to discriminate between the low water content of healthy cells and high water content in tumors to detect malignant breast tissue.	Experimental use (clinical prototype)	—

Electrical Potential Measurement

This technology involves use of electrodes applied to the skin to obtain measurements of electrical potential (differences in electric charge) at various locations on the breast. The difference in electric charge is measured in areas of suspicious findings in comparison with electrodes placed elsewhere on the chest. The abnormal growth of cancer cells may result in an ionic gradient with potassium moving out of the cells and sodium moving into cells. The difference in ionic concentration creates an electrical potential that theoretically could be measured by electrodes placed on the breasts.[d] This approach is proposed for examination of a suspicious finding based on either physical examination or breast imaging. A technician can perform this noninvasive procedure in less than 20 minutes and test results are available for radiologist interpretation within five minutes after the procedure. This technology is currently under clinical investigation to gather data to submit to the FDA. However, initial studies report a sensitivity of 90 to 95 percent and a specificity of 40 to 65 percent for palpable lesions.[8] Additional studies will have to be conducted to verify the detection capability of this device for broad application/adoption.

Electrical Impedance Scanning

Different tissues have different levels of electrical impedance (resistance to conducting electricity). Electrical impedance is lower in cancerous breast tissue than normal breast tissue; therefore, electrical impedance scanning (EIS) devices can be used along with conventional mammography to help detect breast cancer. The electrical impedance scanning device consists of a hand-held scanning probe and a computer screen that displays two-dimensional images of the breast. The device does not emit radiation; rather, a very small amount of electric current, similar to a small battery, is transmitted into the body. The current travels through the breast, where it is measured by the scanning probe. Areas of low impedance, which may correspond to cancerous tumors, show up as bright white spots on a computer screen. The scanner sends the image directly to a computer, allowing the radiologist to move the probe around the breast to get the best view of the area being examined. The device is intended to reduce the number of biopsies needed to determine whether a mass is cancerous. The FDA approved an EIS device called the T-Scan 2000, in 1999, as an adjunct to mammography. However, none of the devices have been sold in the United States to date.[36,e] The scanner is not approved by the FDA as a screening device for

---

[d]See www.biofield.com [Accessed May 9, 2003].
[e]Twenty-five T-Scan units have units been sold internationally.

breast cancer, and is recommended to be used when mammography or other findings clearly indicate the need for a biopsy.

In a separate study comparing EIS to sestimibi scans, the T-scan had 72.2 percent sensitivity and 67 percent specificity in detecting breast cancer and sestamibi had 88.9 percent sensitivity. The T-scan detected one more breast cancer than sestamibi, at the expense of 27 additional false-positive results.[34]

Based on his studies of electrical impedance spectroscopy (the technology on which T-Scan is based), Keith Paulsen concluded that more work needs to be done with this technology. The placement of the electrodes on the breast, which determine the signal, depends on the operator and the impact of this on the test accuracy needs to be tested further. The technique is generally a low resolution, at best detecting tumors that are 1 cm or larger (about pea-sized). Because the technique loses sensitivity as the distance from the electrode increases, lesions deep in the breast will be harder to detect than those close to the skin surface. Finally, although the technique is potentially very high contrast, this remains somewhat controversial. Furthermore, this technology has not been evaluated by any large clinical trials and its lack of widespread acceptance might be due to the extraordinarily high reliability and accuracy of biopsy.

Microwave Imaging

Mapping the differences in the electrical properties can be accomplished by using low-energy electromagnetic waves, known as microwaves. Due to higher water content in tumors as compared with healthy tissue, differences in the electrical-conducting properties of breast tissue can be analyzed. Two to three times the amount of electrical conductivity is observed through microwave imaging of cancerous breast tissue when contrasted with surrounding normal tissue.[5,23,27,48]

While researchers are still years away from clinical trials, they have studied the technique using breast phantoms (test objects that simulate the radiographic characteristics of normal and cancerous breast tissue) and excised breast samples. Researchers were able to identify tumors as small as 6 mm in diameter (comparable to x-ray mammography for masses). But microcalcifications, which are often signs of early breast cancer, can be found much smaller than 6 mm with mammography.

However, breast cancers have the potential to show more contrast at microwave frequencies than at the x-ray frequencies used for mammograms.[12] Also, the sometimes painful breast compression associated with x-ray mammography is not required for the conformal microwave imaging. Women can recline comfortably on their backs during the procedure. Microwaves imaging also avoids the use of radiation (see Harms of Mammography in Chapter 2).

ANATOMICAL TECHNOLOGIES

Approaches Based on Optical Properties

Technology	Description	Developmental Stage	First FDA Approval
Optical	Infrared light is passed through the breast tissue identifying areas of high vascular activity that have been shown to correlate with the rapid growth of tumors.	Experimental use (clinical prototype)	—
Computed Laser Mammography	A modification of conventional optical imaging in which harmless optical lasers penetrate the three-dimensional surface of the breast to identify areas of high vascular activity. Thus, along with the use of a computer program, a three-dimensional image of the breast and the location of possible abnormalities is created.	Experimental use (clinical prototype)	—

Optical Imaging

Optical imaging is a method by which near-infrared light is used to image the hemoglobin content of tissue, identifying possible malignancies. Imaging the absorption of near-infrared light in breast tissue can quantify the hemoglobin content and volume of blood perfusing the tissue, providing contrast between the dense vasculature often associated with cancer and healthy tissue.[21] Since most tumors require an abundance of nutrients delivered through the vasculature of the capillary bed for accelerated growth, the high oxygen content and blood volume has been demonstrated to correlate with malignancy.[21,39] Furthermore, using a technique called diffuse optical tomography, three-dimensional visualizations can be constructed to improve visualization of abnormalities in the tissue.[21,22,39] Only mild breast compression is required for this technique and the breast tissue is not exposed to radiation. This method is favored for its speed, low cost, safety, and noninvasiveness; however, optical imaging has not been validated in large clinical trials and problems of low image resolution and difficulties with image reconstruction will have to be overcome.[21,39] Several companies are in the late stages of development of this technology and are conducting clinical trials for submission to the FDA to obtain marketing approval. Despite the progress made in developing optical imaging, clinical validation of the technology has not occurred to date.

Computed Tomography Laser Mammography

Computed tomography laser mammography (CTLM) visualizes the blood supply of tumors, without the use of x-rays and without breast compression. As with optical imaging, increased blood supply indicates the presence of a tumor, based upon the assumption that the rapid growth of tumor must be supported by increased vascularization. Lasers are used to illuminate the breast in 4-mm increments scanning the breast tissue from the chest wall to the nipple. Algorithms are then used to create three-dimensional cross-sectional images of the breast. The technology is designed to be used as an adjunct to mammography for women who have dense breasts and/or whose mammograms are otherwise difficult to interpret. CTLM can potentially provide additional information to radiologists to guide biopsy recommendations.[f] The technology is not yet available because the FDA has not completed its review for approval of this technology. Research began in November of 1999 at the University of Virginia, yet as of March 2004, no published studies of CTLM indicate the accuracy of detecting breast cancer or the size of the lesions that can be detected.[g]

---

[f]Imaging Diagnostic Systems Press Release. http://www.imds.com/cgi-bin/newspro/viewnews.cgi?newsid1051596000,77709.

[g]UVa Tests New Laser for Breast Imaging. http://www.imds.com/media/harvey_link1.shtml [Accessed March 9, 2004].

ANATOMICAL TECHNOLOGIES

Approaches Based on Magnetic Resonance Properties

Technology	Description	Developmental Stage	First FDA Approval
Magnetic Resonance Imaging	Type of anatomical imaging that involves using an RF pulse-response in a very strong uniform magnetic field. Various tissue types exhibit unique resonance characteristics which can be displayed with differing contrast properties and allow breast lesions to be identified.	Adjunctive clinical use along with mammography	1985

Magnetic Resonance Imaging (MRI)

In MRI, a powerful magnet linked to a computer creates detailed images of the breast without the use of radiation. Each MRI produces hundreds of images of the breast from side-to-side, top-to-bottom, and front-to-back. A radiologist then interprets the images to identify abnormal regions that may require further investigation. During an MRI of the breast, the patient lies on her stomach on the scanning table. The breast hangs into a depression or hollow in the table, which contains coils that detect the magnetic signal. The table is moved into a tube-like machine that contains a powerful magnet. After an initial series of images has been taken, the patient may be given a contrast agent intravenously to enhance the visibility of tissue characteristics. The contrast agent is not radioactive; and can be used to improve the visibility of a tumor. Additional images can be taken after administering the contrast agent. The entire imaging session takes about one hour.

Breast MRI is not FDA approved for routine breast cancer screening, but clinical trials are being performed to determine if MRI is valuable for screening certain women, such as young women at high risk for breast cancer.[h] MRI cannot always accurately distinguish between cancer and benign (noncancerous) breast conditions. Uses of MRI may include assessment of abnormalities that are unclear on a mammogram, determination of the extent of tumor growth after initial diagnosis, and for evaluation of the effectiveness of treatments. MRI may also be useful in imaging augmented breast tissue, dense breast tissue (often found in younger women), and viewing breast abnormalities that can be felt but are not visible with conventional mammography or ultrasound.[43] While contrast-enhanced MRI is statistically significantly more accurate than mammography for detecting multicentric DCIS, it was significantly less specific than mammography for detecting associated invasive disease in one published series.[19] MRI is expensive, about 10 times the cost of conventional mammography and, because it will generate more false-positive results, it generates added costs of additional biopsies and/or other diagnostic follow-up. Ultimately more research on the proper application of MRI is needed. The technique may prove useful for special cases, such as screening women with very high risk of developing breast cancer, examining breast implant integrity, and for determining the extent of disease in women with cancer.[43]

---

[h]American College of Radiology Imaging Network trial 6667. MRI Evaluation of the Contralateral Breast in Women with a Recent Diagnosis of Breast Cancer.

BIOLOGICAL TECHNOLOGIES

Technology	Description	Developmental Stage	First FDA Approval
Ductal Lavage	Involves the collection of cells for microscopic examination by washing the breast ducts with a saline solution. The sample is then analyzed by a pathologist to identify abnormalities.	Limited clinical use	1999
Scinti-mammography (99m Tc-sestimibi)	A harmless radioactive tracer is administered to the patient, which may accumulate differently in cancerous and noncancerous tissue. This accumulation of the tracer can then be imaged using a gamma camera to identify breast lesions.	Adjunctive clinical use along with mammography, but rarely used	1999
FDG-PET	Radioactive compounds are injected into the blood stream and as they are metabolized, the biochemical activity of the tissue can be imaged. Thus, more active tissues may indicate suspicious areas.	Clinical use for monitoring treatment, but not for screening or diagnosis	1976*
Magnetic Resonance Spectroscopy	Type of biological imaging that analyzes the specific molecular components of a tissue by identifying alterations in the biochemistry of the tissue and identifying intrinsic properties of breast cancer.	Experimental use	—

Technology	Description	Developmental Stage	First FDA Approval
Gene Profiling	Characterizes tissue samples based upon the activity of various genes that play a role in developing and invasive breast cancer. The relative activity of thousands of genes on a microarray (glass slide with many spots, each individually representing one gene) is analyzed by computer algorithms to predict the behavior of the tissue.	Experimental use	Not FDA regulated
Genetic Testing	This technique uses a blood test to identify genetic mutations that have been associated with an increased risk of developing breast cancer. To date, the only clinically validated genes have been BRCA1 and BRCA2.	Clinical use for risk assessment	Not FDA regulated
Serum Proteomic Profiling	The relative amounts of various proteins in the blood are measured by mass spectrometry. Computer algorithims are then used to identify patterns that may be indicative of the possible presence of cancer. However, this technique will only indicate the presence of cancer. Another modality will have to be used to image the tissue and determine the locations of the cancer.	Experimental use	—

*PET technology was originally approved in 1976; however, in 2000 the FDA issued a notice that FDG-PET was safe and effective for imaging cancer in patients with a known diagnosis of cancer.

Ductal Lavage

Ductal lavage is a technique for collecting samples of cells from breast ducts for analysis under a microscope. A saline (salt water) solution is introduced into a milk duct through a catheter (a thin, flexible, tube for adding or withdrawing fluids from a cavity) that is inserted into the opening of the duct on the surface of the nipple. The saline solution, which contains cells from the duct, is then withdrawn through the catheter. The breast cells that are washed out are sent to the pathology laboratory for analysis. This technique may be able to identify breast duct cells that have certain abnormal characteristics which may cause them to later develop into cancer. Although the ductal lavage device is approved by the FDA, it is still limited mainly to clinical trials to determine the sensitivity, specificity, and appropriate application in clinical use.[9,10] As of this writing, no federal public health agencies or leading professional medical organizations have recommended ductal lavage as a screening test for women at high risk for breast cancer. Recently published evidence-based guidelines from the American Cancer Society concluded that there are currently insufficient data to recommend the use of ductal lavage either as an independent screening modality or in combination with screening mammography.[47]

Scintimammography

Scintimammography involves injecting a radioactive tracer into the patient, which accumulates differently in cancerous and noncancerous tissues, to help physicians determine the presence of cancer. Currently, the technitium-99m sestamibi compound is the only radioactive tracer approved by the FDA for breast imaging.

This technique may be useful in patients who have dense breast tissue that makes their mammograms difficult to interpret or in patients with palpable abnormalities (i.e., those able to be physically felt) but whose mammograms do not reveal any abnormalities.[17,28,32] Scintimammography may be used to determine whether a patient has a suspicious breast abnormality that would require a biopsy to confirm the presence of breast cancer. The test requires 45 minutes to perform and costs approximately $150 per exam.[6] Nuclear medicine involves the use of radiation, but the dose is very low and presents minimal risk to patients. The half-life of the compound is six hours; thus, most of the compound leaves the body within a day.

To perform the exam, a radioactive tracer (Tc-99m sestamibi) is injected in the patient's arm opposite of the breast being studied. The radioactive tracer travels throughout the body, including the breast under examination, and accumulates in tissue present. Approximately five minutes after the injection, a gamma camera (device that takes pictures of radioactive distribution) is used to capture images of the breast from several angles. Dense breast tissue, common in young women, can obscure x-ray mammograms.[31] Hence, scintimammography, which is less affected by breast density, may have potential as an adjunct to diagnostic mammography by helping to characterize larger lesions.[17,32]

Positron Emission Tomography (PET)

PET is a method by which cellular and molecular events can be evaluated. Radiolabeled molecular probes (radioactive tracers) injected into the blood stream are used to map out the underlying biochemistry.[14] PET scans create live computerized images of chemical changes that take place in tissue. The patient is given an injection of a substance that consists of a sugar attached to a small amount of radioactive material. A common sugar probe used, 2-18F-fluoro-2-deoxy-D-glucose (FDG), is FDA approved and considered safe for administering into the blood stream.

The radioactive sugar is then absorbed at a higher rate by cells with higher metabolism, such as tumors. The radioactivity localized in the tumor acts as a beacon to help radiologists identify suspicious areas. However, clinical use of PET is generally limited to finding metastatic cancer that has traveled from the breast to another location in the body.

After receiving the radioactive drug, the patient lies still for about 45 minutes while the drug circulates throughout the body. The patient then lies on a table, which gradually moves through the PET scanner 6 to 7 times during a 45-minute period to detect the distribution of radiation. A computer translates this information into the images that are interpreted by a radiologist. PET scans are more accurate in detecting larger and more aggressive tumors associated with metastatic cancers than they are in locating tumors that are smaller (less than 8 mm) and less aggressive tumors.[i]

Magnetic Resonance Spectroscopy (MRS)

This spectroscopic technique can measure the metabolism of pathological specimens and identify biochemical changes, which closely correspond with the presence of tumors. For example, breast tissue with a high concentration of choline has been shown to be indicative of invasive breast cancers.[54] Thus, by identifying alterations in the biochemistry of the tissue,

---

[i]National Cancer Institute Fact Sheet. Improving Methods for Breast Cancer Detection and Diagnosis. June 12, 2001. http://cis.nci.nih.gov/fact/5_14.htm [Accessed on April 25, 2003].

MRS is a method of diagnosing breast cancer using biological factors, such as metabolism, that are intrinsic properties of the disease, not possible by imaging the anatomy of the breast. Comparison of the MR spectroscopic technique with the fine-needle aspiration biopsy findings in lymph nodes revealed a sensitivity of 82 percent, specificity of 100 percent, and accuracy of 90 percent.[55]

As with an MRI exam, MRS does not expose the patient to radiation, and takes about 45 minutes to perform. However, this technique is expensive and unproven, and therefore limited to academic medical centers conducting research in this area.

Gene Profiling

Genetic profiling allows for the characterization of a tissue sample based upon the genetic makeup and activity of the sample. For example, tissue samples from an invasive cancer and from a benign cyst will have very different growth characteristics determined by the genetic makeup of the tissue and more importantly the expression of that genetic code (the relative level of gene activity). The relative activity of thousands of genes on a microarray (glass slide with many spots each individually representing one gene) can be analyzed by computer algorithms to predict the behavior of the tissue. A recent study (2002) demonstrated the potential of genetic profiling to predict the clinical outcome of breast cancer.[51] Microarray DNA expression profiles can be used on primary breast tumors to identify a signature expression profile ("poor prognosis signature") of 70 genes strongly predictive of a short interval to distant metastases (<5 years). The "poor prognosis signature" consists of genes regulating cell cycle, invasion, metastasis, and angiogenesis. The gene expression profile outperformed all currently used clinical parameters in predicting outcome of disease, such as lymph node status and histological grade. A large unselected "cohort" of breast cancer patients may be required to validate the findings and bring this approach closer to the clinic. Eventually this technique may be used to select patients who would benefit from adjuvant therapy and avoid ineffective treatments. This approach may also prove useful in assessing prognosis prior to biopsy, helping to reduce the number of open surgical biopsies of benign tissue.

Genetic Testing

Many cases of hereditary breast cancer are due to mutations in either the BRCA1 or the BRCA2 gene. The BRCA genes are tumor suppressor (control the growth of cells) genes that in their mutated forms become cancer susceptibility genes increasing the risks of developing breast and

TABLE A-1 A Mutation-Positive Result May Have Both Benefits and Problems

BENEFITS	PROBLEMS
Resolve uncertainty	Increased fear, anxiety, depression, or guilt
Lead to early diagnosis through increased screening	Make medical decisions more pressing
Identify relatives at increased risk	Affect family relationships (pressure on relatives to get tested, guilt about children, etc.)
Help make decisions about cancer treatment, chemoprevention, prophylactic surgery	Possible employment or insurance discrmination
Decrease risky health behaviors	Fear of screening for fear of finding cancer
Improve healthy behaviors	

SOURCE: Greater Baltimore Medical Center (GBMC) Harvey Institute of Human Genetics. http://www.gbmc.org/genetics/harveygenetics/cra/brcatest.cfm [Accessed May 16, 2003].

ovarian cancer in people that carry the mutation. Women who have BRCA mutations have a 36 to 85 percent lifetime chance of developing breast cancer while the general population has only a 13 percent chance.[j] In testing for these mutations, a small sample of blood is drawn, and the DNA is analyzed for genetic defects in the BRCA1 and BRCA2 genes. The test results can be either mutation-positive or mutation-negative (see Tables A-1 and A-2).

A negative result does not completely eliminate the chance that a genetic mutation exists within a family. Another breast cancer predisposing mutation may be present. Twenty percent of hereditary breast cancer families have mutations in genes other than BRCA1 and BRCA2. The identity of many of these other hereditary breast cancer genes is currently unknown.[k]

Despite the fact that there is no proven approach to prevent breast cancer, there are interventions that may decrease an individual's chance to develop cancer. Major interventions include chemoprevention (use of drugs

---

[j]Breast and ovarian cancer gene testing: Is it right for you? http://www.mayoclinic.com/invoke.cfm?objectid=015A9CD3-3654-4EE8-B8AA87FC0323F818 [Accessed June 10, 2003].

[k]Greater Baltimore Medical Center (GBMC) Harvey Institute of Human Genetics. http://www.gbmc.org/genetics/harveygenetics/cra/brcatest.cfm [Accessed May 16, 2003].

TABLE A-2 A Mutation-Negative Result Also Has Benefits and Problems

BENEFITS	PROBLEMS
Relief	False sense of security, still have background risk for cancer
Cancer risk is similar to general population, normal cancer surveillance	Mary cause some people to stop screening for cancer
Prophylactic surgery may not be needed	Survivor guilt
Children of non-carrier not at increased risk	Altered family relationships

SOURCE: Greater Baltimore Medical Center (GBMC) Harvey Institute of Human Genetics. http://www.gbmc.org/genetics/harveygenetics/cra/brcatest.cfm [Accessed May 16, 2003].

to reduce the risk of cancer) and prophylactic (preventative) surgery. The use of tamoxifen may be offered to reduce the risk of cancer in high risk women.[7] Women at high risk may also be considered for the Study of Tamoxifen and Raloxifene trial,[l] which is evaluating the effectiveness of the drugs tamoxifen and raloxifene together in preventing breast cancer. Increased screening surveillance by mammography to detect cancer at an earlier stage may also increase breast cancer survival. Other changes may include lifestyle changes such as a balanced diet, limiting alcohol consumption, exercising, maintaining a healthy weight, quitting smoking, and avoiding known carcinogens (substances that are known to damage DNA and cause cancer).

Serum Proteomic Profiling

The pattern of proteins in blood serum (protein-containing portion of blood) may prove useful in identifying diseases, such as cancer. The development of cancer may signal a cascade of small changes to the proteins circulating in the blood serum that are detectable through mass spectroscopy (sensitive method for identifying substances by their molecular weight). Using computer algorithms, the relative levels of ionized proteins are measured and can be associated with the possible presence of a disease.

---

[l]Eligible women are 35 years of age or older, postmenopausal and considered at high risk of breast cancer based upon the NCI risk assessment score (>1.66%) or having already had lobular carcinoma in situ. The trial has been open since 3 years and will continue through the end of 2004. National Surgical Breast and Bowel Project. Study of Tamoxifen and Raloxifene. http://www.nsabp.pitt.edu/STAR/Index.html [Accessed June 10, 2003].

Analysis of serum proteomic patterns which comprise many individual proteins, each of which independently were not able to differentiate diseased from healthy individuals, has recently been shown to provide a diagnostic endpoint for cancer detection.[40] For example, certain patterns associated with the presence of cancers are under clinical investigation. From the patient's perspective, the test is as simple as giving blood. Nipple aspirant fluid (fluid secreted through nipple duct openings in a nonlactating breast) is obtained using a noninvasive pump. Using serum proteomic patterns to identify breast cancers from 317 samples showed a sensitivity of 90 percent and specificity of 70 percent. However, even better results were achieved in the detection of ovarian cancer with 99 percent sensitivity and 99 percent specificity.[29]

Although studies have shown progress in this area, clinical proteomics (bedside application of protein pattern diagnostic tests) is not in the near future and large-scale clinical trials will have to be conducted to validate this technique for use as a routine screening tool. In addition, serum proteomics can only reveal that there is high possibility of cancer within the body. It cannot localize the cancer, and therefore must be used adjunctively with some sort of imaging modality. The whole process can take less than a minute from obtaining a sample to interpreting the results.

BIOPSY TECHNOLOGIES

Technology	Description	Developmental Stage
Surgical Biopsy	The gold standard in breast biopsy. Requires a surgical incision to completely remove the lesion (excisional biopsy) or obtain a sample from the lesion (incisional biopsy) to allow the pathologists to make a definitive diagnosis.	Clinical use
Core Needle Biopsy	Larger needle used to obtain tissue samples from a breast lesion. This procedure usually obtains enough tissue to allow a pathologist to make a definitive diagnosis.	Clinical use

Technology	Description	Developmental Stage
Fine Needle Aspiration Biopsy	Small needle used to collect fluid or a small sample of cells from a breast lesion. This minimally invasive procedure allows for a pathologist to make a diagnosis; however, a larger sample size obtained through a more invasive biopsy procedure may be required.	Clinical use
Image Guided Biopsy	Subset of needle biopsy procedures that use imaging techniques to guide needles into lesions and obtain samples from nonpalpable lesions. These imaging techniques typically include mammography, ultrasound, and MRI.	Clinical use
SmartProbe	Real-time tissue identification using a 20-gauge needle probe. The needle incorporates information from three spectroscopic fibers and an impedance microelectrode for breast cancer diagnosis.	Experimental use (clinical prototype)

Biopsy is a procedure that involves obtaining a tissue sample for further analysis to establish a precise diagnosis.

Surgical Biopsy

Traditional open surgical biopsy is the gold standard to which other methods of breast biopsies are compared.[25] Surgical biopsy requires a 1.5- to 2.0-inch incision in the breast to remove suspicious tissue for pathological examination. Surgical biopsy can take the form of either an excisional biopsy (complete removal of the lesion) or an incisional biopsy (only a sample of the lesion is removed for examination).

Surgical biopsy takes place in an operating room. Most often a local anaesthetic (the breast only is numbed) is most often used, as opposed to a general anaesthetic (patient is asleep). The shape of the breast may change after removal of the tissue depending on the size of the lesion. Stitches will be required to close the incision and a scar might be left at the point of incision. If the lesion is nonpalpable, wire localization biopsy will be used with mammography or sonography to locate the area of concern before the operation.

Open surgical biopsy requires a longer period of recovery than percutaneous (performed through the skin) breast biopsy procedures (such as fine needle aspiration or core needle biopsy). Usually, at least one full day of recovery is required and significant bruising can last several months.

Core Needle Biopsy

A core needle biopsy is a percutaneous ("through the skin") procedure that involves removing small samples of breast tissue using a hollow "core" needle. For palpable (able to be felt) lesions, the radiologist or surgeon locates the lesion with one hand and performs a freehand needle biopsy with the other. In the case of nonpalpable lesions (those unable to be felt), image guidance is used most frequently with ultrasound, mammography, or MRI. The core biopsy needle can be from 11 to 16 gauge (outer diameter of 2.77 and 1.65 mm, respectively), while the fine aspiration needle is only 20 or 28 gauge (outer diameter of 0.89 and 0.36 mm, respectively). The core needle biopsy needle also has a special cutting edge. Typically, samples approximately 2.0 cm long are removed. The samples are then sent to the pathology laboratory for diagnosis.

The core needle biopsy procedure typically only takes a few minutes, and most patients are able to resume normal activity the same day. Core needle biopsy usually allows for a more accurate assessment of a breast mass than fine needle aspiration because the larger core needle usually removes enough tissue for the pathologist to evaluate abnormal cells in relation to the surrounding small sample of breast tissue taken with the specimen.[45] Biopsy results are usually available within several days.

Fine-Needle Aspiration Biopsy

Fine needle aspiration (FNA) biopsy is a percutaneous (performed through the skin) procedure that uses a fine-gauge needle and a syringe to sample fluid from a breast cyst or remove clusters of cells from a solid mass.

With FNA, the cellular material taken from the breast is usually sent to the pathology laboratory for analysis. The needle used during FNA is smaller than a needle that is normally used to draw blood. FNA needles are usually 20 or 28 gauge (0.89 and 0.36 mm, respectively), the size of needles typically used to draw blood.

If a breast lump is palpable, the physician will guide a needle into the lesion. If the lump is nonpalpable, the needle will have to be image-guided. The samples are then smeared on a microscope slide, fixed or air dried, stained, and then examined by a pathologist under the microscope, a process similar to the examination of a Pap smear for the early detection of cervical cancer.

FNA is the least invasive method of breast biopsy, and the results are available within minutes if a cytopathologist is available to interpret the results. FNA is a good technique for confirming breast cysts, and since the procedure does not require stitches, patients recover almost immediately. One disadvantage of FNA is that the procedure only removes very small samples of tissue or cells from the breast. If the FNA diagnosis is positive, this procedure can result in an incomplete assessment because the cells cannot be evaluated in relation to the surrounding tissue, which is crucial to establishing the stage of cancer and prognosis. Yet, insufficient sample rates for nonpalpable lesions and lower relative diagnostic accuracy reduce the clinical utility of FNA.[41] Larger samples from a more accurate core needle biopsy or open surgical biopsy may be needed to make a definitive diagnosis.

Image-Guided Biopsy

Imaging techniques play an important role in helping doctors perform breast biopsies, especially of abnormal areas that cannot be felt but can be seen on a conventional mammogram or with ultrasound, such as those DCIS. One type of needle biopsy, the stereotactic-guided biopsy, involves the precise location of the abnormal area in three dimensions using conventional imaging approaches. Stereotactic refers to the use of a computer and scanning devices to gain information about the precise location of parts of the image in three dimensions. A needle is then inserted into the breast and a tissue sample is obtained for a definitive diagnosis from the pathology laboratory.

SmartProbe

Following a suspicious mammogram, a tiny 20-gauge disposable probe connected to a computer is inserted into the suspicious lesion. Measurements of oxygen partial pressure, electrical impedance, temperature, and light scattering and absorption properties are made and instantly displayed on the computer screen. The "smart probe" makes continuous measurements (100 per second) as it moves from the surface of the breast to the center of a suspicious lesion. The entire procedure takes only a few minutes to complete, and the instant display of results will help the physician properly locate the probe within the suspicious tissue. Preliminary clinical investigations are under way at the University of California, San Francisco. Specificity and sensitivity of core needle biopsies are approximately 85 percent, and the gold standard surgical biopsy is 98 percent. The manufacturer of the biopsy probe, Bioluminate, Inc., hopes that the SmartProbe will exceed the accuracy achieved by the core needle procedure and approach the high levels realized by surgical biopsies. However, only a few small studies of the prototype technology have been published.[1,2] Trials of this technology are in very early stages; no evidence of clinical validity has been published as of March 2004.

REFERENCES

1. Andrews R, Mah R, Aghevli A, Freitas K, Galvagni A, Guerrero M, Papsin R, Reed C, Stassinopoulos D. 1999. Multimodality stereotactic brain tissue identification: the NASA smart probe project. *Stereotact Funct Neurosurg* 73(1-4):1-8.
2. Andrews RJ, Mah RW. 2003. The NASA Smart Probe Project for real-time multiple microsensor tissue recognition. *Stereotact Funct Neurosurg* 80(1-4 Pt 1):114-119.
3. Burhenne LJ, Wood SA, D'Orsi CJ, Feig SA, Kopans DB, O'Shaughnessy KF, Sickles EA, Tabar L, Vyborny CJ, Castellino RA. 2000. Potential contribution of computer-aided detection to the sensitivity of screening mammography. *Radiology* 215(2):554-562.
4. Chapman D, Thomlinson W, Johnston RE, Washburn D, Pisano E, Gmur N, Zhong Z, Menk R, Arfelli F, Sayers D. 1997. Diffraction enhanced x-ray imaging. *Phys Med Biol* 42(11):2015-2025.
5. Chaudhary SS, Mishra RK, Swarup A, Thomas JM. 1984. Dielectric properties of normal & malignant human breast tissues at radiowave & microwave frequencies. *Indian J Biochem Biophys* 21(1):76-79.
6. Chen YS, Wang WH, Chan T, Sun SS, Kao A. 2002. A review of the cost-effectiveness of Tc-99m sestamibi scintimammography in diagnosis of breast cancer in Taiwanese women with indeterminate mammographically dense breast. *Surg Oncol* 11(3):151-155.
7. Chlebowski RT, Col N, Winer EP, Collyar DE, Cummings SR, Vogel VG 3rd, Burstein HJ, Eisen A, Lipkus I, Pfister DG. 2002. American society of clinical oncology technology assessment of pharmacologic interventions for breast cancer risk reduction including tamoxifen, raloxifene, and aromatase inhibition. *J Clin Oncol* 20(15):3328-3343.
8. Cuzick J, Holland R, Barth V, Davies R, Faupel M, Fentiman I, Frischbier HJ, LaMarque JL, Merson M, Sacchini V, Vanel D, Veronesi U. 1998. Electropotential measurements as a new diagnostic modality for breast cancer. *Lancet* 352(9125):359-363.
9. Domchek SM. 2002. The utility of ductal lavage in breast cancer detection and risk assessment. *Breast Cancer Res* 4(2):51-53.

10. Dooley WC, Ljung BM, Veronesi U, Cazzaniga M, Elledge RM, O'Shaughnessy JA, Kuerer HM, Hung DT, Khan SA, Phillips RF, Ganz PA, Euhus DM, Esserman LJ, Haffty BG, King BL, Kelley MC, Anderson MM, Schmit PJ, Clark RR, Kass FC, Anderson BO, Troyan SL, Arias RD, Quiring JN, Love SM, Page DL, King EB. 2001. Ductal lavage for detection of cellular atypia in women at high risk for breast cancer. *J Natl Cancer Inst* 93(21):1624-1632.

11. Elmore JG, Miglioretti DL, Reisch LM, Barton MB, Kreuter W, Christiansen CL, Fletcher SW. 2002. Screening mammograms by community radiologists: variability in false-positive rates. *J Natl Cancer Inst* 94(18):1373-1380.

12. Fear EC, Li X, Hagness SC, Stuchly MA. 2002. Confocal microwave imaging for breast cancer detection: localization of tumors in three dimensions. *IEEE Trans Biomed Eng* 49(8):812-822.

13. Freer TW, Ulissey MJ. 2001. Screening mammography with computer-aided detection: prospective study of 12,860 patients in a community breast center. *Radiology* 220(3):781-786.

14. Gambhir SS. 2002. Molecular imaging of cancer with positron emission tomography. *Nat Rev Cancer* 2(9):683-693.

15. Gur D, Sumkin JH, Rockette HE, Ganott M, Hakim C, Hardesty L, Poller WR, Shah R, Wallace L. 2004. Changes in breast cancer detection and mammography recall rates after the introduction of a computer-aided detection system. *J Natl Cancer Inst* 96(3):185-190.

16. Hasnah MO, Zhong Z, Oltulu O, Pisano E, Johnston RE, Sayers D, Thomlinson W, Chapman D. 2002. Diffraction enhanced imaging contrast mechanisms in breast cancer specimens. *Med Phys* 29(10):2216-2221.

17. Houssami N, Irwig L, Loy C. 2002. Accuracy of combined breast imaging in young women. *Breast* 11(1):36-40.

18. Humphrey LL. 2002. Breast cancer screening: a summary of the evidence for the U.S. preventive services task force. *Ann Intern Med* 137:E-347-E-367.

19. Hwang ES, Kinkel K, Esserman LJ, Lu Y, Weidner N, Hylton NM. 2003. Magnetic resonance imaging in patients diagnosed with ductal carcinoma-in-situ: value in the diagnosis of residual disease, occult invasion, and multicentricity. *Ann Surg Oncol* 10(4):381-388.

20. James JJ. 2004. The current status of digital mammography. *Clin Radiol* 59(1):1-10.

21. Jiang H, Iftimia NV, Xu Y, Eggert JA, Fajardo LL, Klove KL. 2002. Near-infrared optical imaging of the breast with model-based reconstruction. *Acad Radiol* 9(2):186-194.

22. Jiang H, Xu Y, Iftimia N, Eggert J, Klove K, Baron L, Fajardo L. 2001. Three-dimensional optical tomographic imaging of breast in a human subject. *IEEE Trans Med Imaging* 20(12):1334-1340.

23. Joines WT, Zhang Y, Li C, Jirtle RL. 1994. The measured electrical properties of normal and malignant human tissues from 50 to 900 MHz. *Med Phys* 21(4):547-550.

24. Keith LG, Oleszczuk JJ, Laguens M. 2001. Circadian rhythm chaos: a new breast cancer marker. *Int J Fertil Womens Med* 46(5):238-247.

25. Kerlikowske K, Smith-Bindman R, Ljung BM, Grady D. 2003. Evaluation of abnormal mammography results and palpable breast abnormalities. *Ann Intern Med* 139(4):274-284.

26. Krishnamurthy S, Sneige N, Bedi DG, Edieken BS, Fornage BD, Kuerer HM, Singletary SE, Hunt KK. 2002. Role of ultrasound-guided fine-needle aspiration of indeterminate and suspicious axillary lymph nodes in the initial staging of breast carcinoma. *Cancer* 95(5):982-988.

27. Li D, Meaney PM, Tosteson TD, Jiang S, Kerner TE, McBride TO, Pogue BW, Hartov A, Paulsen KD. 2003. Comparisons of three alternative breast modalities in a common phantom imaging experiment. *Med Phys* 30(8):2194-2205.

28. Liberman M, Sampalis F, Mulder DS, Sampalis JS. 2003. Breast cancer diagnosis by scintimammography: a meta-analysis and review of the literature. *Breast Cancer Res Treat* 80(1):115-126.

29. Liotta LA, Kohn EC, Petricoin EF. 2001. Clinical proteomics: personalized molecular medicine. *JAMA* 286(18):2211-2214.

30. Liu HT, Sun LZ, Wang G, Vannier MW. 2003. Analytic modeling of breast elastography. *Med Phys* 30(9):2340-2349.

31. Lumachi F, Ferretti G, Povolato M, Marzola MC, Zucchetta P, Geatti O, Brandes AA, Bui F. 2001. Accuracy of technetium-99m sestamibi scintimammography and X-ray mammography in premenopausal women with suspected breast cancer. *Eur J Nucl Med* 28(12):1776-1780.

32. Lumachi F, Zucchetta P, Marzola MC, Ferretti G, Povolato M, Paris MK, Brandes AA, Bui F. 2002. Positive predictive value of 99mTc sestamibi scintimammography in patients with non-palpable, mammographically detected, suspicious, breast lesions. *Nucl Med Commun* 23(11):1073-1078.

33. Mainiero MB, Gareen IF, Bird CE, Smith W, Cobb C, Schepps B. 2002. Preferential use of sonographically guided biopsy to minimize patient discomfort and procedure time in a percutaneous image-guided breast biopsy program. *J Ultrasound Med* 21(11):1221-1226.

34. Melloul M, Paz A, Ohana G, Laver O, Michalevich D, Koren R, Wolloch Y, Gal R. 1999. Double-phase 99mTc-sestamibi scintimammography and trans-scan in diagnosing breast cancer. *J Nucl Med* 40(3):376-380.

35. National Cancer Institute. 2004. *Fifth National Forum on Biomedical Imaging in Oncology Meeting Summary.* Bethesda, MD.

36. Neugebauer J. 2003. T-Scan: Post-Script on a 1999 "Medical Breakthrough." *Institute of Medicine Workshop on New Technologies for the Early Detection and Diagnosis of Breast Cancer.* Washington, DC: Institute of Medicine Committee on New Approaches to Early Detection and Diagnosis of Breast Cancer.

37. Newcomer LM, Newcomb PA, Trentham-Dietz A, Storer BE, Yasui Y, Daling JR, Potter JD. 2002. Detection method and breast carcinoma histology. *Cancer* 95(3):470-477.

38. Niklason LT, Christian BT, Niklason LE, Kopans DB, Castleberry DE, Opsahl-Ong BH, Landberg CE, Slanetz PJ, Giardino AA, Moore R, Albagli D, DeJule MC, Fitzgerald PF, Fobare DF, Giambattista BW, Kwasnick RF, Liu J, Lubowski SJ, Possin GE, Richotte JF, Wei CY, Wirth RF. 1997. Digital tomosynthesis in breast imaging. *Radiology* 205(2):399-406.

39. Ntziachristos V, Chance B. 2001. Probing physiology and molecular function using optical imaging: applications to breast cancer. *Breast Cancer Res* 3(1):41-46.

40. Petricoin EF, Zoon KC, Kohn EC, Barrett JC, Liotta LA. 2002. Clinical proteomics: translating benchside promise into bedside reality. *Nat Rev Drug Discov* 1(9):683-695.

41. Pisano ED, Fajardo LL, Caudry DJ, Sneige N, Frable WJ, Berg WA, Tocino I, Schnitt SJ, Connolly JL, Gatsonis CA, McNeil BJ. 2001. Fine-needle aspiration biopsy of nonpalpable breast lesions in a multicenter clinical trial: results from the radiologic diagnostic oncology group V. *Radiology* 219(3):785-792.

42. Pisano ED, Johnston RE, Chapman D, Geradts J, Iacocca MV, Livasy CA, Washburn DB, Sayers DE, Zhong Z, Kiss MZ, Thomlinson WC. 2000. Human breast cancer specimens: diffraction-enhanced imaging with histologic correlation—improved conspicuity of lesion detail compared with digital radiography. *Radiology* 214(3):895-901.

43. Schnall MD. 2003. Breast MR imaging. *Radiol Clin North Am* 41(1):43-50.

44. Simpson HW, Wilson D, Griffiths K, Mutch F, Halberg F, Gautherie M. 1982. Thermorhythmometry of the breast: a review to 1981. *Prog Clin Biol Res* 107:133-154.

45. Singh HK, Kilpatrick SE, Silverman JF. 2004. Fine needle aspiration biopsy of soft tissue sarcomas: utility and diagnostic challenges. *Adv Anat Pathol* 11(1):24-37.

46. Sinkus R, Lorenzen J, Schrader D, Lorenzen M, Dargatz M, Holz D. 2000. High-resolution tensor MR elastography for breast tumour detection. *Phys Med Biol* 45(6):1649-1664.

47. Smith RA, Cokkinides V, Eyre HJ. 2004. American Cancer Society guidelines for the early detection of cancer, 2004. *CA Cancer J Clin* 54(1):41-52.

48. Surowiec AJ, Stuchly SS, Barr JB, Swarup A. 1988. Dielectric properties of breast carcinoma and the surrounding tissues. *IEEE Trans Biomed Eng* 35(4):257-263.

49. Szebeni A, Rahoty P, Besznyak I. 2002. Clinical validity of new ultrasound methods in the differential diagnosis of breast diseases. *Breast* 11(6):489-495.

50. Van Houten EE, Doyley MM, Kennedy FE, Weaver JB, Paulsen KD. 2003. Initial in vivo experience with steady-state subzone-based MR elastography of the human breast. *J Magn Reson Imaging* 17(1):72-85.

51. van't Veer LJ, Dai H, van de Vijver MJ, He YD, Hart AA, Mao M, Peterse HL, van der Kooy K, Marton MJ, Witteveen AT, Schreiber GJ, Kerkhoven RM, Roberts C, Linsley PS, Bernards R, Friend SH. 2002. Gene expression profiling predicts clinical outcome of breast cancer. *Nature* 415(6871):530-536.

52. Wilson DW, George D, Mansel RE, Simpson HW, Halberg F, Griffiths K. 1984. Circadian breast skin temperature rhythms: overt and occult benign and occult primary malignant breast disease. *Chronobiol Int* 1(2):167-172.

53. Wu T, Stewart A, Stanton M, McCauley T, Phillips W, Kopans DB, Moore RH, Eberhard JW, Opsahl-Ong B, Niklason L, Williams MB. 2003. Tomographic mammography using a limited number of low-dose cone-beam projection images. *Med Phys* 30(3):365-380.

54. Yeung DK, Cheung HS, Tse GM. 2001. Human breast lesions: characterization with contrast-enhanced in vivo proton MR spectroscopy—initial results. *Radiology* 220(1):40-46.

55. Yeung DK, Yang WT, Tse GM. 2002. Breast cancer: in vivo proton MR spectroscopy in the characterization of histopathologic subtypes and preliminary observations in axillary node metastases. *Radiology* 225(1):190-197.

Appendix B

Workshop Agendas

**NEW APPROACHES TO BREAST CANCER DETECTION
(WORKSHOP #1)**

National Academy of Sciences Building
Washington, DC
January 7, 2003

9:00   **Welcome and Introduction**
        Ed Penhoet, Committee Chair

9:10   **Overview of Current Options in Breast Cancer Detection**
        Laura Esserman, University of California San Francisco

9:40   **Comparisons of Multiple Modalities: US, PET, MRI, Optical**
        Mitchell Schnall, University of Pennsylvania

10:10   **Technical Advances in Mammography: Digital Mammography
        and DEI**
        Etta Pisano, University of North Carolina

10:40   **Comparison of Four Breast Imaging Techniques**
        Keith Paulsen, Dartmouth

11:10   **Computer Assisted Diagnosis**
        Maryellen Giger, University of Chicago

11:40   **DISCUSSION**

12:00   **LUNCH**

12:45   **Introduction to Tumor Markers**
          Jeff Marks, Duke University Medical Center

12:50   **The Search for Breast Cancer Biomarkers**
          Sara Sukumar, Johns Hopkins Oncology Center

1:20   **Deciphering the Molecular Signatures of Breast Cancer**
          Lance Liotta, Laboratory of Pathology, National Cancer
          Institute

1:50   **Molecular Imaging**
          David Piwnica-Worms, Washington University

2:20   **DISCUSSION**

2:30   **BREAK**

2:45   **Making Sense of the Mountains of Data: Bioinformatics and**
          Breast Cancer Detection
          Michael Vannier, National Cancer Institute/University
          of Iowa

3:15   **SmartProbe: Spin-off Technology from NASA**
          Richard Hular, BioLuminate, Inc.

3:30   **TransScan: Post-Script on a 1999 "Medical Breakthrough"**
          John Neugebauer, TransScan Medical, Inc.

3:45   **Optical Scanning, Almost Approved**
          Phillip C. Thomas, DOBI, Inc.

4:00   **DISCUSSION**

4:15   **WRAP-UP**

4:45   **ADJOURN**

FROM DEVELOPMENT TO ADOPTION OF NEW APPROACHES TO BREAST CANCER DETECTION AND DIAGNOSIS (WORKSHOP #2)

Keck Center of the National Academies
Washington, DC
February 18, 2003

9:00   **Welcome and Introduction**
        Ed Penhoet, Committee Chair

9:10   **Marketing Strategies: How Companies Work to Encourage Adoption of New Medical Technologies**
        Laura Shapiro, Siemens Medical Solutions

10:00   **The Role of Innovative Not-for-Profits in Medical Innovation: Lessons from CaP CURE**
        Howard Soule, CaP CURE

10:50   **The Role of Breast Cancer Philanthropies in Developing New Approaches to Breast Cancer Detection**
        Susan Braun, Susan G. Komen Foundation

11:40   DISCUSSION

3:00   ADJOURN

FROM DEVELOPMENT TO ADOPTION OF NEW APPROACHES TO BREAST CANCER DETECTION AND DIAGNOSIS (WORKSHOP #3)

National Academy of Sciences Building
Washington, DC
March 25, 2003

9:30   **Welcome and Introduction**
        Ed Penhoet, Committee Chair

9:35   **NCI Programs to Support Development of New Approaches to Breast Cancer Detection**
        Ed Staab, Branch Chief, Diagnostic Imaging, NCI

10:15   **Regulatory Challenges for *In Vitro* Diagnostics**
Joseph Hackett, Special Projects Officer, Office of *In Vitro* Diagnostics, FDA

10:55   **Challenges in Assessing the Safety and Efficacy of Cancer Detection Devices**
David Feigal, Director, Center for Devices and Radiological Health, FDA

11:35   **DISCUSSION**

12:30   **LUNCH**

1:15   **CMS Perspective on Adoption of New Breast Cancer Detection Technologies**
Sean Tunis, Acting Chief Medical Officer, CMS

1:55   **Private Health Payers' Perspective on Adoption of New Breast Cancer Detection Technologies**
Alan Rosenberg, Vice President of Medical and Credentialing Policy, WellPoint Health Networks

2:35   **DISCUSSION**

2:50   **BREAK**

3:10   **Better Information and Decision Tools: The Needs of the Consumer**
Mary Ropka, University of Virginia Medical School

3:50   **Decision Support in Breast Cancer Detection Options: Health Systems Perspective**
Nananda Col, Brigham & Women's Hospital

4:30   **DISCUSSION**

4:45   **ADJOURN**

Appendix C

ROC Analysis: Key Statistical Tool for Evaluating Detection Technologies

ROC analysis provides a systematic tool for quantifying the impact of variability among individuals' decision thresholds. The term receiver operating characteristic (ROC) originates from the use of radar during World War II. Just as American soldiers deciphered a blip on the radar screen as a German bomber, a friendly plane, or just noise, radiologists face the task of identifying abnormal tissue against a complicated background. As radar technology advanced during the war, the need for a standard system to evaluate detection accuracy became apparent. ROC analysis was developed as a standard methodology to quantify a signal receiver's ability to correctly distinguish objects of interest from the background noise in the system.

For instance, each radiologist has his or her own visual clues guiding them to a clinical decision as whether the pattern variation of a mammogram indicates tissue abnormalities or just normal variation. The varying decisions make up a range of decision thresholds.

SENSITIVITY AND SPECIFICITY DEPEND ON INDIVIDUAL READER'S DECISION THRESHOLDS

Sensitivity and specificity are the most commonly used measures of detection accuracy. Both depend upon the decision threshold used by individual readers, and thus vary with each reader's determination of what to call a positive test and what to call a negative test. Measures of sensitivity and specificity alone are insufficient to determine the true performance of a diagnostic technology in clinical practice.

For example, cases are classified as normal or abnormal according to a specific reader's interpretation bias. As the decision point for identifying an abnormal result is shifted to the left or right, the proportions of true positives and true negatives change. Thus, the relationship reveals the tradeoff between sensitivity and specificity. For instance, using an enriched set of data with 100 exams that includes 10 true cancers, if a reader correctly identifies 8 cancers while missing 2 cancers (a sensitivity rating of 0.8 or 80 percent) of the 90 true negatives, the reader only correctly identified only 72 as normal (a specificity of 0.8 or 80 percent). However, a reader with more stringent criteria for an abnormal test may have a higher false-negative rate, increasing the number of missed cancers and decreasing the number of false alarms. For example, using the same distribution of 100 cases, the reader would correctly identify 6 cancers (a sensitivity of 0.7 or 70 percent). However, the reader would now correctly identify 85 true negatives as normal (a specificity of 0.94 or 94 percent). The opposite effect could also be obtained for a reader with less stringent criteria. Such a reader would have a higher false-positive rate but would find more cancers. Therefore, this example shows that these measures that depend on the true-positive rate and true-negative rate respectively are reader specific. In the case of interpreting mammograms, different radiologists with different decision thresholds can affect the clinical outcome in the assessment of non-obvious mammograms.

ROC CURVES ARE NECESSARY TO CHARACTERIZE DIAGNOSTIC PERFORMANCE

The ROC curve maps the effects of varying decision thresholds, accounting for all possible combinations of various correct and incorrect decisions.[4] A ROC curve is a graph of the relationship between the true-positive rate (sensitivity) and the false-positive rate (1-specificity) (see Figure C-1). For example, a ROC curve for mammography would plot the fraction of confirmed breast cancer cases (true positives) that were detected against the fraction of false alarms (false positives). Each point on the curve might represent another test, for instance each point would be the result of a different radiologist reading the same set of 20 mammograms. Alternatively, each point might represent the results of the same radiologist reading a different set of 20 mammograms.

The ROC curve describes the overall performance of the diagnostic modality across varying conditions. Sources of variation for these conditions can include different radiologist's decision thresholds, different amounts of time between interpreting mammograms, or variation within cases due to the inherent imprecision of breast compression. ROC analysis allows one to average the effect of different conditions on accuracy. There-

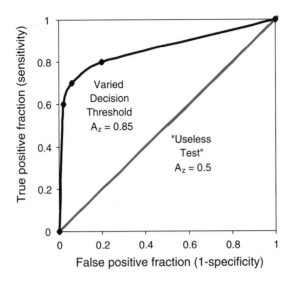

FIGURE C-1 Receiver operating characteristic (ROC) graph of a varying decision threshold compared with a "useless test." The three decision thresholds discussed in the previous section are represented on this graph. The best-fit curve drawn through these points is the ROC curve, which represents the overall performance of the diagnostic test across all possible interpretations (decision thresholds). The overall accuracy of this test under varying conditions is determined by the area under the complete curve, 0.85.

The leftmost point shows low sensitivity and high specificity. The middle point shows moderate sensitivity and specificity. The rightmost point shows high sensitivity and low specificity. Yet because they all lie on the same curve they have the same overall statistical accuracy, which is quantified by A_Z.

The 45-degree-angle line represents a series of guesses between two choices, as in a coin toss. This would be considered a "useless test" if the outcome of the test was dichotomous (for example cancer vs. no cancer) for diagnostic purposes. For instance, radiologists reading mammograms with their eyes closed would tend to fall on this line. The number of true positives would approach the number of false negatives.

The area under such a curve, 0.5, represents 50 percent accuracy of the test. In contrast, the ROC curve for a test with 100 percent accuracy will trace the Y-axis up at a false-positive fraction of zero and follow along the top of the graph at a true-positive fraction of one. The area under such a curve would be 1.0 and represent a perfect test.

fore, the area under the ROC curve can be viewed as the diagnostic accuracy of the technology.

There is often ambiguity in comparing diagnostic modalities when one has only a single sensitivity-specificity pair measure on one modality and a single sensitivity-specificity pair measured on a competing modality.[5]

Since there is no unique decision threshold used by radiologists, there is no reason to single out specificity and sensitivity values. Radiologists adjust their decision thresholds as a function of context and available information, such as whether a patient is known to be at high risk for breast cancer, the presence of signs or symptoms, or the likelihood of being sued for a missed cancer.

There are many situations in which relying on single estimates of specificity and sensitivity would distort the ranking of competing systems. Different sensitivity-specificity pairs on the ROC curve can arise from many ambiguities beyond variability among radiologists, such as patient variation, use of different machines, and different image processing software.

The ROC approach can be used to accurately compare breast cancer diagnostic tests. The ROC plot provides a visual representation of the accuracy of a detection test, incorporating not only the intrinsic features of the test, but also reader variability.

Figure C-2 shows an example of how ROC curves were used to analyze

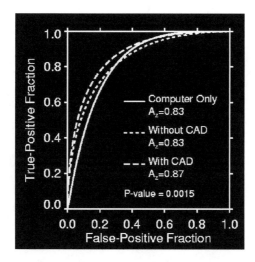

FIGURE C-2 Example of ROC curve analysis for computer-assisted detection. A comparison of the ROC curves for computer only, without CAD, and with CAD, show the value of ROC curves in evaluating diagnostic technologies. The area under the curves, corresponding to overall diagnostic accuracy, illustrates that a radiologist "with CAD" will maximize sensitivity and specificity as compared with the other two approaches. In addition, comparison of the computer alone with the unassisted radiologist shows the same overall accuracy; however, the curve for the radiologist alone is shifted to the left indicating a slightly higher specificity. Yet, if ROC curves cross and the areas are the same the result would suggest that one test provides the optimal strategy for certain cases and the other test may be better with another set of cases.

the value of a computer-assisted detection (CAD) system.[3] The curves represent the accuracy, in terms of sensitivity and specificity, of a modality across the varying conditions of the study. At a true-positive fraction of 80 percent, radiologists who used CAD outperformed those who did not use CAD in terms of sensitivity and specificity. Nevertheless, data based on a single decision threshold are insufficient to rank competing systems, because they fail to account for the various decision thresholds that will be applied using the modality. The area under the ROC curve is the best way to rank competing systems, because it integrates the essential measures of sensitivity, specificity, and decision threshold. Figures C-3 and C-4 demonstrate the ability of ROC curves to differentiate the benefits and limitations of two tests over a range of conditions that may occur in clinical practice. The greater area under the ROC curve in the example indicates that computer-assisted mammography increases a radiologist's ability to correctly identify neoplastic breast tissue, as well as to avoid false alarms.

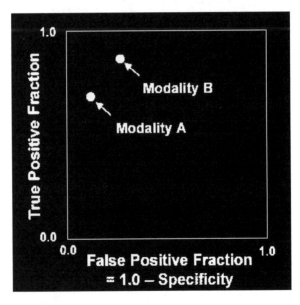

FIGURE C-3 Comparison of two diagnostic modalities without ROC curves. Without the help of ROC curves it is difficult to reach a conclusion as to which modality is more accurate.
SOURCE: Adapted from Metz C. Methodologic Issues. Fourth National Forum on Biomedical Imagining in Oncology. Bethesda, MD. February 6, 2003.

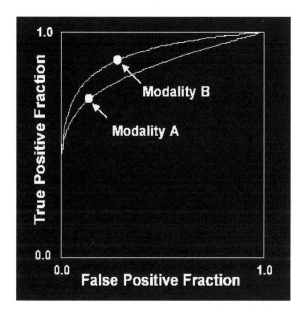

FIGURE C-4 Comparison of two diagnostic modalities utilizing ROC curves. After drawing ROC curves it is easy to see that modality B is better. Modality B achieves a higher true-positive fraction at the same false-positive fraction as modality A. Modality B also results in a lower false-positive fraction with the same true-positive fraction as modality A.
SOURCE: Adapted from Metz C. Methodologic Issues. Fourth National Forum on Biomedical Imagining in Oncology. Bethesda, MD. February 6, 2003.

MULTIPLE-READER MULTIPLE-CASE ROC

The findings of clinical studies are insignificant unless the results can be applied to some sort of clinical use. Therefore, in the case of breast cancer diagnostic modalities, the reader in the study must represent all radiologists and the case set must also closely resemble all mammograms that can be generated in the clinic. It may be impossible to exactly replicate the full variability of mammography findings in clinics nationwide. However, clinical studies that incorporate more case variation to measure the diagnostic accuracy of a modality will have significantly more clinical value than studies based on little case variation.

Variability in cancer detection tests has two main components, reader variability and case-sample variability. The first was described in the discussion of ROC analysis. The latter results from subtle differences in mammograms that, when spanning the continuum from definitely revealing cancer to definitely not revealing cancer, may influence a reader's decision. Methodological solutions to account for these sources of variability can maximize the amount of information that can be gathered from data sets.

The combination of ROC analysis and a study design with multiple readers and multiple cases provides a possible solution to the components of variance. In multiple-reader multiple-case (MRMC) ROC analysis, all readers interpret every mammogram in the case set. The readers in a study represent the diverse readership that might use a specific technology. The representative case-set population allows one to generalize the findings to the diverse breast cancer cases that may appear in nationwide clinics. This allows for significant findings to be generalized to widespread clinical practice.

The MRMC study design has several advantages over the collection of single-reader ROC analyses because MRMC analysis provides a quantitative measure of the performance of a diagnostic test across a population of readers with varying degrees of skill. Even though having more than one reader increases variability in the measurement, MRMC studies can be designed so that the statistical power of differences between competing modalities will be greater than if only one reader's interpretation is used.[1] When using MRMC methodology, statistical models can be used to account for both case variability and reader variability. The results of a study in which readers interpret different mammogram case sets cannot account for case-sample variation. Therefore, single-reader studies can only be generalized to the cases that each reader interpreted. Conversely, the results of an MRMC study can be generalized to all radiologists as well as all mammograms.[6]

The practical result of MRMC methodology is saving time and money. The concept of design of pivotal studies using results from pilot MRMC studies offers an opportunity for the development of imaging technology assessment with some degree of coherence and continuity. MRMC studies during the research phase of imaging system development can provide the information to design and size studies for the demonstration of safety and effectiveness required for Food and Drug Administration (FDA) approval.[6] MRMC methods yield more information per case, which translates into smaller sample sizes for trials. Reducing the size of trials makes it easier to recruit patients. Smaller trials also require less money. This procedure can also be used to help design clinical trials by estimating the size of future studies. For instance, the FDA approval of the first digital mammography technology was based on only 44 breast cancers across 5 readers in a pilot study using the MRMC paradigm. The results of this study can be generalized to a pivotal trial of 200 cancers and 6 readers, or 78 cancers with 100 readers.[7] According to the 2001 FDA guidance on digital mammography systems, ROC estimates that take into account uncertainties are an essential part of a clinical study. The FDA also presents several methodologies that have been used in the past to measure uncertainties in ROC estimates; however, it is noted that MRMC methodology is the only approach that accounts for reader and case variability.[2] As a result, through November 2002, all successful submissions to the FDA of a system for digital mammography utilized the MRMC ROC paradigm.

REFERENCES

1. Beiden SV, Wagner RF, Doi K, Nishikawa RM, Freedman M, Lo SC, Xu XW. 2002. Independent versus sequential reading in ROC studies of computer-assist modalities: analysis of components of variance. *Acad Radiol* 9(9):1036-1043.
2. Center for Devices and Radiological Health. 2001. Premarket Applications for Digital Mammography Systems; Final Guidance for Industry and FDA. Washington, DC: Food and Drug Administration.
3. Giger M. 2003. Computer Assisted Diagnosis. *Workshop on New Technologies for the Early Detection and Diagnosis of Breast Cancer*. Washington, DC: Institute of Medicine of the National Academies.
4. Metz CE. 1978. Basic principles of ROC analysis. *Semin Nucl Med* 8(4):283-298.
5. Wagner RF, Beiden SV. 2003. Independent versus sequential reading in ROC studies of computer-assist modalities: analysis of components of variance. *Acad Radiol* 10(2):211-212; author reply 212.
6. Wagner RF, Beiden SV, Campbell G, Metz CE, Sacks WM. 2002. Assessment of medical imaging and computer-assist systems: lessons from recent experience. *Acad Radiol* 9(11):1264-1277.
7. Wagner R. 2003. CDRH Research Perspectives. *Fourth National Forum on Biomedical Imaging in Oncology*. Bethesda, MD: National Cancer Institute.

Appendix D

Common Weaknesses in Study Designs

The following section describes some of the most common weaknesses in study design seen by medical technology evaluators.

Poorly Described Patient Populations. Unless the criteria used to determine patients' eligibility for a study are clearly outlined, and the characteristics of the patients who actually get enrolled are clearly described, it is impossible to know to which populations of patients the results of the study can be confidently applied, or whether the results from two different studies are truly comparable. If the experience of particular subgroups of patients is important and likely to vary, then enrollment should be stratified on the basis of those patient subgroup characteristics.

Too Narrow a Patient Population. The patients enrolled in a study of a new technology should be similar to the patients in whom the technology is most likely to be used. The enrolled population should include individuals without the target disease of interest, such as patients with risk factors for the disease but without the disease itself, patients with different, but commonly confused conditions, and patients with other types of pathology in the same organ systems.[a] Failure to enroll the appropriate spectrum of patients in a study of a new diagnostic technology can lead to overestimates

---

[a]For example, different breast cancer detection technologies vary in their ability to detect microcalcifications, which are not cancerous lesions but are significant breast cancer risk factors. For instance, ultrasound is highly sensitive to lesions but does a poor job of detecting microcalicifications.

of both the sensitivity and specificity of the new technology. Similarly, failure to enroll an appropriate spectrum of patients in a study of a new therapy can lead to an overestimate of the effectiveness of that therapy. This particular failure lies at the root of countless headlines announcing new breakthrough procedures or therapies that kindle excitement, but deliver only false hopes—and leave the public wondering why there are so few breakthroughs in their own treatment.

Failure to Use Appropriate Controls or Comparison Groups. The purpose of a control group is to allow the observer to conclude that any change observed in the "active treatment group" is due to the treatment being studied, rather than to other factors. Control groups are particularly important when factors in addition to the intervention under study can affect the outcome of interest, when the new technology of interest and some established technology are both effective, and when the natural course of untreated disease is not clear or consistent, as is the case with breast cancer. Failure to use a control group, or use of an inappropriate control group, can make it impossible to draw meaningful conclusions from a study.

Failure to Demonstrate the Comparability of Patients in Treatment and Control Groups. Given the purpose of a control group, it is important that patients in the treatment and control groups be similar in terms of baseline characteristics that can influence the outcome of the intervention under study. For example, if one study group included more women at high risk for breast cancer than another group, then a detection technology tested in the high-risk group would likely detect more cancer cases than a technology tested in the low-risk group, leading to the perception that the detection system was more sensitive than a system tested in lower risk patients.

Unclear Definition of Study Endpoints. Medical technologies can be assessed a multiple levels, depending upon whether they are diagnostic or therapeutic. The most basic level at which a diagnostic technology can be assessed is definition of its performance characteristics—sensitivity and specificity. Even this basic level of assessment is not easy to perform. It requires comparison of the performance of the new technology with that of a gold standard. And true gold standards (such as tissue obtained during surgery) are not always available.

Bias. The confidence that you can have that the results of using a technology described in a study are the same results you would get if you used the technology in a similar fashion depends on the absence of bias. Bias is systematic sources of variation that distort the results of a study in one direction or another. There are many types of bias that have been described including those that are especially problematic in cancer screening. The most common general sources of bias in clinical trials are:

Confounding. A confounding variable is one that falsely obscures or accentuates the relationship between two factors, such as the effect of a treatment on patient outcome. Confounding occurs when a factor other than the interventions being compared is not distributed equally in the study groups being assessed and affects the outcome of interest.

Systematic Errors or Differences in Measurement. Selection bias can occur inadvertently if there are systematic errors or differences in the way particular patient characteristics (e.g., eligibility criteria) are measured or in the way a determination is made of the intervention to which a patient was exposed. (The latter could be a problem when exposure to the intervention is ascertained from insurance claims data, which may or may not be comprehensive or accurate.) The most common sources of bias due to measurement error, however, arise in evaluation of the outcomes of patients in two arms of a study. Ascertainment of patient outcomes by an "unblinded'" investigator who knows what intervention each patient received poses a serious risk of bias. An unblinded investigator, for example, may interpret particular findings differently, or look for particular findings with varying efforts, if she or he has preconceived notions about the comparative effects of the two technologies under study. Finally, although it may seem obvious that measurements of the outcomes of patients in two arms of a study should be performed in an identical manner and at the same point in time (relative to the interventions under study), this important aspect of study design is not always followed.

Loss of Patients to Follow-Up. Anyone who has conducted an observational study knows how difficult it is to follow patients over time. Loss of patients to follow-up becomes a threat to the internal validity of a study when it occurs in a substantial proportion of patients and at differential rates in the various arms of a study. Failure to account for all patients who were initially enrolled in a study is particularly problematic. In one study submitted to the Food and Drug Administration (FDA), for example, data on patients who had received a new device were reported only for those patients who were followed for at least one year. Many patients dropped out of the study prior to the one-year endpoint, however, due either to side effects of to ineffectiveness of the device. Consequently, the results reported to the FDA exaggerated the effectiveness and tolerability of the device. All enrolled patients thus must be accounted for. If some patients withdraw or are lost to follow-up, the number of withdrawals and losses in each arm should be reported with specification of the reasons for withdrawal.

Inappropriate Statistical Analysis and Planning. On occasion, statistical analyses reported in published studies are not performed correctly, or the most appropriate statistical analyses are not performed. In other instances, statistical issues, such as statistical power to detect a difference between two arms of a study if one really existed, do not seem to have been adequately considered in planning the study, or had to be compromised for practical reasons (such as study cost or patient availability). As a result, the results reported in some studies are misleading and have a significant probability of being wrong. Investigators should report the statistical significance of their results, and provide 95 percent confidence intervals around group differences or main effects. In addition, if relative risks or odds ratios are reported (such as reporting that a particular outcome is twice as likely to occur with treatment A as with treatment B), the absolute rate with which the outcome occurs also should be reported.

Poorly Described Techniques. Diagnostic and therapeutic techniques are often employed using very specific protocols or techniques that affect the effectiveness or safety of the interventions. For example, different pulse sequences can be used in magnetic resonance imaging studies and different software might base comparisons of digitized mammography images on different calculations. Unless the technology under study, and the technologies to which it is being compared, are clearly described, it is not possible to meaningfully compare the results of one study to those of other studies of what appears to be the same technology. Without such descriptions it also may be difficult or even impossible to judge the relevance of the study results.

Glossary

Absolute risk—a measure of risk over time in a group of individuals; may be used to measure lifetime risk or risk over a shorter time period.

Accuracy—the degree to which a test measures the true value of the attribute it is testing.

Adjuvant therapy—the use of another form of therapy in addition to the primary surgical therapy. It usually refers to hormonal therapy, chemotherapy, or radiation.

Allele—any one of a series of two or more different genes that occupy the same position (locus) on a chromosome.

Amplification—a process by which genetic material is increased.

Analytical validity—the accuracy of a test in detecting the specific characteristics that it was designed to detect, often measured by sensitivity and specificity. However, this accuracy does not imply any clinical significance, such as diagnosis.

Angiogenesis—the formation of new blood vessels.

Antigen—a substance that induces the immune system to produce antibodies that interact specifically with it.

Atypical hyperplasia—proliferation of cells showing atypical nuclear form, especially as scattered cells.

Autosomal—a non-sex-linked form of inheritance (the gene is not found on the X or Y chromosome).

Bias—in general, any factor that distorts the true nature of an event or observation. In clinical investigations, a bias is any systematic factor other than the intervention of interest that affects the magnitude of (i.e., tends to increase or decrease) an observed difference in the outcomes of a treatment group and a control group.

Bioinformatics—use of computers and specialized software to organize and analyze biological information and data.

Biomarker—A substance sometimes found in the blood, other body fluids, or tissues. A high level of biomarker may mean that a certain type of cancer is in the body. Examples of biomarkers include CA 125 (ovarian cancer), CA 15-3 (breast cancer), CEA (ovarian, lung, breast, pancreatic, and gastrointestinal tract cancers), and PSA (prostate cancer). See also *Tumor marker.*

Biopsy—refers to a procedure that involves obtaining a tissue specimen for microscopic analysis to establish a diagnosis; can be done surgically or with needles.

Blind study—a study in which the identity and relevant characteristics of the study subjects are concealed from the investigators.

BRCA1—a gene located on the short arm of chromosome 17; when this gene is mutated, a woman is at greater risk of developing breast or ovarian cancer, or both, than women who do not have the mutation.

BRCA2—a gene located on chromosome 13; a germ-line mutation in this gene is associated with increased risk of breast cancer.

Breast self-examination—monthly physical examination of the breasts with the intent of finding lumps that could be an early indication of cancer.

Cancer—a general term for more than 100 diseases in which abnormal cells divide without control. Cancer cells can invade nearby tissues and can spread through the bloodstream and lymphatic system to other parts of the body. There are several main types of cancer. Carcinoma is cancer that begins in the skin or in tissues that line or cover internal organs. Sarcoma is cancer that begins in bone, cartilage, fat, muscle, blood vessels, or other connective or supportive tissue. Leukemia is cancer that starts in blood-forming tissue such as the bone marrow, and causes large numbers of abnormal blood cells to be produced and enter the bloodstream. Lymphoma is cancer that begins in the cells of the immune system.

Carcinogen—any substance or agent that produces or incites cancer.

Carcinoma in situ—Cancer that involves only the cells in which it began and that has not spread to nearby tissues.

Case-control study—a study that compares two groups of people—those with the disease or condition under study (cases) and a very similar group of people who do not have the disease or condition (controls). Researchers study the medical and lifestyle histories of the people in each group to learn what factors may be associated with the disease or condition. For example, one group may have been exposed to a particular substance that the other was not. Also called a retrospective study. Results from this type of study are generally less reliable than a well-designed randomized controlled clinical trial.

Case report—a description of a single case, typically describing the manifestations, clinical course, and prognosis of that case.

Case series—a descriptive, observational study of a series of cases, typically describing the manifestations, clinical course, and prognosis of a condition.

Catheter—a tube passed through the body for evacuating or injecting fluids into body cavities.

cDNA—complementary DNA synthesized by RNA-directed DNA polymerase using RNA as a template; may be used as a probe for the presence of a gene code.

Cell culture—the growth of cells in vitro, generally for experimental purposes.

Chemoprevention—the use of natural or laboratory-made substances to prevent cancer.

Chemoprophylaxis—drug treatment designed to prevent future occurrences of disease.

Chemotherapy—the treatment of disease by means of chemicals that have a specific toxic effect on the disease producing microorganisms (antibiotics) or that selectively destroy cancerous tissue (anticancer therapy).

Chromosome—chromosomes carry the genes, the basic units of heredity. Humans have 23 pairs of chromosomes; one member of each pair is from the mother and the other is from the father. Each chromosome can contain hundreds or thousands of individual genes.

Clinical breast examination—a physical examination of the breasts, performed by a health care provider, with the intent of finding lumps that could be an early indication of cancer.

Clinical outcome—the end result of a medical intervention, such as survival or improved health.

Clinical trial—a formal study carried out according to a prospectively defined protocol that is intended to discover or verify the safety and effectiveness of procedures or interventions in humans. The term may refer to a controlled or uncontrolled trial. Randomized controlled clinical trials are considered the gold standard for clinical evidence.

Clinical utility—identifying the clinical and psychological benefits and risks of positive and negative results of a given technique.

Clinical validity—the accuracy of a test in diagnosing or predicting risk for a disorder, often measured by sensitivity and specificity.

Cohort study—an observational study in which outcomes in a group of patients that received an intervention are compared with outcomes in a similar group, that is, the cohort, either contemporary or historical, of patients that did not receive the intervention. In an adjusted- (or matched-) cohort study, investigators identify (or make statistical adjustments to provide) a cohort group that has characteristics (e.g., age, gender, disease severity) that are as similar as possible to the group that experienced the intervention.

Composition of matter patent—proprietary claim on an actual substance that is isolated and properly characterized (i.e., BRCA1 or 2 gene sequence).

Computed tomography—a special radiographic technique that uses a computer to assimilate multiple x-ray images into a two-dimensional, cross-sectional image, which also can be reconstructed into a three-dimensional image. This can reveal many soft tissue structures not shown by conventional radiography.

Computer-aided detection—use of sophisticated computer programs designed to recognize patterns in images and provide assistance to interpreters to detect the presence of disease. This approach has been used along with mammography for the detection of breast cancer.

Confidence interval—a range within which an estimate is deemed to be close to the actual value being measured. In statistical measurements, estimates cannot be said to be exact matches, but, rather, are defined in terms of their probability of matching the value of the characteristic being measured.

Confounding factors—factors for which data adjustment is needed because they are entangled with other factors related to the disease or condition of interest.

Contralateral—originating in or affecting the opposite side of the body.

Contrast agent—a substance that enhances the image produced by medical diagnostic equipment such as ultrasound, x-ray, magnetic resonance imaging, or nuclear medicine or an imaging-sensitive substance that is ingested or injected intravenously to enhance or increase contrast between anatomical structures.

Controlled observational studies—An experiment or clinical trial that includes an experimental group and a comparison (control) group that are not blindly assigned into their respective groups. These studies included those that compare outcomes among those who do or do not receive screening, but in which the subjects are not blindly assigned to a specific group.

Core-needle biopsy—procedure in which a hollow needle is used to remove small cylinders of tissue from a suspected cancer.

Cost-benefit analysis—a comparison of alternative interventions in which costs and outcomes are quantified in common monetary units.

Cost-effectiveness analyses—methods for comparing the economic efficiencies of different therapies or programs that produce health outcomes.

Cross-sectional comparison—an observational study in which both risk factor(s) and disease are ascertained at the same time.

Cytogenetics—the study of cytology in relation to genetics.

Cytological screening—examination of cells for changes indicative of a disease or risk of disease, for example, Papanicolaou test (Pap smear) for cervical cancer.

Cytology—The study of cells using a microscope to examine the characteristics of formation, structure, and function of cells.

Deoxyribonucleic acid—the genetic material of all cells and many viruses that is a polymer of nucleotides. The monomer consists of phosphorylated 2-deoxyribose N-glycosidically linked to one of four bases—adenine, cytosine, guanine, or thymine. The sequence of these bases encodes genetic information.

Detection—identifying disease. Early detection means that the disease is found at an early stage, before it has grown large or spread to other sites.

Diagnosis—definitive confirmation of a specific disease usually by imaging procedures and from the use of laboratory findings.

Diagnostic mammography—x-ray-based breast imaging undertaken for the purpose of diagnosing an abnormality discovered by physical exam or screening mammography. Also known as problem solving mammography.

Diagnostic testing—the evaluation of patients with signs or symptoms associated with a disease.

Digital mammography—see *full-field digital mammography*.

DNA—abbreviation for deoxyribonucleic acid. DNA holds genetic information for cell growth, division, and function. See also *deoxyribonucleic acid.*

Dose-response—the relation between the dose of a drug or other chemical and the degree of response it produces, as measured by the percentage of the exposed population showing a defined effect.

Dosimetry—measurement of the amount of x-rays and radioactivity absorbed.

Duct—a hollow passage for gland secretions. In the breast, a passage through which milk passes from the lobule (which makes the milk) to the nipple.

Ductal carcinoma in situ—a lesion in which there is proliferation of abnormal cells within the ducts of the breast, but no visible evidence of invasion into the duct walls or surrounding tissues; sometimes referred to as "precancer" or "pre-invasive cancer."

Ductal lavage—a procedure in which a small catheter is inserted into the nipple and the breast ducts are flushed with fluid to collect breast cells.

Effectiveness—the extent to which a specific test or intervention, when used under *ordinary* circumstances, does what it is intended to do.

Efficacy—the extent to which a specific test or intervention produces a beneficial result under *ideal* conditions (e.g., in a clinical trial).

Elastography—the measurement of the elastic properties of tissue.

Electrical impedance imaging—a procedure by which images are generated by transmitting a low-voltage electrical signal through the tissue.

Electrical potential measurements—compares altered electrical gradients on various locations on the breast to potentially help identify cancer.

Electronic palpation—use of pressure sensors to quantitatively measure palpable features of the breast such as the hardness and size of lesions.

Epidemiology—science concerned with defining and explaining the interrelationships of factors that determine disease frequency and distribution.

Epigenetics—the study of changes producing phenotypic effects in which gene activity is altered without modifying the nucleotide sequence.

Epithelial tissue—those cells that form the outer surface of the body and that line the body cavities and the principal tubes and passageways. They form the secreting portions of glands and their ducts and important parts of certain sense organs. The cells rest on a basement membrane and lie close to each other, with little intercellular material between them.

Etiology—the study of the causes of a disease.

Exon—the portions of the DNA sequence in a gene that specify the sequence of amino acids in a polypeptide chain, as well as the beginning and end of the coding sequence.

False-negative result—a test result that incorrectly indicates that the abnormality or disease being investigated is not present when in fact it is present.

False-positive result—a test result that indicates that the abnormality or disease being investigated is present when in fact it is not.

Familial clusters—a disease occurring in a family more frequently than would be expected in random distribution; however, some clusters may be due to chance.

Fine-needle aspiration—a procedure by which a thin needle is used to draw up (aspirate) cell samples for examination under a microscope.

Full-field digital mammography—similar to conventional mammography (film-screen mammography) except that a dedicated electronic detector system is used to computerize and display the x-ray information.

Gel electrophoresis—a method for separating proteins or nucleic acid fragments that is carried out in a silica or acrylamide gel under the influence of an electric field.

Gene—a functional unit of heredity made up of a sequence of nucleotides that occupies a specific place or locus on a chromosome.

Genetic marker—a genetic change in cells that is indicative of cancer or malignant potential, or a piece of DNA that lies on a chromosome so close to a gene that the marker and the gene are inherited together. A marker is thus an identifiable heritable spot on a chromosome. A marker can be an expressed region of DNA (a gene) or a segment of DNA with no known coding function.

Genome—an organism's entire complement of DNA, which determines its genetic makeup.

Genotype—the genetic constitution of an organism or cell, as distinct from its expressed features known as the phenotype.

Germ-line mutation—an inherited mutation found in all cells in the body.

Health Maintenance Organization (HMO)—organized system for providing comprehensive prepaid health care that has five basic attributes: (1) provides care in a defined geographic area; (2) provides or ensures delivery of an agreed-upon set of basic and supplemental health maintenance and treatment services; (3) provides care to a voluntarily enrolled group of persons; (4) requires their enrollees to use the services of designated providers; and (5) receives reimbursement through a predetermined, fixed, periodic prepayment made by the enrollee without regard to the degree of services provided.

Heterogeneous—exhibiting variable characteristics.

Heterozygosity—the state of having different alleles at a specific locus in the genome.

High-throughput technology—any approach using robotics, automated machines, and computers to process many samples at once.

Histology—the study of the microscopic structure of tissue.

Hyperplasia—an increase in the number of cells in a tissue or organ, excluding tumor formation.

Imaging agent—any substance administered to a patient for the purpose of producing or enhancing an image of the body; includes contrast agents used with medical imaging techniques such as radiography, computed tomography, ultrasonography, and magnetic resonance imaging, as well as radiopharmaceuticals used with imaging procedures such as single-photon emission computed tomography (SPECT) and positron emission tomography (PET).

Immunocytochemistry or immunohistochemistry—a laboratory test that uses antibodies to detect specific biochemical antigens in cells or tissue samples viewed under a microscope; can be used to help classify cancers.

Immunology—the study of immunity to diseases.

In situ—in position, localized. In breast cancer usually either ductal carcinoma is situ (DCIS) or lobular carcinoma in situ (LCIS), in which early cancer that has not spread to neighboring tissue.

Incidence—the number of new cases of a disease that occur in the population per unit of time.

Infiltrating ductal carcinoma—breast cancer that has spread out of the breast ducts. See also *invasive ductal carcinoma.*

Inflammatory breast cancer—A type of breast cancer in which the breast looks red and swollen and feels warm. The skin of the breast may also show the pitted appearance called peau d'orange (like the skin of an orange). The redness and warmth occur because the cancer cells block the lymph vessels in the skin.

Intermediate outcomes—findings that are not health outcomes in themselves (e.g., cellular atypia) but that precede or may increase the risk of such outcomes.

Invasive cancer—cancers capable of growing beyond their site of origin and invading neighboring tissue.

Invasive ductal carcinoma—a cancer that starts in the ducts of the breast and then breaks through the duct wall, where it invades the surrounding tissue; it is the most common type of breast cancer, and accounts for about 80 percent of breast malignancies, also known as infiltrating ductal carcinoma.

Invasive lobular carcinoma—a cancer that starts in the milk-producing glands (lobules) of the breast and then breaks through the lobule walls to involve the surrounding tissue; accounts for about 15 percent of invasive breast cancers.

Lead-time bias—overestimation of survival time because of the backward shift in the starting point for the measurement of survival as a result of early detection.

Length bias—overestimation of survival benefit due to the detection of slowly growing lesions by screening tests, perhaps including lesions that will never cause mortality.

Lesion—an abnormal change in structure of an organ or other body part due to injury or disease; especially one that is circumscribed and well defined.

Lifetime probability—the probability of being diagnosed with a specified cancer during an entire lifetime of a certain amount of years.

Linkage analysis—study aimed at establishing linkage between genes by analyzing the tendency for two or more nonallelic genes to be inherited together, because they are located more or less closely on the same chromosome.

Lobular—of or pertaining to the lobes of an organ, such as the liver, lung, breast, thyroid, or brain.

Lobular carcinoma in situ—abnormal cells within a breast lobule that have not invaded surrounding tissue. Not cancer *per se*, but can serve as a marker of future cancer risk.

Localized cancer—a cancer that is confined to the place where it started; that is, it has not spread to distant parts of the body.

Loss of heterozygosity (LOH)—loss of one allele at a specific genetic locus, usually accompanied by a point mutation in the remaining allele.

Magnetic resonance imaging (MRI)—method by which images are created by recording signals generated from the excitation (the gain and loss of energy) of elements such as the hydrogen of water in tissue when placed within a powerful magnetic field and pulsed with radio frequencies.

Magnetic resonance spectroscopy (MRS)—A noninvasive imaging method that provides information about cellular activity (metabolic information). Can also be used along with magnetic resonance imaging (MRI) which provides information about the shape and size of the tumor (spatial information). Also called magnetic resonance spectroscopic imaging and proton magnetic resonance spectroscopic imaging.

Malignant—a tumor that has the potential to become lethal through destructive growth or by having the ability to invade surrounding tissue and metastasize.

Malignant transformation—changes that a cell undergoes as it develops the ability to form a malignant tumor.

Mammogram—x-ray image of the breast.

Mammography—the practice of imaging breast tissue with x-rays for screening or diagnostic purposes in detecting or diagnosing cancer.

Mass spectroscopy—a method for separating ionized molecular particles according to mass by applying a combination of electrical and magnetic fields to deflect ions passing in a beam through the instrument.

Medicaid—federal- and state-funded health insurance program for certain low-income people. It covers approximately 36 million individuals including children; aged, blind, and/or disabled people; and people who are eligible to receive federally assisted income maintenance payments.

Medicare—a program that provides health insurance to people age 65 and over, those who have permanent kidney failure, and people with certain disabilities.

Menarche—onset of menstruation at puberty.

Menopause—permanent cessation of menstrual activity.

Messenger RNA—the molecule, also called mRNA, that carries the information from the DNA genetic code to areas in the cytoplasm of the cell that make proteins.

Meta-analysis—systematic methods that use statistical techniques for combining results from different studies to obtain a quantitative estimate of the overall effect of a particular intervention or variable on a defined outcome. This combination may produce a stronger conclusion than can be provided by any individual study (also known as data synthesis or quantitative overview).

Metaplasia—the change in the type of adult cells in a tissue to a form that is not normal for that tissue.

Metastasis—the ability of cancer cells to move from one part of the body to another, resulting in the growth of a secondary malignancy in a new location.

Method-of-use patent—proprietary claim on the specific use of a characterized substance or invention (i.e., the genetic test for mutation).

Methylation—the attachment of a methyl group (CH_3) to cytosine residues of eukaryotic DNA to form 5-methylcytosine.

Microarray—thousands of different oligonucleotides spotted onto specific locations on glass microscope slides or silicon chips, which are then hybridized with labeled sample DNA or RNA.

Microcalcifications—tiny calcium deposits within the breast, singly or in clusters; often found by mammography. They may be a sign of cancer.

Microsatellite(s)—stretches of DNA consisting of short, repeated sequences showing a higher spontaneous mutation rate than coding DNA, which makes them useful markers for DNA stability.

Modality—method of application or use of any therapy or medical device.

Molecular epidemiology—a science that focuses on the contribution of potential genetic and environmental risk factors, identified at the molecular level, to the etiology, distribution, and prevention of disease within families and across populations.

Molecular markers—changes in cells, at the molecular level, that are indicative of cancer or malignant potential.

Monoenergetic x-rays—a beam of x-rays whose photon energy is found to lie within a very narrow band. Currently, these types of x-rays can only be produced at a synchrotron.

Morbidity—a diseased condition or state; the incidence of a disease or of all diseases in a population.

Morphology—science of structure and form without regard to function.

Mortality rate—the death rate; expresses the number of deaths in a unit of population within a prescribed time and may be expressed as crude death rates or as death rates specific for diseases and, sometimes, for age, sex, or other attributes.

Mutation—a change either in the nucleotide sequence of DNA or in the order, number, or placement of genes on or across chromosomes that may result in a change in the structure or function of a protein and possibly the lack of expression of a protein altogether.

Neoplasm—An abnormal mass of tissue that results from excessive cell division. Neoplasms may be benign (not cancerous), or malignant (cancerous). Also called tumor.

Nipple aspiration—use of suction to collect breast fluid through the nipple of nonlactating women.

Observational studies—A type of study in which individuals are observed or certain outcomes are measured. No attempt is made to affect the outcome (for example, no treatment is given).

Occult tumors—undetected and without symptoms.

Odds ratio—a comparison of the presence of a risk factor for disease in a sample of diseased subjects and nondiseased controls.

Oligonucleotide—a small DNA or RNA molecule composed of a few nucleotide bases.

Oncology—branch of medicine dealing with the treatment of cancer.

Optical imaging—use of light, usually in the near-infrared range, to produce an image of tissue.

p value—the probability that an outcome as large as or larger than that observed would occur in a properly designed, executed, and analyzed analytical study if in reality there was no difference between the groups; often used to define statistical significance of results.

p53—a tumor suppressor gene commonly mutated in cancer.

Paget's disease of the nipple—A form of breast cancer in which the tumor grows from ducts beneath the nipple onto the surface of the nipple. Symptoms commonly include itching and burning and an eczema-like condition around the nipple, sometimes accompanied by oozing or bleeding.

Palpable tumor—a tumor that can be felt during a physical examination.

Pap smear—a cytological test developed by George N. Papanicolaou for the detection of cervical cancer.

Penetrance—the proportion of individuals with a specific genotype who express the associated characteristic in the phenotype.

Phenotype—the physical characteristics or makeup of an individual.

Photonics—the technology of generating and harnessing light and other forms of radiant energy whose quantum unit is the photon. The science includes light emission, transmission, deflection, amplification, and detection by optical components and instruments, lasers and other light sources, fiber optics, electro-optical instrumentation, related hardware and electronics, and sophisticated systems.

Polymerase chain reaction—a process for amplifying a DNA molecule from 10^6 to 10^9 fold.

Polymorphism—the regular and simultaneous occurrence in a population of two or more alleles of a gene in which the frequency of the rarer of the alleles is greater than can be explained by recurrent mutation alone.

Positional cloning—cloning a gene simply on the basis of knowing its position in the genome without any idea of the function of that gene.

Positive predictive value—a measure of accuracy for a screening or diagnostic test; indicates what portion of those with an abnormal test result actually have the disease; formula (PPV = TP/ TP + FP).

Positron emission tomography—use of radioactive tracers such as labeled glucose to identify regions in the body with altered metabolic activity.

Premalignant—changes in cells that may, but that do not always, become cancer. Also called "precancer."

Prevalence—the number of cases of disease, infected persons, or persons with some other attribute, present at a particular time and in relation to the size of the population from which they are drawn.

Primary cancer prevention—prevention the development of cancer.

Prognosis—prediction of the course and end of disease and the estimate of chance for recovery.

Progression—the growth or advancement of cancer, indicating a worsening of the disease.

Prophylactic bilateral mastectomy—surgical removal of both breasts with the intent of reducing the risk of developing breast cancer later in life.

Prophylaxis—the prevention of disease, preventive treatment.

Proprietary rights—exclusive rights held by a private individual or corporation under a trademark or patent.

Prostate-specific antigen (PSA) testing—used to screen for cancer of the prostate and to monitor treatment by measuring the amount of PSA in the blood. PSA is a protein produced in the bloodstream.

Proteome—all of the proteins produced by a given species, just as the genome is the totality of the DNA possessed by that species.

Proto-oncogene—A normal gene which, when altered by mutation, becomes an oncogene that can contribute to cancer. The defective versions of proto-oncogenes, known as oncogenes, can cause a cell to divide in an unregulated manner. This growth can occur in the absence of normal growth signals such as those provided by growth factors.

Randomization—a method that uses chance to assign participants to comparison groups in a trial by using a random-numbers table or a computer-generated random sequence. Random allocation implies that each individual being entered into a trial has the same chance of receiving each of the possible interventions.

Randomized controlled trial—a true prospective experiment in which investigators randomly assign an eligible sample of patients to one or more treatment groups and a control group and follow patients' outcomes (also known as randomized clinical trial). This is the gold standard for evidence in a clinical trial.

Relative risk—compares the risk of disease among people with a particular risk factor to the risk among people without that risk factor. If the relative risk is above 1.0, then risk is higher among those with the risk factor than those without. Relative risks below 1.0 reflect an inverse association between a risk factor and the disease, that is, a protective effect, or lower risk, associated with the exposure.

Reliability—the consistency of the result when a test is repeated. Also known as reproducibility.

Risk—a quantitative measure of the probability of developing or dying from a particular disease such as cancer.

Scintimammography—use of radioactive tracers to produce an image of the breast.

Screen-film mammography—conventional mammography in which the x-rays are recorded on film.

Screening—systematic testing of an asymptomatic population to determine the presence of a particular disease.

Screening mammography—x-ray-based breast imaging in an asymptomatic population used to detect breast cancers at an early stage.

Secondary cancer—cancer that has spread from the site where it first appeared to another site.

Sensitivity—a measure of how often a test correctly identifies women with breast cancer. Calculated as the number of true-positive results divided by the number of true-positive results plus the number of false-negative results; formula ($Se = TP/[TP + FN]$).

Signal transduction—the biochemical events that conduct the signal of a hormone growth factor from the cell exterior, through the cell membrane, and into the cytoplasm. This involves a number of molecules, including receptors, proteins, and messengers.

Soft copy—image display on a computer screen rather than on film.

Somatic mutation—an alteration in DNA that occurs after conception. Somatic mutations can occur in any of the cells of the body except the germ cells (sperm and egg) and therefore are not passed on to children. These alterations can (but do not always) cause cancer or other diseases.

Sonography—a technique in which high-frequency sound waves are bounced off internal organs and the echo pattern is converted into a two-dimensional picture of the structures beneath the transducer. See also *Ultrasound*.

Specificity—the proportion of persons without disease who correctly test negative; formula (Sp = TN/[TN +FP]).

Specimen bank—stored patient tissue samples that are used for biomedical research (also tumor or tissue banks).

Spectroscopy—analytical use of an instrument that separates radiant energy into its component frequencies or wavelengths by means of a prism or grating to form a spectrum for inspection.

Spiral computed tomography—a detailed cross-sectional picture of areas inside the body. The images are created by a computer linked to an x-ray machine that scans the body in a spiral path. Also called helical computed tomography.

Squamous cell carcinoma—a malignant growth originating from a squamous cell. This form of cancer can be seen on the skin, lips, and inside the mouth, throat, or esophagus.

Statistical power—the likelihood that a study will find a particular effect if the effect exists; usually varies with sample size and other factors.

Stereotactic breast biopsy—use of breast images (x-ray or ultrasound) taken at various angles to generate a three-dimensional image for plotting the exact position of the suspicious lesion and for guiding the placement of a biopsy needle.

Surrogate endpoints—short-term, intermediate endpoints in a clinical study that are thought to be representative or predictive of longer-term outcomes.

Surveillance—close and continuous observation, screening, and testing of those at risk for a disease.

Survival—average period of time from diagnosis to death.

Systemic therapy—treatment involving the whole body, usually using drugs.

Telemammography—the process of satellite or long-distance transmission of digital mammography for consultation.

Thermography—use of a device that detects and records the heat produced by tissues to generate an image.

Thermotherapy—use of lasers or high-intensity ultrasound to heat and destroy tumor cells.

Tissue array—small cylinders of tissue punched from 1,000 individual tumor biopsy specimens embedded in paraffin. These cylinders are then arrayed in a large paraffin block, from which 200 consecutive tissue sections can be cut, allowing rapid analysis of multiple arrayed samples by immunohistochemistry or in situ hybridization.

Tomography—any of several techniques for making x-ray pictures of a predetermined plane section of a solid object by blurring out the images of other planes.

Tomosynthesis—a variation of tomography in which several radiographs of a patient are taken at different angles, and back-projection of the resulting images produces a light distribution in a chosen three-dimensional volume of space that replicates the same volume in the patient.

Transcription—synthesis of RNA by an enzyme called RNA polymerase that uses a DNA template; the first step in protein biosynthesis.

Transcriptome—the complete collection of transcribed elements of the genome. In addition to mRNAs, it also represents noncoding RNAs which are used for structural and regulatory purposes. Alterations in the structure or levels of expression of any one of these RNAs or their proteins can contribute to disease.

Translational research—the research needed to move the fruits of basic research into clinical practice.

Tumor—an abnormal mass of tissue that results from excessive cell division that is uncontrolled and progressive, also called a neoplasm. Tumors perform no useful body function. They may be either benign (not cancerous) or malignant.

Tumor marker—any substance or characteristic that indicates the presence of a malignancy.

Tumor suppressor genes—genes that slow cell division or that cause cells to die at the appropriate time. Mutations in these genes can lead to uncontrolled cell growth and the development of cancer.

Tumorigenesis—the induction of the malignant growth of abnormal cells.

Ultrasound—use of inaudible, high-frequency sound waves to create an image of the body.

Venipuncture—the puncture of a vein (usually in the arm) with a hollow bore needle for the purpose of obtaining a blood specimen.

X-ray—a type of ionizing radiation used for imaging purposes that uses energy beams of very short wavelengths (0.1 to 1000 angstroms) that can penetrate most substances except heavy metals.

Index

A

AAC Consulting Group, Inc., 223
Access to breast imaging
  cultural factors, 78
  financial factors, 2, 4-5, 21, 69, 76, 78, 100, 103-106
  legislation promoting, 80
  patents and, 257
  as quality assurance component, 4, 75-79
  race/ethnicity and, 76
  of risk assessments, 8
  social factors, 76, 78
  socioeconomic status and, 5, 76
  and survival rates, 66-67
  uninsured women, 5, 76, 78-79
  waiting times, 7, 101
  workforce issues, 4, 7, 21, 100, 101-102, 103-106, 115
Accuracy. *See also* Analytical validity; Sensitivity of technologies; Specificity
  of biological technologies, 156, 160, 161
  biopsies, 161, 290, 299
  CAD technology and, 202, 281
  clinical trials of, 202-204
  defined, 326
  digital mammography, 21, 93
  molecular profiling, 170
  MRI, 32, 45, 92, 96-98, 294
  of radiation technologists, 111-112

screen-film mammography, 21, 92
  of specialists vs. generalists, 86, 89, 94-95, 101, 281
  standards for reporting, 202
Adjuvant therapy, 1, 55, 299, 326
AdvaMed, 196
Advanced Mammography Systems, Inc., 223
Advanced Medical Laboratories, Inc., 222
Advocacy groups, 12-13, 79, 82, 210-211, 277
African Americans, 45, 76, 77, 78, 128, 133, 208
Age factors
  at birth of first child, 8, 127
  DCIS, 51, 52
  density of breast tissue, 45, 86
  efficacy of mammography, 42
  incidence of breast cancer, 43, 50, 51, 142
  menarche, 127
  menopause, 127
  mutations, 128
  radiation sensitivity, 48
  risk of breast cancer, 8, 20, 30, 31, 124, 125, 126, 127, 130, 137, 143-144, 199
  sensitivity of mammography, 85, 87, 281
  standard of care, 7, 40, 281
  utilization of mammography, 20, 64